The Revolution Will Not Be Microwaved

The Revolution Will Not Be Microwaved

Inside America's Underground Food Movements

Sandor Ellix Katz

Chelsea Green Publishing
White River Junction,
Vermont

Editor: Ben Watson
Managing Editor: Marcy Brant
Project Editor: Collette Leonard
Copy Editor: Nancy Ringer
Proofreader: Collette Leonard
Designer: Peter Holm, Sterling Hill Productions
Design Assistant: Daria Hoak, Sterling Hill Productions

Printed in the United States
First printing, October 2006
10 9 8 7 6 5 4 3 2 1

Our Commitment to Green Publishing
Chelsea Green sees publishing as a tool for cultural change and ecological stewardship. We
strive to align our book manufacturing practices with our editorial mission, and to reduce
the impact of our business enterprise on the environment. We print our books and catalogs
on chlorine-free recycled paper, using soy-based inks, whenever possible. Chelsea Green is
a member of the Green Press Initiative (www.greenpressinitiative.org), a nonprofit coalition
of publishers, manufacturers, and authors working to protect the world's endangered forests
and conserve natural resources.

The Revolution Will Not Be Microwaved was printed on Enviro 100 Natural, a 100 percent
post-consumer-waste recycled paper supplied by Maple-Vail.

Library of Congress Cataloging-in-Publication Data

Katz, Sandor Ellix, 1962-
  The Revolution will not be microwaved : inside America's underground food
movements / Sandor Ellix Katz.
      p. cm.
  Includes bibliographical references and index.
  ISBN-13: 978-1-933392-11-0
  1. Food. 2. Food supply—United States. 3. Food habits—United States.
I. Title.

  TX357.K38 2006
  641.3–dc22

2006026616

Chelsea Green Publishing Company
Post Office Box 428
White River Junction, VT 05001
(802) 295-6300
www.chelseagreen.com

To people everywhere practicing cultural survival
by keeping food traditions alive.

Contents

List of Recipes

Acknowledgments

This book has been inspired by many people, starting with my father, who has always had a garden and a compost pile, and fed us vegetables like kohlrabi, celeriac, parsnips, and brussels sprouts. I thank him and all the other farmers, gardeners, and plant lovers in my life—there are lots of you!—for sharing your abundant bounties, plant medicine, and green fervor. I thank the animal tenders and beekeepers, and the ones with courage to slaughter. I thank the bakers, brewers, cheesemakers, miso makers, and sauerkraut makers. I thank the urban gardeners and the forest homesteaders. I thank the seed savers and skill sharers. I thank the dumpster divers, gleaners, and foragers. I thank the co-ops, farmers' markets, and CSA farms. I thank the crusaders, protesters, and watchdogs. I thank the cooks, chefs, and kitchen magicians everywhere who find creative expression in keeping people well fed. I also thank the dishwashers and those who do the grimy tasks that keep the kitchens clean and safe. This book, and my life, are rich in inspiration.

For the title of this book, I thank Gil Scott-Heron, who wrote and performed the song "The Revolution Will Not Be Televised." For sharing their stories or recipes or pointing me toward helpful information as I worked on this book, I thank Buffy Aakaash, Etain Addey, Roberta Bailey, Allan Balliet, Peter Bane, Blue Bayer, Hector Black, Derrick Blaylock, Maggie Brown, Cailen Campbell, Jok Church, Christopher Cogswell, Frank Cook, Patrick Crouch, Cindy and Ed Curran, Shawn Dady, Michaela DeSoucey, Pattie Eakin, Murray Edelman, Alex and Max Edelstein, Krista Eikmann, Tanya Einhorn, Leif Forer, Morag Gamble, Kehben Grifter, Mike Hartman, Gabby Haze, David Holmgren, Ashley and Patrick Ironwood, Aresh Javadi, Barbara and Jim Joyner, Janell Kapoor, Jonathan Katz, Ann Tindell Keener, Bill Keener,

Carol Kimmons, Greg King, Izzy Klatzker, Nance Klehm, Steve Koch, Albert Kregs, Gary Lawless, Tim Low, Lapis Luxury, Forrest Martin, Mark McAfee, Leroy Miller, Merril Mushroom, Alan Muskat, Richard Osborne, Jeff Poppen, Jessica Prentice, Nancy Ramsey, Lynn Razaitis, Markiss Sagee, Franklin Sanders, Mark Shipley, Tom Strong, Michael Szuberla, Brian Thomas, Michael Thompson, Antanas Vainius, MaxZine Weinstein, B. Whiting, Adam Wilson, Cleo Woelfle-Erskine, Valencia Wombone, Leppard Zeppard, and, from the realm of the strictly first name, Buck, Didi, Greg, Jordan, Junebug, Kokoe, Les, May, Natalie, Nettles, Orchid, River, Ruebix, Silverfang, Simmer, Socket, Spark, and Xtn. I thank Jai Sheronda for sharing his photographs. For allowing me to reproduce their graphics, I thank the Beehive Collective and Phil Howard of the Center for Agroecology and Sustainable Food Systems. I thank Anna Salzano for translating. I thank Neal, Garth, Mikee, and By the Way for sharing their offices. I thank Buffy, Jordan, Silverfang, Tanya, Meka, Janell, MaxZine, Merril, Nettles, Leopard, Alan, Anu Bonobo, and Ed for reading this manuscript as it evolved and offering me feedback. I thank Valencia for invaluable research assistance. I thank my editor Ben Watson and all the other wonderful folks at Chelsea Green, especially Margo Baldwin and Alice Blackmer, for their enthusiasm and unwavering encouragement.

For facilitating the explorations that took my life on the paths that led me to and through this book, I thank all my lovely fellow communards and co-stewards of Short Mountain Sanctuary: Boxer, Daz'l, Goneaway, Hush, Jai Sheronda, "snacktivist" Kelly Bella, Lapis Luxury, Laurel Anne Honey Lamb, Leopard, Lucky, Markiss, River, Simmer, Soami, Socket, Valencia, and Weeder, along with the Idahoes and the rest of our ever-growing extended family, and all the amazing people who have been part of this special place through the years. Thank you for all your love and support.

Introduction

I was inspired to write this book by two years of traveling around the United States and Australia talking to people about fermentation, following the publication of my previous book, *Wild Fermentation: The Flavor, Nutrition, and Craft of Live-Culture Foods* (Chelsea Green, 2003). Mostly we discussed the incredible array of wonderful foods and drinks that result from the miraculous actions of microorganisms, but inevitably the conversation would stray into other realms of fermentation, specifically social ferment. The word *ferment*, along with the words *fervor* and *fervent*, comes from the Latin verb *fervere*, to boil. Just as fermenting liquids exhibit a bubbling action similar to boiling, so do excited people, filled with passion and unrestrained. Revolutionary ideas, as they spread and mutate, ferment the culture. Agitation of fermenting liquids stimulates the process and quickens fermentation, as evidenced by increased bubbling action. Agitation similarly stimulates social ferment.

The kinds of places I have visited to talk with groups and teach workshops have often been food co-ops, farmers' markets, community spaces, and farms. I've met people who are reclaiming their connection to food in many exciting and hopeful ways: folks dedicated to growing food using methods that build soil fertility and raising animals with compassion; gardeners and farmers reviving nearly abandoned seed-saving practices as a critical link in food independence; urban community gardeners creating green oases and bringing the cityscape back to earth; people organizing around themes of food justice, food security, and food sovereignty; scavengers who glean from orchards, fields, and dumpsters; caring folks who redistribute discarded food to hungry people; healers who use food as medicine; passionate advocates of whole, traditional, slow, and raw foods; people fueling cars with used

deep-frying oil—the list goes on. The diverse activists I meet everywhere make me feel part of a broad movement to build alternatives to
the dominant food system and transform the world one bite at a time.

From there is a small glimpse of the revolution I see happening: It's not a
militant confrontation at all but rather a quiet culinary mutiny. It's
what's known as "the bread club" in a Western town of about eight
thousand people, which I cannot identify without jeopardizing the
club's continued existence. The club started in 2002 as the pickup site
for bread baked by B., a fellow fermentation enthusiast I met in my
travels.

From the start there was an underground aspect to the bread distribution. "I would gladly bake the way I do legally if I could," says B.
"The fact is it is impossible on my scale. For me to build a certified
kitchen with attached oven, I would have to go greatly into debt and
then bake my ass off just to pay off that debt, probably seven days a
week, and then I'd grow to hate baking and hire other people to bake,
and then I would just be a business owner. And so I bake underground,
every other week, because I love to, and after two and a half years I still
love it, and I actually make a little bit of money doing it. I just imagine
all the underemployed people I know being able to do something like
this, and be proud of it, and make a little money, and not be a minimum-
wage slave, but it's not legal. And that's wrong."

In the current regulatory environment, the rules make small-scale
traditional food production and distribution almost impossible. Selling
home-baked bread, or any food prepared in a home kitchen, is prohibited by most, if not all, health codes in the United States. Livestock for
sale (with the exception of poultry, in most places) may not be slaughtered by the farmers who raise them; instead they must be trucked to
anonymous factory-like commercial slaughterhouses. Milk and other
dairy products may not be sold without pasteurization, which diminishes nutritional quality, digestibility, and flavor. Cider, too, is nearly
always required to be pasteurized or irradiated. In other words, *real*
food, increasingly illegal, is being replaced by processed food products.
Laws dictating food standards are driven by the model of mass production, where sterility and uniformity are everything, rendering much of
the trade in local food technically illegal. Eating well has become an act
of civil disobedience. The bread club is political resistance.

"The first few weeks it was just a pickup spot for my sixty loaves of bread," B. continues, "but as the weeks went on, people would pick up their bread and stick around for a while, visiting, especially after T. and M. started bringing their homemade goat cheeses to sell." In addition, the bread club now features raw milk, free-range eggs, and seasonal produce from several gardeners. Occasionally, locally caught salmon, locally gathered seaweed, wild-harvested mushrooms, and honey are available, as well as glasses of homemade wines for an optional donation. People also bring prepared dishes such as quiche, muffins, cheesecake, cinnamon rolls, and pie.

"It evolved on its own without any real agenda by any of us," reflects B. "It wasn't long before it became a two-hour social and market gathering that has continued ever since. There is no advertising, just word of mouth, and it seems every week there are at least a couple of new faces. It seems there are always at least fifteen to twenty people there, and throughout the two hours, I would say that at least sixty people come through. Everyone who comes knows someone, although now there are people who know someone who knows someone. Most are from our town, but some come from a bigger town thirty minutes away." Food always brings people together, and the production and marketing of local food offers great opportunities for community organizing.

"We've always wondered if or when the health department might pay us a visit, but none of us are overly worried about it. If it happens, it happens. I secretly envision everyone nicely but forcefully throwing the poor person out on the street, telling him that this is none of his business. We think about different ways to describe it, like a 'private food buying club,' but we haven't really needed to defend it yet. I wonder whether such a visit might be inevitable as the club gets more well known. I also wonder to what extent they can prosecute us. What if we just refuse to stop gathering? Would they try to fine us, or would they have to come in and arrest all of us and cart us away? Hopefully we can just remain under the radar, but in other ways, if they do crack down, I almost hope for confrontation, because I think this is a rebellion that might explode in their faces if they try. You just don't mess with people's food. We will see. I think that although we are breaking the letter of the law, we are actually honoring the spirit of the law, and that gives us a certain righteous power."

The bread club is not an isolated phenomenon. Many different people—in many different places and motivated by many different concerns—are building resistance movements that reject dead, industrialized, homogenized, globalized food commodities in favor of real, wholesome, local, unadulterated food. In these pages, you will meet a few of them.

Of course, political ideology is hardly the first thing that motivates most individuals' food decisions. Around the world, including here in the United States, many people are not lucky enough to have choices concerning the type, quality, variety, or sources of the food they eat. Access to food and available resources are major factors in most people's daily decision making. So are their concepts of good nutrition, and the insidious sway of marketing.

For me, food is above all a sensual experience. I love the smells, flavors, textures, and colors of food, and how satisfied it can make me feel. I salivate just thinking of harvesting fresh fruit in the summertime. In technicolor odorama, I can vividly recall the tastes of the sweet succession of fruits as the season progresses: juicy sweet mulberries that inspire me to climb trees in their pursuit, black raspberries, wineberries, plums, peaches, blackberries, blueberries, cherry tomatoes, pears, apples, figs, passionfruit, persimmons, pawpaws. . . . Being in a plentiful patch of ripe fruit always forces me to surrender to my greedy desire. I literally stuff my mouth with berries, then crush them and luxuriate in the juicy rush of sensations. Yummm!

The food-related political activism that I feel most passionate about is an extension of this sensual pursuit in that it seeks to revive local food production and exchange, and to redevelop community food sovereignty. There is no sacrifice required for this agenda because, generally speaking, the food closest at hand is the freshest, most delicious, and most nutritious. This revolution will not be genetically engineered, pumped up with hormones, covered in pesticides, individually wrapped, or microwaved. This is a revolution of the everyday, and it's already happening. It's a practice more of us can build into our mundane daily realities and into a grassroots groundswell. This revolution is wholesome, nurturing, and sensual. This revolution reinvigorates local economies. This revolution rescues traditional foods that are in danger of extinction and revives skills that will enable people to survive the inevitable collapse of the unsustainable, globalized, industrial food system.

The production and exchange of local food is not the only way people are protesting the corporate, chemical, and genetically modified (GM) food agenda. Other important food-related activist work is being undertaken in the arenas of policy and regulation: there are campaigns that oppose GM foods and demand that they be labeled as such; that support meaningful organic standards, pesticide limits, fair trade, and farm worker rights; and that challenge the fast-food industry.

People are also confronting the forces of globalization directly, wherever the transnational entities such as the World Trade Organization (WTO) or the World Economic Forum hold their international meetings. These global corporate alliances promote "free trade" as the ultimate good, imposing it upon people around the globe. "WTO has become a global constitution based on the logic and primacy of trade and commerce," writes Vandana Shiva. "The right to trade without limits, without barriers has been elevated to the supreme right. The right to protect living resources, livelihoods, and lifestyles has been reduced to a 'barrier to free trade.'"[1] Protests and civil-disobedience actions have been a continual presence at the meetings of these globalizing entities, along with escalating repression and aggression by authorities. Many more people are engaged in activism around the larger universe of related issues, such as control of indigenous lands, economic justice, war, environmental destruction, cultural survival and cultural appropriation, access to health care, and so on.

With so much to be done, it's easy to feel overwhelmed by it all. When you're feeling overwhelmed, or even just busy, constant convenience consumerism is at your service. Most people in our culture are overworked and stressed. Convenience is our consolation, but the ever-increasing expectation of it also drives very destructive societal choices. Convenience is insidious, inviting us always to fall back into fast food and all the other alluring empty promises of globalized corporate food.

Taking care of ourselves, producing good-quality food, and supporting local producers and markets have to be recognized as activist work. To me, activism is an attitude: emboldened and empowered. I like the quote attributed to Gandhi: "Be the change you want to see in the world." It's important to hold social institutions accountable because they exert so much power, but ultimately no institution can bestow upon us the worlds we dream. Nothing is more revolutionary than actively seeking to embody and manifest the ideals we hold.

The vision of transformation that informs my activist impulse is an ideal, a dream that sustains me and gives me some small sense of hope and belief in the future. It is an abstraction that guides me. But my passion for food is not at all abstract. Food is the stuff of our most basic material reality. Food nurtures us, comforts us, and structures our lives. Our daily habits and routines revolve around it. It is fully sensual, composed of smells, flavors, textures, and aftertastes. Eating is a full-body experience, involving the nose, the mouth, the hands, the teeth, the tongue, the throat, the vast array of internal sensations relating to digestion, and the renewing pleasure of defecation.

Although food is such a fundamental need, most of us are dangerously disconnected from its source. In the United States in 2002, fewer than 2 percent of people were involved in direct agricultural production.[2] Supposedly we have been freed from such drudgery to pursue higher callings. But what some disparage as drudgery is in truth the rhythm of basic sustenance and survival. This rhythm, defined by the seasons and the specificity of place, gives shape to different cultures and provides the context for building community.

Throughout time, most people have been directly involved in obtaining food through wild-food gathering, hunting, and subsistence agriculture. How to feed oneself is among the most vital skills that each generation imparts to its offspring. The essence of empowerment, it is an integral aspect of any organism's integration into its environment. The mass disconnection of human beings from the harvesting and cultivation of our own food reflects a broader disconnection from the natural world, our physical environment, the land, wild plants and animals, the cycles of life and death, even our very bodies. This disconnect is a source of spiritual longing, leaving us searching for reconnection and yearning for meaning.

Our food system desperately demands subversion. We face unprecedented environmental and nutritional crises. Chemical monocrop agriculture is not only depleting the soil of nutrients and producing nutritionally impaired crops but also eroding the topsoil, breeding resistant pests, and poisoning our food and water supplies. GM crops and the "life industry" of patented genetic material raise the stakes, increasing chemical use, farmer dependence on large corporations, the loss of bio-diversity, and the potential for huge-scale health and environmental disasters.

Our system of transporting even the most basic of foods across vast distances requires petroleum, control of which has been at the center of global political conflict in recent times, and sources of which are finite and likely to become scarcer in the near future. This petroleum-based global transport system is also, of course, a driving force behind global warming. Livestock produced by the twisted logic of economies of scale is not only treated cruelly but pumped up with synthetic hormones, antibiotics, and other chemicals that pose numerous health risks, not only to meat eaters and milk drinkers but to everyone who drinks water. Fish too are toxic, containing in their flesh alarming levels of mercury and other heavy metals absorbed from our polluted waters. And as a result of all this ingestion of toxic chemicals, human cancer rates are soaring. Diseases directly related to diet, such as diabetes and obesity, have also reached epidemic proportions, especially among children.

All these crises of our postagrarian, postindustrial, postmodern time converge in the food we eat. Food is among our most basic daily needs. We can get it—cheaply and in great variety and abundance—at any of dozens of huge retail chain stores. We can choose from literally tens of thousands of products that have been shipped across the globe and packaged in wasteful, polluting marketing wraps: meat raised in truly gruesome conditions; produce grown with toxic chemicals; and exotic tropical specialties from places where the legacy of colonialism leaves people growing luxury export crops instead of food they can eat. Food in the supermarket is anonymous, detached from its origins, lacking history, nutrient density, and life force. It is food as pure commodity, and we need better food than that.

Activists all around the world are devoting themselves to the creation of better food choices. The chapters of this book explore ten different themes of food-related issues and activist projects. Far from comprehensive, this book aims to inspire you to become a food activist yourself, and in that process to become more connected to the sources of your food and water. The food system on whose fringes we all are doing our work may seem monolithic and indomitable, but we are nourishing ourselves and one another by our actions, and creating exciting alternatives. To continue with the fermentation metaphor: we are seed cultures, agents of continuity and change, working now and in the future to thrive and proliferate as conditions allow, liberating ourselves and one another and all who will join us from the perils of dependence on dead, anonymous, industrialized, genetically engineered, and chemicalized corporate food.

The Revolution Will Not Be Microwaved

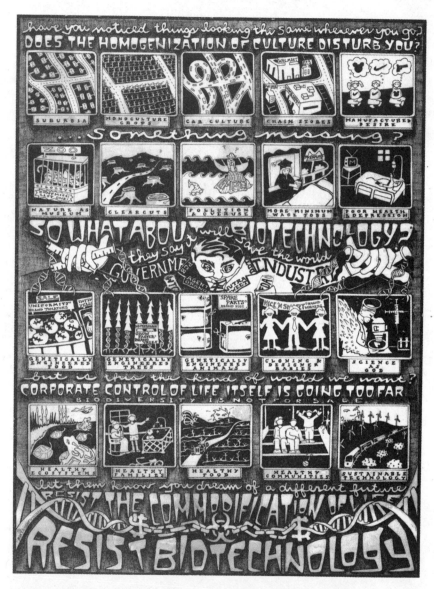

Poster by the Beehive Design Collective. *"Our mission is to cross pollinate the grassroots, by building connections between activists who use words, and those who speak in pictures, to help create more accessible, powerful campaigns for the important issues of our time."* The bees are currently at work on a Food System Map illustrating the contrasts between corporate monoculture and traditional polyculture food systems. www.beehivecollective.org. Used by permission.

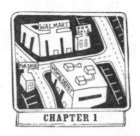

CHAPTER 1

Local and Seasonal Food versus Constant Convenience Consumerism

onvenience is great. We all love it because, by definition, it makes our lives easier: "suited to one's personal ease or comfort." Supermarkets in the middle of the night are calm, can be fun, and make us feel secure because we can satisfy any whim at any moment. And the right yummy treat, in the right place, at the right time, can be a godsend. We all know how easy it is to become accustomed to ready access to familiar foods regardless of time (season) and space (location). But at what price? What's wrong with catering to the convenience of the consumer? Why can't we just enjoy the fact that most members of our affluent society have an unprecedented range of food products to choose from, including those labeled organic, free range, grass fed, and fair trade?

Follow the money. In a traditional local food system, wealth (in the form of food) is created locally, from the land worked by the people. The money people spend on food in that context gets recirculated locally, and food production is a significant generator of economic activity: it supports local mechanics, babysitters, craftspeople, and other local food producers. In economics, this phenomenon is called the *multiplier effect*. A dollar spent on a local grower's produce will continue to circulate locally and multiply its benefits through economic stimulation.

In sharp contrast to the simple and visible exchanges that characterize the path of locally produced food, globalized corporate food follows a long and largely inscrutable chain of transactions, most of which is invisible to the consumer. In this food system, only a tiny proportion of what consumers spend on food at the store goes to the people who grow it. The bulk of our food spending immediately departs from our local communities into the unfathomably huge infrastructures of the shipping and trucking, food-processing, marketing, and retailing industries. Frances Moore Lappé, author of *Diet for a Small Planet*, whose food activism has had tremendous influence since the 1970s, describes this phenomenon as "a colossal transfer of income and capital from producers to middlemen—to the agricultural equivalents of Wall Street arbitrageurs and bond sellers."[1] Rather than paying for food itself, we are paying for an elaborate system for getting it to the right place, at the right time, in the right processed form, and in the right package.

The U.S. Department of Agriculture (USDA) annually publishes the *Agriculture Fact Book*, which contains a figure of a dollar bill broken into segments to represent the allocation of each dollar we spend on food. The *2001–2002 Fact Book* showed that farmers received nineteen cents per food dollar; the remaining eighty-one cents went toward everything else, subsumed under "marketing."[2] This shocking statistic reveals the distorted values of our consumerist culture.

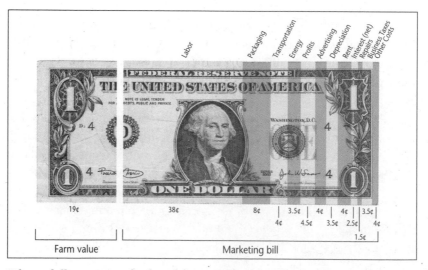

What a dollar spent on food paid for in 2000. Source: USDA.

The Globalization of Food

The multinational corporations that drive the globalized food industry always talk in benevolent terms of feeding the world. "As the global population grows, the challenge to feed the increasing numbers becomes more difficult," begins the "Monsanto Pledge." But thinking of food in terms of feeding millions or billions of people renders it far too abstract and impersonal. Food production on such a scale is the province of experts, specialists, and people with accumulated capital—that is, capitalists. They promote the lie that without their expertise and technology, there would not be enough food for everybody. In their worldview, small-scale, low-tech farming systems may be quaint, but they are certainly inadequate and unrealistic for feeding the mass of humanity. "Very few scientists have the guts to tell activists what this game of producing food for 6.4 billion people is all about," claims Norman Borlaug, the Nobel Prize–winning agronomist who is credited with exporting hybrid varieties and chemical-input agriculture to the Third World in the "Green Revolution" of the 1960s.[3]

But is food production really a game? It is if you're thinking about it at the scale of 6.4 billion people. A roll of the dice determines global price levels, disease vulnerability, and crop failures. "I'll trade you two blight-resistant hybrid varieties for one new genetically modified crop." Power and scale make anything into a game.

Meanwhile, we must sustain ourselves, as we have always been able to do. We are all inherently capable of growing food. We do not have to be dependent on the nutritionally deficient food produced by a global corporate system that is neither stable nor sustainable. In order to eat well and live healthy lives, we must revive and encourage food production in every local community, not further abdicate it to huge economic entities that are driven by profit rather than our well-being. "For most of the history of this country our motto . . . has been Think Big," writes agrarian essayist Wendell Berry. "The citizen who is willing to Think Little, and, accepting the discipline of that, to go ahead on his own, is already solving the problem."[4]

The conventional wisdom in mainstream agriculture is that large-scale crops are more "efficient," yielding efficiencies of scale—more food produced by fewer people. Yet efficiency can be measured in different ways.

Production per unit of labor is only one analysis. Production per unit of land is another. Fertile land is much more scarce than the people needed to work it. And actually, holistic, diversified, sustainable farming systems—"the farm organism," in the language of biodynamic agriculture—can be far more productive than conventional agribusiness models in terms of yield per unit of land.

Small farms and gardens can be planted densely, producing food on many levels—underground, on the ground, and in the air—simultaneously. Typical large-scale farms, in contrast, grow fields of just one crop at a time ("monocropping"), using the land far less intensively. If the true objective were to maximize total agricultural production from limited land resources, then small, dense, diversified farms could certainly produce more food than huge monocrop farms. More people would be required to grow the food, and it wouldn't be as uniform, as easy to amass for global marketing, or as cheap.

In our consumer culture, we expect food to be extremely cheap. The average proportion of household income that Americans spend on food is under 10 percent, half what it was fifty years ago.[5] This is often trumpeted as a triumph of the American economic miracle. The front page of our local newspaper recently reported that the Tennessee Farm Bureau had declared January 29 to February 5, the fifth week of the year, as "Food Checkout Week" because "in just five weeks, the average American will have earned enough disposable income to pay for his or her food supply for the entire year."[6] This less than 10 percent compares to more than 70 percent of household income spent on food in Tanzania, 55 percent in the Philippines, and 20 percent in Japan.[7] I love a bargain as much as anyone, and I'm sure glad I don't need to spend 70 percent of my income on food, but where we direct our resources reflects what we value. Food is this cheap in our country because the people whose labor is involved are paid virtually nothing, and many of food's true costs are hidden.

Hidden costs include fuel for transportation—subsidized in the United States—as well as the military and political costs of maintaining control of the land, sea, and sky, and labor and energy supplies. Then there are the environmental costs of chemical agriculture, including every kind of pollution, groundwater and ozone depletion, global warming, soil erosion, mineral depletion, and species extinctions—as well as the health-care costs for treating the diseases created by the pollution and chemical residues in food. Many of these "externalized" costs are too huge for us to fully comprehend and impossible to calculate. But we need to acknowledge them and start finding ways to factor them in. "It's like a bad TV ad," observes the anticonsumerism magazine *Adbusters*. "Price does not include the $1 billion spent yearly by the U.S. military to secure Mideast shipping lanes; the $1 billion spent on air-pollution-related illness in Ontario, the $1.8 billion the UK will spend to 'adapt' to global warming, the $15 billion cleanup for every record-breaking hurricane that spins out of the changing climate."[8]

As the system of international trade of globalized food commodities grows, the average food item travels farther between producer and consumer than ever before. This means more transportation energy is embedded in the food and greater time elapses between harvest and consumption, during which nutrients are diminished. One often-cited Iowa State University analysis created a hypothetical shopping cart containing only foods grown within the state. It calculated the distances from local growers to the university and found that the local food traveled an average of 56 miles. It then "sourced" the same foods through conventional institutional systems and, by investigating the sources of each item, found that the food had traveled an average of 1,494 miles, nearly twenty-seven times farther.[9]

Of course, the limitation of this study is that it focused just on raw agricultural produce that can be locally grown, in season. The true average distance from farm to plate is actually much greater than 1,500 miles, because only a miniscule proportion of the food Americans buy is unprocessed agricultural products. Most food—70 percent of U.S. agricultural production[10]—is industrially processed, often at multiple locations. Also, much of it is imported. Until recently, the United States always exported far more food than it imported; now for the first time we are teetering at the edge of an agricultural trade deficit.[11]

In some of its details, food shipping can be downright ridiculous. My friend Les, who is a trucker, had a job driving between Idaho and Maine, back and forth, hauling frozen Idaho potato products to Maine and frozen Maine potato products to Idaho. Go figure. It must make business sense for whoever is paying to have it moved. I came across a news report that a Seattle-based salmon marketer is shipping Alaskan salmon and crab to China for labor-intensive processing, then shipping it back to the United States, a total of 8,000 miles. "Something that would cost us one dollar per pound labor here, they get it done for twenty cents in China," says Charles Bundrant, founder of Trident Seafoods.[12] This is the logic of global capital, and it is shortsighted because it ignores, or externalizes, the depletion of nonrenewable resources and the grave environmental costs of all these extraneous food miles. Barbara Kingsolver calls this "the energy crime of food transportation."[13] It is truly decadent.

I don't want to come across as holier-than-thou. I love pineapples (by some calculations, the single most energy-guzzling food) and coconuts and tea and chocolate and lychees and many other food commodities that are available to me only by the grace of the global transportation system. I do not categorically reject foreign trade. It broadens our horizons and potentially enables everybody to enjoy treats from faraway places. But it also increases everyone's dependence on huge economic players, the only ones with the resources to move mass cargo. The scandal of our contemporary food system is that not just a few exotic luxuries but virtually *everything*—including the most basic and mundane staples—is transported such vast distances, traveling thousands of miles from producers to consumers.

In my explorations I came across a fascinating book called *Tangled Routes: Women, Work, and Globalization on the Tomato Trail*, by educator and activist Deborah Barndt. Barndt investigates the people and places, and traces the complex web of power relations, along the transcontinental route of tomatoes from Mexican fields, across the United States, and into Canadian supermarkets and fast-food outlets. She removes the tomato from the realm of abstraction ("imported tomato") and breaks the journey down into discrete steps performed by specific individuals with personal details. Products that travel thousands of miles have stories to tell, few of them pretty.

The tomato trail begins in the historical context of five hundred years of tangled roots: the brutal Spanish conquest of Central America, the Spanish "discovery" of this new fruit, and struggles for control of land. In the Mexican tomato fields, Barndt finds that many of the pickers are women and their children, not uncommonly breast-feeding mothers with babies on their backs. "In breast-feeding her child, Reyna [a

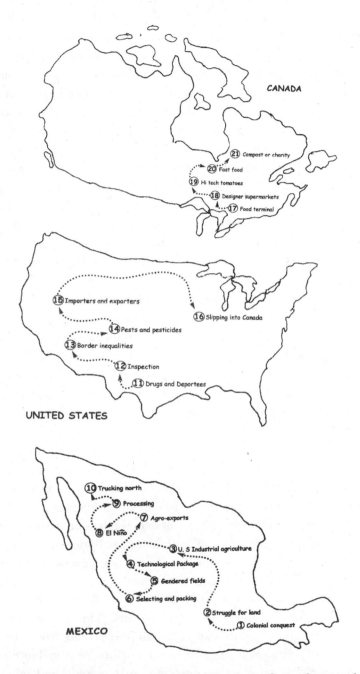

The transcontinental tomato trail, as depicted by Margie Adams of Art Work in Deborah Barndt's *Tangled Routes: Women, Work, and Globalization on the Tomato Trail* (Rowman & Littlefield, 2002). Used by permission.

tomato picker] passed the pesticides from the plants to her hands, which then got into his mouth, and almost poisoned him," reports one of the tomato pickers she interviewed. "Indigenous women and children are clearly in the most precarious position of all who bring us the corporate tomato," observes Barndt.[14] The long-distance truckers who haul the tomatoes across the continent are also part of the story behind those imported tomatoes, as are the families from whom they are separated most of the time and the people who work as cashiers in supermarkets and fast-food joints where the tomatoes end their journey. Each step along the tomato trail is performed by underpaid wage slaves who are desperate for jobs in order to feed themselves and their families. The convenient and alluring out-of-season tomato, like many other foods, is cheap at the expense of the people "on the ground" who bring it to us.

Another part of the reason why food is so cheap is that in the United States the major agricultural commodities are heavily subsidized through a byzantine and hypocritical system that favors monocropping and larger-scale operations. Between 1995 and 2004, the U.S. government paid $144 billion in agricultural subsidies. Seventy-two percent of these subsidies were granted to just 10 percent of U.S. farms, which means big industrial farms received far more money than the smaller operations.[15]

The U.S. farm subsidy program is as confusing as the tax code: indecipherable to most lay generalists, it is designed for and understood primarily by its major beneficiaries. Among the subsidies is the U.S. Milk Income Loss Contract program. To encourage surplus production and make large-scale dairy farming profitable, the federal government guarantees a minimum price for milk. If the market price is at or above that level, then market forces reign; but if the price dips below the set minimum, the USDA compensates the farmer a portion of the difference.

For all the rhetoric about "free trade," milk prices in the United States are set by government technocrats. This news report from Denver in 2005 sounds like it could have come from the Soviet Politburo Central Planning Office: "The price of a gallon of milk is likely to rise by at least seventy cents in Colorado and other states between now and May 1 as the government adjusts prices to reflect a worldwide shortage of dairy products."

What makes this system so grossly unfair and hypocritical is that the U.S. government then dumps surplus milk (as well as other food commodities) into poorer nations, underselling local production. Compliance with the regulations of the International Monetary Fund (IMF), the World Bank, and other international financial institutions doesn't allow these nations to levy tariffs on the imported milk or to subsidize their own food-production industries. They are not free to similarly guarantee a price to their dairy farmers (who cannot compete with the cheap American surplus milk powder), so local production capacity suffers.

Double standards like these make a mockery of "free trade." What's so free about it if the world's richest and most powerful governments can subsidize their favorite food industries, but the less powerful cannot? The United States is not alone in subsidizing milk; a typical cow in the European Union is subsidized to the tune of US$2.20 per day, more than what many of the world's poorest people live on.[16] The hypocrisy of rules forcing poor nations to abandon subsidies and tariffs is far from free trade—it's forced trade. "Free trade is the protectionism of the powerful," says Indian food activist Vandana Shiva.[17]

Free is just a word, like *natural* or even *organic*, used to legitimize and glorify the business practices of huge, profit-driven, amoral, transnational corporate entities that would rather see all six billion of us dependent on them than able to feed ourselves and each other. "The international trading system is not a force of nature beyond human control," writes the international antipoverty agency Oxfam. "The way in which it operates, the way in which it distributes costs and benefits, and the opportunities that it provides or destroys are the consequences of political choices."[18]

The film *Life in Debt* (2001) documents the agricultural-policy double standard over milk and its impact in Jamaica. Dairy farmers there couldn't sell their milk after the IMF required the Jamaican government to end trade barriers and agricultural subsidies. As cheap American milk powder (the surplus encouraged by price guarantees in the United States) flooded the market, Jamaican dairy farmers couldn't compete and ended up discarding massive quantities of milk as their industry shriveled up and died. "We have no national food security," reflects former president Michael Manley in the film. "Give us back our market." Policies ostensibly designed to integrate debtor nations into the global economy have the result of discouraging self-reliance. "It's an insult to our dignity," says Manley.

Globalization actually contributes to world hunger rather than alleviating it. Large-scale global food producers undersell local producers, thereby undermining community food security and creating dependence. In the West African nation of Ghana, frozen chicken imports jumped 500 percent after import tariffs were removed as a condition for debt forgiveness by the IMF and the World Bank. Local chicken sales plummeted, unable to compete, and domestic food-production capacity suffered. Kenneth Quartey, head of Ghana's National Association of Poultry Farmers, says, "What you're breeding is a culture of dependency."[19]

Even if it's not as cheap as mass-producing food thousands of miles away, producing food locally is the only way to have true food security. Anywhere in the world, food production is essential for survival. Global surpluses can certainly help sustain people through droughts and crop failures, but our primary dependence on a globalized food system makes us all vulnerable. Farming everywhere needs to be reoriented toward local needs rather than commodity mass production. We need to bring food production back to earth, making it production we can see and be part of, production based in the community and sustaining the community.

Building Local Food Systems

Buying food directly from the farmers who grow it not only ensures that your food is as fresh as can be; it also means that those farmers are receiving not nineteen cents on the consumer food dollar but the full dollar. That makes farming a far more viable means of earning a living. "Food quality depends on consumers who respect agricultural labor and educate their senses, thus becoming precious allies for producers," says Carlo Petrini, the Italian founder of the Slow Food movement (for more on Slow Food, see chapter 4).[20] The farmer's prosperity is not isolated. Each farmer's success at tapping into local markets inspires others to take up the hoe.

Farmers' markets are growing all around the United States, with more than 3,700 markets registered with the USDA in 2004, more than double the number registered a decade earlier.[21] Food co-ops and buyers' clubs are thriving in some places and disappearing in others; not every bold experiment lasts forever. One problem small, decentralized food retailers face is obtaining products to sell. The food buying club we are part of can no longer obtain many items we used to buy because the largest retailers demand exclusive contracts with manufacturers and distributors and prohibit sales to competitors. At every level, we find "free trade" constrained by the actions of the most powerful economic actors. But the impulse to experiment endures. Marketing food locally is experimental because it flies in the face of all the dominant trends, such as global trade, corporate food marketing, and one-stop shopping. Innovators are inventing unconventional business models as they go.

One form of local food system that has seen a dramatic rise in popularity in the United States and around the world is community-supported agriculture (CSA). CSA farms operate by subscription, linking producers directly to consumers. Subscribers prepurchase a share in the farm's production and receive boxes of mixed seasonal produce each week throughout the growing season. CSAs benefit consumers by giving them fresh, seasonal food, as well as a direct personal connection to a farm. They benefit farmers by giving them predictable income and reducing the time they must spend marketing their produce. CSAs also spread the risk of crop failures, traditionally borne by the farmer alone, among all the CSA members. For instance, if the eggplant crop fails, the farmer will not lose a portion of the year's income; members simply won't get any eggplants and will enjoy other vegetables instead.

Jeff Poppen runs a CSA out of his Long Hungry Creek Farm in Red Boiling Springs, Tennessee. Jeff's farm is one of the most gorgeous and productive I have ever seen, and it has inspired me and many other gardeners and farmers. He's been farming here for nearly thirty years, using biodynamic methods for the past twenty. Biodynamics refers to a farming practice articulated by Rudolf Steiner, an early-twentieth-century Austrian thinker whose ideas about both education (upon which Waldorf schools are based) and agriculture have had enduring influence around the world. Biodynamic farming is a holistic approach involving basic natural processes enhanced by methods such as using homeopathic herbal composts and harmonizing with lunar and celestial influences. "Matter is never without spirit," explains Jeff, "and spirit is never without matter." Biodynamics is a somewhat esoteric practice, but the results are quite consistently compelling. Jeff's farm is a vision of abundance and fertility, as are the other biodynamic farms I've visited.

Jeff is a charismatic fellow who loves to talk about growing food. He views farming as an alchemical art, using earth, air, and water to create food; it's "like manna from heaven," he says. Whenever I've seen him out in the world, he's been giving food away, sharing both his bounty and his passion. Jeff also shares his food-growing zeal on public television in Nashville, through a weekly gardening column ("The Barefoot Farmer") in the *Macon County Chronicle*, and online at www.barefoot-farmer.com. He really puts it out there, and I admire that. Jeff personifies the activist farmer. For him, making the world a better place begins with building soil fertility, and that pursuit is what drives his farming practice.

Jeff started selling his farm produce to a Nashville health food store in 1980, and until the late 1990s he continued selling to it and other area health food stores. Then, he says,

> a national corporation bought one of the stores, which had been a major outlet for us, and it made corporate sense to ship California potatoes to Nashville in late July. . . . A box of garlic was turned down not because of quality or price, but because there was no room on their computer for another garlic item. Next, I received a letter requesting a $2 million insurance policy (in case someone got ill eating garlic?) and was instructed to ship the produce to their Cincinnati warehouse, to then be trucked back to Nashville. My ideal of local agriculture was fading fast. When a few folks from the city offered to help organize a CSA, we jumped on it. Now, as we wind up our fourth year, a community of sixty families around Nashville cares about the farm. I'm not concerned about how to market produce, crop failures, or budget blues, and I make my decisions based on what is best for the farm as a whole.[22]

Shares in the Long Hungry Creek Farm CSA are $25 per week, $100 per month, or $650 for the whole thirty-week season (May through December). Half shares are available as well. The weekly baskets change as the season progresses, and they include bouquets of flowers.

"CSAs offer hope for rural America, not only in a practical, financial way, but on a deeper level, too," says Jeff. "CSA members enjoy many of the pleasures of a farm without having to own one. They can bring their family out for a picnic, see animals and gardens, and eat fresh organic food all week. They are reestablishing a connection to the land, reuniting a lost tie between the city and the country, developing a mutual trust and friendship with a farmer, and helping wealth to be created locally."

The CSA concept (known in some other English-speaking lands as "box schemes") developed in Japan in the 1970s and was first tried in the United States in the mid-1980s. By 1990 there were an estimated 60 CSAs in the United States; fifteen years later there were some 1,700.[23] This same period also saw tremendous growth in farmers' markets. The USDA's 2002 Census of Agriculture documented a 37 percent increase from 1997 to 2002 in the value of agricultural products sold "directly to individuals for human consumption."[24]

The revival of local markets for agriculture doesn't happen spontaneously. It takes more than one farmer's efforts to make it happen. It takes organizing and networking to bring producers and consumers together. One organization I've encountered, the Appalachian Sustainable Agriculture Project (ASAP), that creates such linkages in mostly rural western North Carolina has produced a seventy-two-page local food guide listing seventeen CSAs, thirty-six farmers' markets and tailgate markets, 128 family farms, and dozens of orchards and U-pick farms, as well as restaurants and grocers featuring local produce. The ASAP area, the region around Asheville, North Carolina, is notable for how well developed its local food systems are; however, it is not unique. All around the country there similar local food initiatives. More and more regions can now boast of extensive farmers' markets, CSAs, and other innovative connections between local growers and local consumers. Linkages like this take work, but the potential for them exists everywhere.

Regulating the Taste and Nutrients Out of Food

Where sanctioned markets exist for local food, the range of what they can sell is quite limited. The free exchange of food at the local level is virtually nonexistent; laws enacted in the name of hygiene require expensive facilities, licensing, and processing. Yes, sanitation and hygiene are important. But expensive facilities do not guarantee safe practices. And simply by virtue of scale, smaller production facilities do not carry the same risk potential as large facilities, for even a worst-case scenario has limited impact. Scale is everything in risk assessment.

No matter how many farmers' markets there are in western North Carolina, Cailen Campbell can't sell his fresh-pressed sweet apple cider at any of them. I met Cailen at the Southeast Permaculture Gathering at Earthaven Ecovillage in Black Mountain, North Carolina. He brought with him his wooden cider-press-on-wheels and crates and crates of apples gleaned from unharvested local orchards. He was providing a participatory demonstration, accepting donations for the cider but not selling it. Cailen told me that the local health authorities wouldn't permit him to sell apple cider without processing it by pasteurization or irradiation, which would destroy important nutrients and enzymes. In other words, an accomplished fruit gleaner with a human-powered mechanical press can't set up a small-time occasional cider stall at a farmers' market without diminishing his product and investing in expensive equipment to do so.

How real is the raw cider threat? Pasteurization or irradiation of cider has become the norm in the aftermath of a 1996 outbreak of *E. coli* 0157:H7 attributed to a large-scale juice producer, Odwalla, in which sixty-six people were reported sick and a sixteen-month-old baby died. Contamination was presumed to be from manure on apples harvested from the ground, though it could have occurred in the production facility. After several years of debate, in 2002 the U.S. Food and Drug Administration began requiring pasteurization or irradiation for large-scale juice producers and warning labels on untreated juices from small producers. Many states and localities have prohibited the sale of any unpasteurized juices.

Without minimizing the death of that baby, we have to assess risk as a relative phenomenon. We live with a certain level of risk every time we get into a car. We live with the risk of crime, violence, and bites from venomous creatures. We live with the risk of heart disease and cancer. We may do things to limit our risk, but then again, we may not. That decision is generally regarded as the prerogative of the individual. Real food, from the earth, is fraught with potential biological risks. The more we sterilize our food to eliminate all theoretical risk, the more we diminish its nutritional quality. Can't we reasonably decide to accept those risks that can accurately be described as "one in a million"? Do we have to demonize every food that ever becomes contaminated and declare it unsafe without sterilization?

The health risks of apple cider beg a popular beverage comparison: At the time of U.S. independence from Britain, cider (mostly hard) was the nation's most popular drink, with consumption topping thirty-five gallons per person in 1767 Massachusetts.[25] Today the drink that Americans consume in such mega-quantity is soda, with each of us drinking an average of nearly fifty-four gallons in 2004.[26] Though probably not a single person's death has ever been directly attributed to soda (drowning in a vat in a factory, perhaps?), soda consumption does contribute to obesity, diabetes, and even cancers (see chapter 6). We're whipped up into a panic about the freak incidents of contamination while the real risk factors in the food supply achieve "global ubiquity" (the Coca-Cola Corporation's stated goal).

The apple orchard near my father's home in New York State, where I have enjoyed raw apple cider all my life, has been irradiating its cider since the new rules came into effect. Some states, however, still allow unprocessed cider to be sold directly from producers to consumers. In Farmington, Maine, I stopped at a cider stand in the parking lot of an ice cream shop, and I was thrilled to learn that the cider was not only fresh but still raw. I learned this from a label on the cider jugs: "Warning: This product has not been pasteurized and, therefore, may contain harmful bacteria that can cause serious illness in children, the elderly, and persons with weakened immune systems."[27]

Warn people if you must. My immune system, tenuous as it might be, is not so weak as to believe that juice squeezed out of an apple is better after it's been heated or irradiated. Raw nutrients and enzymes are important (see chapter 5). The owner of the stand told me that most people are more enthusiastic about the cider after they read the warning label. They know it's real and prepared in the traditional way. They do not think they are risking their lives. And they feel good about giving their money directly to a producer rather than into an impersonal system in which the producer receives very little.

Applying requirements that make sense for industrial-scale production to small producers renders small-scale production prohibitively expensive. In the industrializing nineteenth century, when food processing at an unprecedented scale was creating contamination problems, "food science became obsessed with purity," writes cultural historian Felipe Fernández-Armesto in *Food: A History*. "Far-sighted food producers realized that purity legislation, by driving up unit costs, would favour economies of scale and bring more business to the heavily capitalized reaches of the industry. Hygiene was a selling point which would enhance any brand."[28]

This industrial-scale global trade system requires uniformity and standardization. We sacrifice quirks of flavor, texture, nutrition, biodiversity, and the specificity of local culture in exchange for convenience, predictability, and a plethora of empty choices. French Situationist theorist Guy Debord calls this

> the logic of the commodity in all of its abstract purity. . . . The food that has lost its taste presents itself in every case as perfectly hygienic, dietary, and healthy in comparison to the risky adventures of pre-scientific food preparation. . . . For the qualitative, one substitutes various ideological claims—State laws that are supposedly imposed in the name of hygiene or simply to guarantee the appearance of it—that favor the concentration of production. . . . All historical traditions must disappear and the abstraction rules in the absence of quality.[29]

The rallying cry of pro-globalization forces is *Free Trade! Free Trade!* Why then do many people who wish to buy or sell food at the local level find it prohibited? Isn't simple exchange the origin and essence of Free Trade™? How could "free trade" preclude small-time neighborly buying and selling of basic foods? This is a theme that will come up throughout the disparate topics covered in this book.

Many of these restrictions on free local trade disappear if we can redefine the transaction as purchasing a share in an endeavor rather than purchasing particular products. Thinking "outside the box," inventing new structures to support local food production, enables people to circumvent and subvert laws restricting what can be sold. CSAs radically restructure the relationship between producer and consumer, eliminating sales transactions. "I don't sell anything from my farm anymore," says Jeff Poppen with irrepressible glee. "I give it all away to our members." The CSA concept is gradually expanding beyond vegetables into other foods. I've heard about a grain, bean, and seed CSA project and another offering wool, alpaca, and llama fibers, and in subsequent chapters we will see how the "farm-share" model is being used to similarly build community support for farm operations producing milk (chapter 5) and meat (chapter 8).

What about Organic?

Food raised and prepared without reliance on synthetic chemicals is *absolutely* better to eat than the products of the chemical-driven agricultural mainstream, for many reasons. Chemical agriculture pollutes our water, air, and earth, impairs the web of life in the soil, erodes biodiversity, and requires high levels of "inputs" such as irrigation, the chemicals themselves, and fuel, and its products contain toxic residues. Chemical agriculture is an unmitigated disaster, and a relatively new phenomenon: prior to World War II, virtually all food was produced without chemicals, by what we now call "organic" methods.

Theories about chemical fertilization had been bandied about since the nineteenth century, but production of agricultural chemicals first developed around World War I, and really swung into high gear after 1945, when war-driven factory output needed to be redirected to other uses. "We are eating the leftovers of the Second World War," says Vandana Shiva. "The chemicals of warfare have been deployed as pesticides and herbicides."[30] Some of the chemicals were developed with multiple uses in mind. The neurotoxic properties of organophosphate chemicals caught the attention of Bayer Corporation chemists in Germany in the 1930s, and they proceeded to develop organophosphates "simultaneously as agricultural pesticides and as nerve gases for

military use,"[31] including the notorious Zyklon-B used for mass extermi-
nations in Nazi gas chambers.[32] The postwar production and marketing
of chemicals in agriculture was remarkably successful; in just a few
decades, chemical-driven agricultural practices and their toxic-residue-
laden products became so widespread that they came to be referred to
as "conventional."

Agricultural chemicals kill—and not only plants and insects and
worms and birds and fungi and the vast universe of soil organisms; they
kill people as well. The World Health Organization reports that three
million cases of pesticide poisoning occur every year, resulting in more
than 250,000 deaths.[33] As one example, three women who were
employed as tomato pickers during their pregnancies by a firm called
Ag-Mart in North Carolina gave birth to severely deformed babies.
Records showed that Ag-Mart illegally sent workers into freshly sprayed
fields as a regular practice.[34] The same dangerous chemicals enter our
bodies in smaller doses whenever we eat "conventional" produce. We all
get to face the effects of chronic pesticide exposure as we grapple with
growing incidences of cancer, reproductive disorders, developmental
deformities, various degenerative neurological disorders, and a host of
other diseases.

That said, I still have my doubts about the organic label. What something *isn't* (full of chemicals) doesn't tell us much about what that thing
is. Whether a food is "organic" or not, the same food-chain questions of
origin, distance traveled, and connection apply.

Where I live, the nearest commercial source of organic food is the
local Piggly Wiggly supermarket, which carries exactly three organic
products—butter, low-fat milk, and lettuce, all from brands in national
distribution. Nobody selling at the local farmers' market describes their
produce as organic, though a few folks, in response to my questions
(not in their signage), say they use no chemicals. Our friends who
operate a local produce stand, Andy and Judy Fabri of A&J Produce,
sell chemical-free vegetables from their own garden and other small-
scale local producers, as well as "conventional" produce from the
Nashville wholesale market. At our request, they have sometimes procured organic produce for us, but they think it's throwing money away.
Not that they don't appreciate the superiority of food grown without
chemicals—their own garden is organic—it's just that their experiences

with unscrupulous distributors in the wholesale market leads them to the conclusion that just because a box or bag of produce says it is organic does not make it so. "I've watched them take boxes marked 'organic' and fill them with regular produce," Andy says. "Organic is great, but the whole system is corrupt."

For a selection of organic produce, we can go twenty-five miles to Wal-Mart, or twice as far to Wild Oats (and soon Whole Foods). These national chains purchase produce in quantities sufficient for national distribution. Even though that produce is grown in accordance with the USDA standards (or maybe not, as Andy points out), it has nothing to do with community-based food production. A dollar spent on organic plums at Wal-Mart goes to corporate headquarters in Bentonville, Arkansas, to the real-estate developer who owns the land the store is built on, to the truckers who brought it there, and, as a small fraction of that dollar, to the grower and the cashier. Wal-Mart is the largest private employer in the United States and represents an astounding 2 percent of the entire U.S. economy.[35] "While charging low prices obviously has some consumer benefits," states a congressional report on Wal-Mart, "mounting evidence from across the country indicates that these benefits come at a steep price for American workers, U.S. labor laws, and community living standards."[36]

Organic products in national distribution are an upscale market niche available through the desire-gratifying magic of constant convenience consumerism and produced by factory-style monocultures. Ironically, although the organic movement began as an act of resistance against the trend toward factory farming in mainstream agriculture, its success has aroused the interest of the major global agribusiness corporations to which the organic movement originally defined itself as an alternative.

The market for organic foods is expanding rapidly. According to the USDA, demand for organic products has increased by 20 percent or more each year since the early 1990s, and the trend continues.[37] Most of the nationally distributed organic food products are now owned by major food conglomerates. "Now that organic food has established itself as a viable alternative food chain," writes Michael Pollan, "agribusiness has decided that the best way to deal with that alternative is simply to own it."[38]

Organic Industry Structure
August 2006*

*This structure is constantly changing. For example, Anheuser-Busch (#6) is currently test marketing Wild Hop and Stone Mill organic beer, and Kraft is expected to introduce organic versions of some of its products, including Nabisco Oreos, in late 2006.

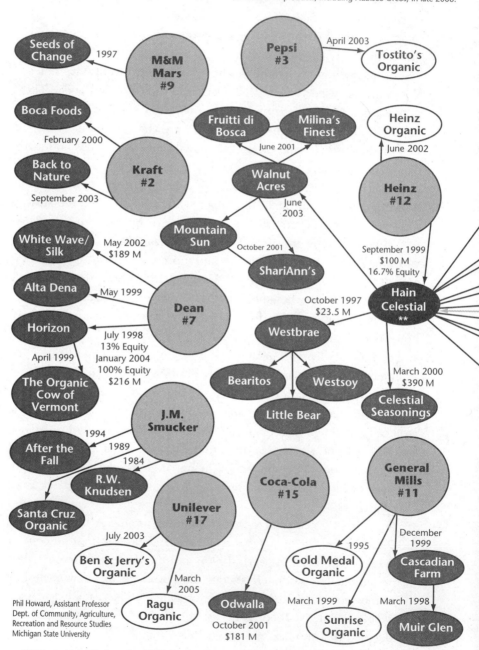

Phil Howard, Assistant Professor
Dept. of Community, Agriculture,
Recreation and Resource Studies
Michigan State University

**Heinz announced in December, 2005, that the company would begin selling all of its shares in Hain Celestial.

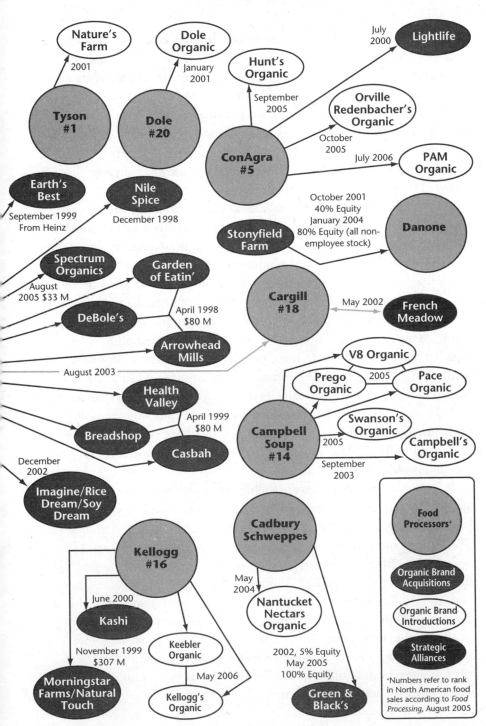

Nature's Farm
2001
Tyson #1

Dole Organic
January 2001
Dole #20

Hunt's Organic
September 2005

Orville Redenbacher's Organic
October 2005

July 2000 Lightlife

ConAgra #5

July 2006 PAM Organic

Earth's Best
September 1999 From Heinz

Nile Spice
December 1998

Stonyfield Farm

October 2001 40% Equity
January 2004 80% Equity (all non-employee stock)

Danone

Spectrum Organics
August 2005 $33 M

Garden of Eatin'

Cargill #18

May 2002 French Meadow

DeBole's

April 1998 $80 M

Arrowhead Mills

August 2003

V8 Organic

Prego Organic 2005 Pace Organic

Health Valley

April 1999 $80 M

Breadshop

Casbah

Campbell Soup #14

Swanson's Organic

2005

September 2003

Campbell's Organic

December 2002

Imagine/Rice Dream/Soy Dream

Kellogg #16

June 2000
Kashi

November 1999 $307 M

Keebler Organic

Morningstar Farms/Natural Touch

May 2006

Kellogg's Organic

Cadbury Schweppes

May 2004

Nantucket Nectars Organic

2002, 5% Equity
May 2005
100% Equity

Green & Black's

Food Processors⁺

Organic Brand Acquisitions

Organic Brand Introductions

Strategic Alliances

⁺Numbers refer to rank in North American food sales according to *Food Processing*, August 2005

Periodically updated online at www.certifiedorganic.bc.ca/rcbtoa/services/corporate-ownership.html

Organic certification rules were originally self-generated—through organic processes, as it were—from grassroots associations of farmers committed to growing food without chemicals. In 2002, after years of discussion, drafts, and controversy, the USDA adopted a national organic standard. In the process, some voices argued for a "principle of proximity" to factor locality into organic standards; however, such calls have thus far gone unheeded. In its translation from a motley patchwork of peer-review standards to a USDA regulatory category, "organic" has changed from an ethic of holistic thinking and eco-integration to a law subject to lobbying and loopholes. A 2005 congressional backroom deal inserted amendments to the federal organic standards into an agricultural appropriations bill. The amendments, permitting manufacturers to use nonorganic ingredients and synthetic additives and processing aids in certified organic products, were supported by the Organic Trade Association, an industry group of manufacturers of organic products.

Sleazy political manipulations serve to undermine organic credibility. "Many growers feel that organic certification serves only agribusiness," reports Michael Sligh, director of sustainable agriculture policy at the Rural Advancement Foundation International (RAFI). "It's not so important for direct marketing; it's more important for interstate and global trade."[39] Indeed, many growers I've talked with who are selling their produce directly to local consumers, Jeff Poppen included, are opting out of the USDA "organic" labeling system because it is expensive and irrelevant.

It's irrelevant because growers selling directly to consumers can use alternative language to explain or demonstrate their eco-friendly farming methods. They don't require the expensive "organic" branding. The farmers and their stories are part of the appeal of the produce. The greater the distance between production and consumption, between the farmer and the consumer, the more important the organic label becomes. In this context, "organic" is a brand, a label, a market niche, far removed from ideals of community-based eco-farming and the roots of the organic movement. One thing "organic" doesn't mean is local. People wishing to resist corporate control and eat fresh, healthy food have to move beyond organics and into the foodshed,[40] thinking about where our food actually comes from.

Expanding Access

Some people have the idea that food marketed as organic or locally grown is inherently elitist. We must acknowledge that to be in the position to be selective about the food we eat is to hold a privileged position. "We who are systematically privileged—whether by virtue of race, class, education, or gender—cannot escape the fact that, in every choice we make, every action we take, we exercise that privilege," writes philosopher Lisa Heldke, author of *Exotic Appetites: Ruminations of a Food Adventurer*. "The question we must ask is not 'How can we avoid privilege?' but 'How can we work to undermine the structures that give me privilege in the first place?'"[41]

Many people who are not in a position to be selective would also prefer to eat food that is not a repository of toxic wastes. In places where most people have little disposable income, both urban and rural, consumers generally have far fewer choices than consumers in more affluent locales. "One of the great, often unspoken, forms of oppression that low- and moderate-income communities suffer through is the lack of access to healthy food," writes community activist Mark Winston Griffith of Brooklyn, New York.[42] Ironically, many things, food among them, cost more in these areas, too. There is nothing fair about poverty and the gross inequalities of resources and opportunities that are reflected in every aspect of our society, food choices included. Some activists are working, and many more are needed, to bring access to fresh, wholesome food to poor people and underserved neighborhoods, as part of a movement for food justice.

Food production and distribution do not have to be driven by profit. West Oakland, California is a community of twenty-five thousand people served by thirty-six convenience stores and only one supermarket. These stores give residents easy access to overprocessed, overpriced junk food, but few choices for produce and other healthy foods. Community organizers have created an exciting, innovative, shopping alternative for West Oakland residents: the People's Grocery, a mobile market. The market-on-wheels makes five stops along a regular route three days per week, selling healthy food at affordable prices, with an emphasis on locally grown produce. The People's Grocery grows much of the produce it sells in community gardens at a local YMCA, a land trust, and an elementary school. The nonprofit organization has grown to include two youth programs: the Collards 'n Commerce Youth Entrepreneurship Program, which involves fifteen- to eighteen-year-olds in all aspects of the operation, from food production to marketing, and the Urban Rootz Food & Justice Camp for younger kids. "Because the universal and intimate nature of food makes it a natural springboard for addressing many issues, People's Grocery is focusing on the basic human right to food as an organizing tool for justice and health in West Oakland," the organization's Web site declares. "We combine grassroots and street-level marketing/organizing techniques with socially responsible business practices and sustainable agriculture to create new approaches to addressing food justice."[43]

In Detroit, a group called Earth Works has gardens on several large city lots. When I visited in 2005, we had to climb up four stories in order to take in the full scale of Earth Works' largest garden. Under the brilliant summer sun, a crew of about eight people—some students performing community service requirements—was harvesting box after box of squash, beans, tomatoes, peppers, and more. Earth Works distributes the vegetables at a local soup kitchen and to mothers at a local WIC office (Women, Infants, and Children is a federal program that provides basic nutrition to mothers and their young children). When local, chemical-free produce is made available to people with few resources, they respond enthusiastically.

Another strategy that some activists have used to integrate local food access into the mainstream is to compel local institutions to seek out local seasonal produce. In 2004 the Seattle school board adopted broad new nutrition policies, including a directive that school meal programs "offer fresh, local, organic, non-genetically modified, non-irradiated, unprocessed food, whenever feasible."[44] "Whenever feasible" remains to be seen, but a buying policy is a great place to start. Parent activists in many places are demanding healthier food in schools, and policies are in flux. Enough school districts, universities, and other institutions have become interested in buying local food that an annual Farm to Cafeteria Conference is now being held. *Time* magazine reports that 200 U.S. universities have adopted local-food purchasing policies,[45] and a 2005 survey of 130 of them found them spending an average of $162,000 per year on local food.[46] Because they govern the purchase of food to feed large numbers of people, institutional food policies can have a powerful stimulating effect on local food systems.

At the Carolina Farm Stewards Association conference in Asheville, North Carolina, I attended a presentation by representatives of the Small Farmer Distribution Network, which organizes cooperatives of mostly African-American farmers in Alabama, Georgia, and the surrounding region to market their crops to area school districts. At another conference, Acres USA, I heard about a project in Appleton, Wisconsin, in which a whole-grain bakery, Natural Ovens, sponsored and designed a healthy school lunch program for an alternative high school. Project staff report that cutting sugar and other highly processed foods out of the school lunch menus and serving primarily fresh, locally grown food dramatically improved student behavior and performance.

Beyond serving healthy food and stimulating the local food economy, school lunch programs can be valuable educational opportunities. Encouraging local food means weaving food production back into the web of community life. School gardens can be integrated into the curriculum, used to teach kids practical life skills while also allowing them to explore basic concepts of biology, nutrition, economics, design, teamwork, and problem solving and to produce some of their own food. This is experiential education, a radical break from the educational monoculture of our age in which standardized tests reign supreme.

Without farm-to-school linkages, many young people grow up without a clear idea of where food comes from. Farmer Michael Ableman describes a visit from a group of city kids: "I let them loose within the rows of the tall cherry tomato vines and watched their brain cells exploding with new information as they harvested and ate vine-ripe tomatoes for the first time in their lives. . . .This was real education . . . the experience of seeing and eating food in context."[47]

Quite a few schools have established excellent gardening programs, spurring advocacy, funding, and curriculum development efforts. Alice Waters's Edible Schoolyard Program, based at a middle school in Berkeley, California, is one such program. "Make lunch a mandatory subject," she says. The international Slow Food movement has undertaken a Slow Food in Schools initiative, in which local chapters are adopting schools and helping them start gardens and weave gardening into their curricula.

Schools are not the only local institutions that need food. How about getting hospitals to buy and serve local food? Imagine how much more healing that would be compared to the overprocessed junk most hospitals serve now. Gardens at hospitals and other healing centers can be put to therapeutic use as well. The fastest-growing public institution in American society is prisons, with more than two million people incarcerated in the United States at present. At least a few prisons have gardens as part of their therapeutic programs. I'm certainly not advocating that prisoners be forced to farm; however, more prisons could be institutionally encouraged to start gardening programs and also to purchase local food to serve to their populations.

Some people have made a conscious choice to eat only local foods. Gary Paul Nabhan restricted himself for a year to foods from within a foodshed of 250 miles from his Tucson, Arizona, home, and he documented the experience in a book, *Coming Home to Eat* (Norton, 2002). As he purged his kitchen of long-distance foods at the beginning of his adventure, it "revealed that the bulk of my diet had been brought to me by just a handful of food processors and distributors. The contents of my cupboard, fridge, and pantry in Arizona were dominated by agricultural commodities that had been bred, produced, processed, and distributed by the same companies, active everywhere from Argentina to Zaire."[48]

Nabhan's self-imposed restriction led him to meet many neighbors engaged in small-scale food production. It also broadened his awareness of local foraging possibilities:

> There were plenty of wild greens growing along the roadside: amaranths, lamb's-quarters, and purslane, known locally as *verdolagas*. Collectively, Sonorans called these greens *quelites de los agues*, the wild spinaches of the summer rainy season. I harvested several garbage bags full of their tender growth tips, avoiding the older, more fibrous leaves and stems.
>
> Tonight I entered *quelite* heaven, enjoying the freshest greens I could imagine. I grilled some scallions and poblano chiles, then added a mound of hand-washed greens to the saucepan. They wilted as the moisture on their leaves sizzled on the bottom of the pan. I served them immediately. Their fla-

vors were so fresh, so buzzed with their recent photosynthetic surge that my meal sizzled with sunshine. Within minutes of devouring them, I felt greener, as if I were on some folic acid high. I dreamed that night of having chlorophyll in my skin, as if I had become green as the Green Giant himself.[49]

Another local food quest that has been well documented is the Hundred-Mile Diet undertaken by Alisa Smith and J. B. MacKinnon in Vancouver, British Columbia. "This may sound like a lunatic Luddite scheme, but we had our reasons," they write. "The short form would be: fossil fuels bad." In a Vancouver weekly and online, they recounted stories of their experiences. "Eating locally is a grand adventure," they conclude. "The persistent idea that a local diet can't be varied is an indication of how disconnected most of us are from the reality of living in one of the planet's richest ecological regions."[50]

Different groups have been encouraging people to try local eating experiments. Slow Food USA invites its members to organize groups for the Local Food Challenge, in which members spend a month eating only local foods. In August 2005, in the San Francisco Bay Area, hundreds of people participated in a program called Locavores, in which they pledged to eat only foods from within a one-hundred-mile distance. The Locavores movement (in some groups spelled Localvores) is rapidly spreading to different regions. Another organized effort, the Buy Local Challenge, posted blog diaries from participants. One District of Columbia resident who took up the challenge recounts his interactions at a local natural foods supermarket:

> **Cheese Section:**
> **Me:** Um, excuse me. I'm trying to find a locally produced cheese?
> **Worker:** From where?
> **Me:** Um, like Maryland or Virginia, close . . .
> **Worker:** Sorry, we have a Cheddar from New York, everything else is from Wisconsin.
> **Me:** Really, nothing closer than New York?
> So I bought New York cheddar. . . .

Bread Section:

Me: Um, hi, I was looking for a bread that was made with local products.

Worker: (mute . . . points to a rack of bread)

Me: (*all these breads are from Texas* . . . so I move to the next worker behind the counter)

Me: Hi, do you have any Maryland produced bread?

Worker: What is that?

Me: I'm part of a month-long challenge to buy local and eat local, so I want sandwiches for lunch and need local bread.

Worker: You might try a local bakery. All our breads are produced from Whole Foods products, not sure where they come from.

Me: I look up at the sign, hanging above her head that reads . . . Bakery, and say "Thank you." So much for a local grilled cheese sandwich.[51]

Local and seasonal eating usually requires that we adjust our expectations. Some foods we are used to eating on a daily basis may simply not be possible in this scheme. For instance, unless you live in Florida, you might have to let go of that morning glass of orange juice. But other foods, no less delicious or nutritious (in fact generally far more so), will replace them. We can learn to love what grows abundantly and easily around us and reorient our tastes and our habits. Another completely different take on the idea of a local food challenge a "land fast," a period of eating only what can be harvested in the immediate vicinity, in the gardens and the woods. In certain seasons, one could be very satisfied.

Relatively few people have voluntarily chosen to make the switch to exclusively local foods. But in some cases circumstances have resulted in the abrupt disappearance of global trade, and it has been demonstrated that people *can* survive and restore food sovereignty. Take, for example, Cuba. Until 1989 Cuba's major trading partners were the Soviet nations of Eastern Europe. Cuba exported sugar and imported most other foods, as well as fuel, machinery, and chemicals. In 1989 about three times as much Cuban land was planted in sugar cane than was planted in all other food crops combined. Fifty-seven percent of the calories in the Cuban diet were imported.[52] But the abrupt disintegration of the Soviet-allied governments and the Soviet Union itself resulted in the sudden loss of these trading partners.

The loss of its trade partners meant a loss of two-thirds of Cuba's food supply, as well as the fuel, machinery, and chemicals upon which its agricultural system depended. Compounding the shortages was a tightening of the U.S. economic blockade of Cuba in the early 1990s. The food shortage was so acute that diseases of malnutrition became widespread.

Lacking the "inputs" (such as chemicals, fuel, and hybrid seeds) required for industrial-style monoculture, Cuba was forced to transform its farming system. Food production was decentralized, and farmers in each region were encouraged to diversify rather than specialize. Urban, family, and community gardening, which had always been features of Cuban life, were officially encouraged, and a program of public education and model farms was undertaken to spread knowledge about biological farming methods. The Ministry of Agriculture even replaced its front lawn with vegetable gardens.[53]

By 1999, Cuba had become a nation of food producers. Urban gardens alone produced more than eight hundred thousand tons of food, mostly vegetables.[54] There is no way to compare this sector to pre-1989 levels, because until then this sector was considered insignificant and not counted. However, this remarkable statistic shows that cities *can* produce food, though not in the style of acres upon acres of grain fields; instead, intensive cultivation of yards and parks and rooftops can ensure a steady supply of fresh produce to urbanites (for more on urban gardening, see chapter 3).

The prospect of a crisis is obviously not the only compelling reason to revive local food production. There are many benefits of local food, starting with flavor, continuing through nutrition, and definitely including community economic stability. But it's good for us who live in a culture of constant convenience consumerism to be reminded that the time-honored methods of producing food can still feed people perfectly adequately.

For most people in most places throughout time, the food available has been organic and local. Organic was all there was until the mid-twentieth century, and anything beyond local, to the extent that it was available at all, was an expensive luxury, out of daily reach for average people. Abundant globalized food may not always be available to us either. It is easy for me to imagine the United States, or the whole world, in suddenly different economic circumstances, with an abrupt halt to all international trade, as Cuba faced in 1989, that forces a transition to greater dependence on community-based food production. The skills and practice of food production are important to revive and to prevent from disappearing.

Growing Your Own: The Most Local Agriculture

Reading about the achievements of Cuba's populist agriculture, I recalled stories of the American "victory garden" movement during the World Wars of the twentieth century. My grandfather Isadore Katz, whom I never knew, started a victory garden at his home in Englewood, New Jersey, when he was a teenager during World War I. He won an award for having the best garden in northern New Jersey. For the rest of his life Isadore kept a garden, and he passed his passion for growing food on to my father, who loves his garden, organizes lavish feasts around its bounty, and who evidently has passed that passion on to me. What a cultural sea change we have undergone in two generations, such that in moments of national crisis our leaders encourage us no longer to produce but rather to consume, as President Bush did in urging people to go shopping as an expression of patriotism in the fall of 2001. Becoming a producer subverts the consumerist paradigm.

I say "becoming a producer" as if it were easy, and I know it isn't. Growing food is hard work, and it takes time to learn. That's why the time to start is now. It's tempting to romanticize the growing of food or to see the garden as utopia. Charles Fourier, a nineteenth-century French social theorist who is remembered as a utopian socialist, considered horticulture to be "attractive labor" and envisioned a society in which the growing of food would be "orgiastically pleasurable."[55] In my own experience, growing food definitely has its orgiastically pleasurable and ecstatic moments—for instance, witnessing the miracle of germination or tasting the first ripe tomato of the season—but gardening is also hard work requiring perseverance. Time is a precious commodity in our culture. Most of us feel like we don't have enough of it. Yet some busy, overworked people find contemplation, relaxation, and peace in the garden.

The garden can be quite a bewildering place if you're not tuned in to plants and their rhythms. I can see that it's a completely alien idea for most people to go out and harvest and, even more so, to base their food preparation and eating on what's growing. The allure of convenience has severed us from the rhythms of what grows when and where. I feel so lucky to have grown up in a household with a garden, to have watched meals form around ripe vegetables and not just shopping lists generated from abstract desires. I meet so many people—people who love food and cooking—who are utterly clueless about what grows when and are completely disempowered in the green world of the garden.

It's very challenging for people used to constant convenience consumerism to adapt to a bioregional and seasonal approach to food. The garden is nothing like the supermarket. Snow peas have their moment, and a glorious moment it is, but you can't walk into the garden in mid-August looking for snow peas just because that's what the recipe calls for. Nor peppers in May. The seasonality of food—the fact that most fruits and vegetables come into season for a very limited period—makes it all the more special. The luscious, fleeting ripeness becomes something to anticipate, something to savor, something to eat more of while you can, something to preserve for future enjoyment, something to remember, and something to look forward to again when the cycle repeats itself. The experience of the food itself is enriched by its seasonality.

Unlike some communities, which define themselves by high ideals like "sustainability" or "self-sufficiency," Short Mountain Sanctuary, the community where I have lived for the past thirteen years, is above all else a safe space for queer folks. We also try to be ecologically sustainable, of course, but we are a haven for all sorts of interesting people for whom growing food is not necessarily a central priority. Just a few of us are involved in vegetable gardening on a regular basis. Though the community at large certainly appreciates our garden's bounty, and many are willing to pitch in on big planting or harvesting projects, most people do not seem to familiarize themselves with what's growing or avail themselves of it, unless it's harvested for them.

One of the recurring annoyances for me in my life here has been the whine of "we don't have any food" because we are running out of store-bought produce in the kitchen, when meanwhile the garden is full of fresh vegetables. Maybe not eggplant in May or radishes in August; but in our climate, with our cold-frames, there's something fresh to be had year-round. The worst insult to the gardeners is to buy in town a vegetable that we have growing here in great profusion. My former fellow-communard Kasha will always be remembered for his vegetable-stomping temper tantrum when someone came home from town with a bag of okra, while our garden okra was going unharvested. People simply don't think to look. Eating out of the garden requires an education, which most of us in the twenty-first century lack. But if you seriously want to resist the global food system, start getting yourself that education.

Growing food yourself and learning about wild foods that grow nearby are absolutely the best ways to have ready access to the freshest, chemical-free food. For me, like many other people across space and time, getting to know plants—working with them, developing ongoing relationships with them—has been a deeply transformative experience. Seed germination and plant growth are ecstatic bursts of life that can energize, affirm, and inspire our own lives.

Harvesting from the garden is my favorite part of the process. Every season I learn about more ways to enjoy plants in different stages of their growth. For instance, the preflowering stalks of garlic, called scapes, are delicious, and cutting off the top before it fully develops redirects the energy of the plant down into the underground bulb, whose harvest follows shortly thereafter, as the plant dies back. Some radish varieties develop lovely tender seedpods on the plants not harvested for their succulent young roots. As the roots mature and become woody, the stalks grow tall and go to flower, and green, juicy, spicy seedpods develop, which are delicious raw as well as cooked. All plants (like all humans) go through different stages of development, and when you grow (with) them, you are forced to notice them.

Anyone can grow plants. There's lots of information out there, more than you could possibly ever read, more than you would want to, and many of the sources contradict each other. Don't worry! Start however you can, find mentors, and let your experience with the plants be your guide. If you stick with it, each year will bring you greater abundance.

Certain foods (fruits and nuts) require years to produce; others (such as radishes) take only a few weeks. Plant what suits your tastes and your circumstances. You can grow plants in a tiny yard, in a plot in a community garden, on the roof or fire escape, or guerilla-style in public spaces (see chapter 3). Be creative. With a little luck, you may grow old enjoying fruit from trees and bushes you plant now. My friend Hector Black, who recently celebrated his eighty-first birthday, glows with pride at the (literally) tons of blueberries the bushes he planted thirty-some years ago now produce, and my father loves to take his grandchildren out to pick blueberries from the bushes his father planted sixty-some years ago.

I came across a do-it-yourself gardening zine written by Chris and Laura, two new gardeners bursting with enthusiasm about what they learned in their first season of gardening and eager to share their discoveries. In it, they reflect on the fact that our culture teaches people no skills for providing for the most basic necessities of life: "Instead we are submersed in a culture of restaurants, real estate, and retail. We are taught not to provide nor to make but to consume." Chris and Laura's first season of gardening was a profound step in their education: "Just the feeling of food that we had grown ourselves made us feel powerful. It made us feel like we could escape this consumerist culture and maybe provide a sane alternative."[56] Growing food for yourself and those you love is profoundly empowering. Try it and you'll see.

Cleo Woelfle-Erskine is a gardener and activist in Oakland, California, who has traveled extensively visiting and documenting urban community gardening projects and edited the book *Urban Wilds: Gardeners' Stories of the Struggle for Land and Justice*. "Everyone's got to eat," Cleo declares. "And while gardens aren't a cure-all to the problems of economic racism and environmental injustice, unequal access to resources and an exploitative profit system, they can help us get by a little easier, give us space to breathe, to learn from the earth, and to begin to reweave relationships based on respect for the land and for the people around us."[57] Gardens can also be a willful act in defiance of mainstream norms and values. Cultural theorist Peter Lamborn Wilson writes, "Growing a garden has become—at least potentially—an act of resistance. But it's not simply a gesture of refusal. It's a positive act. It's praxis."[58]

Growing food, with its huge (and endless) learning curve, is a tangible step toward a healthier, more just, and more sustainable world. "This is not exactly a hobby," explains novelist and essayist Barbara Kingsolver about her family's garden. "It's more along the lines of religion, something we believe in the way families believe in patriotism and loving thy neighbor as thyself."[59] Bring a spirit of solidarity and outreach into your gardening practice by sharing your bounty, sharing your skills, and building community around the rewards and challenges of small-scale local food production.

Recipe: Chickweed Pesto

With or without a garden of your own, weeds are a great source of nourishment. Weeds are everywhere. My dictionary says a weed is "an economically useless or unsightly plant, especially of wild growth."[60] In practice, weeds are anything other than plants being intentionally cultivated. Ironically, in many cases the weeds growing in a garden are more nutritious than the cultivated plants you have to work for. They're

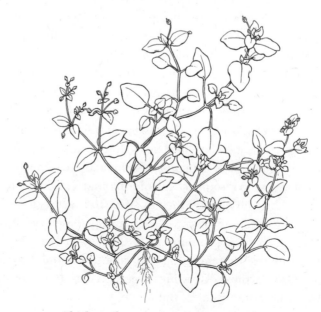

Chickweed. ©Bobbi Angell. Used by permission.

delicious, too. I am a weed forager. I love to eat weeds. They taste strong, and I wish to share in their powerful adaptive qualities.

Chickweed is an old friend that has sustained me through thick and thin. I pick it and usually eat it on the spot. I look for the most succulent patches, with fresh flowers. Often I talk to the chickweed as I harvest. When the chickweed is at its most lush (late March and early April where I live in Tennessee) I harvest big bowlfuls with scissors and make it into pesto with other weeds.

Ingredients (for 4 cups of pesto)
1 cup seeds or nuts, soaked in water for four to eight hours
8 cups chickweed and other tasty edible weeds
1 head garlic, peeled
1/4 to 1/2 cup olive oil
salt to taste
1/8 to 1/4 cup parmesan cheese (optional)

As soon as you think about making pesto, before you go out harvesting weeds, soak seeds or nuts. I sure do love pine nuts, the classic pesto nuts, but, alas, they are quite expensive and I most often use sunflower seeds. You could just as well use walnuts (try harvesting black walnuts) or pumpkin seeds, or whatever you have around or especially like. Soaking seeds and nuts makes them swell, initiates enzymatic transformations that make them more digestible, and gives the pesto a creamier texture. To make 4 cups of pesto, soak 1 cup of seeds or nuts.

Harvesting is what weed pesto is all about. Try to collect a lot; a half pound of weeds, about 8 cups densely packed, will halve in volume as it is pureed into pesto. To do this, you need to get to know the common weeds around you. Perhaps local gardeners or other knowledgeable people could point out the ones they know. Watch for weed walks or wild-foods foraging outings organized by local naturalists, herbalists, and plant lovers, or consult a good plant identification book. I'm adventurous about tasting plants (though not fungi) that I don't know. I bite off just a tiny bit, chew it well, and mix it with my saliva. If the flavor is unpleasant I spit it out before I swallow. If the flavor is agreeable, I'll swallow and try a bit more.

Many common edible and medicinal weeds are bitter. Chickweed is ideal for culinary use because it is not at all bitter; it has a rich, green herby flavor, and in its youthful stages, its fibers are easily broken down. It also contains saponins, soaplike compounds that emulsify when blended, giving chickweed pesto an especially creamy texture. In our bodies, these saponins "emulsify and increase the permeability of all membranes," writes herbalist Susun S. Weed. "By creating permeability chickweed encourages the shifting of boundaries at all levels, from cellular to cosmic."[61]

When I harvest chickweed, I go for the growing ends, using my fingers to stretch out the chickweed tops as if they were hairs being trimmed, and then clip with scissors. I clean as I go, discarding grass and any discolored parts. Inevitably as I harvest I come across stands of other weeds I love that thrive in the same spring exuberance as chickweed. Cleavers is juicy and has a pleasant mild flavor, and medicinally it is associated with lymphatic circulation, which is critically important for good health. I also add wild onions, garlic chives, and any of a number of abundant spring wildflowers such as toothwort, which has a horseradish-like flavor. I even add roots to the pesto—earthy-flavored burdock roots, which blend right in. Sometimes I add stinging nettles, but these I steam with just a bit of water for not even a minute, just enough to wilt the leaves and deactivate the stinging hairs. You can augment the weeds with herbs such as cilantro, parsley, or anything green.

Once you've harvested your weeds, blend them with the soaked seeds or nuts, lots of garlic (a whole head of peeled cloves), and olive oil. Usually I use a food processor, though with a bit of patience you can do it with a sharp knife and cutting board or a big mortar and pestle. Grind the ingredients into a paste, adding additional oil or water as necessary to achieve a smooth, creamy texture. (Many pestos are oily, but I prefer to use just a little oil and more water.) Add salt to taste and, if desired, Parmesan cheese (cutting back the salt accordingly). The classic way to serve pesto is over pasta, but it also makes a very versatile spread or sauce. Try it in an omelet, on a sandwich or nori roll, or with rice. This pesto is bursting with the flavors and energy of spring. It's a great way to get kids—or anyone—to eat lots of greens, and it will enhance whatever it is served upon.

Action and Information Resources

Books

Ableman, Michael. *Fields of Plenty: A Farmer's Journey in Search of Real Food and the People Who Grow It.* San Francisco: Chronicle Books, 2005.

———. *On Good Land: The Autobiography of an Urban Farm.* San Francisco: Chronicle Books, 1998.

Barndt, Deborah. *Tangled Roots: Women, Work, and Globalization on the Tomato Trail.* Lanham, MD: Rowman & Littlefield, 2002.

Belasco, Warren. *Appetite for Change: How the Counterculture Took on the Food Industry 1966–1988.* New York: Pantheon Books, 1989.

Berry, Wendell. *The Art of the Commonplace: The Agrarian Essays of Wendell Berry.* Washington, DC: Shoemaker & Hoard, 2002.

———. *A Continuous Harmony: Essays Cultural and Agricultural.* New York: Harcourt Brace Jovanovich, 1974.

Brown, Lester R. *Eco-Economy: Building an Economy for the Earth.* Washington, DC: Earth Policy Institute, 2001.

Clark, Robert, ed. *Our Sustainable Table.* San Francisco: North Point Press, 1990.

Fern, Ken. *Plants For A Future: Edible and Useful Plants for a Healthier World.* Clanfield, Hampshire (England): Permanent Publications, 1997.

Fernández-Armesto, Felipe. *Food: A History.* London: McMillan, 2001.

Flores, Heather C. *Food Not Lawns: How to Turn Your Lawn into a Garden and Your Neighborhood into a Community.* White River Junction, VT: Chelsea Green, 2006.

Fromartz, Samuel. *Organic, Inc.: Natural Foods and How They Grew.* New York: Harcourt, 2006.

Funes, Fernando, Luis Garcia, Martin Bourque, Nilda Perez, and Peter Rosset, eds. *Sustainable Agriculture and Resistance: Transforming Food Production in Cuba.* Oakland, CA: Food First Books, 2002.

Groh, Trauger, and Steven McFadden. *Farms of Tomorrow Revisited: Community Supported Farms, Farm Supported Communities.* Kimberton, PA: Biodynamic Farming and Gardening Association, 2000.

Halweil, Brian. *Home Grown: The Case for Local Food in a Global Market.* Washington, DC: Worldwatch Institute, 2002.

Heldke, Lisa M. *Exotic Appetites: Ruminations of a Food Adventurer.* New York and London: Routledge, 2003.

Krebs, A. V. *Corporate Reapers: The Book of Agribusiness.* Washington, DC: Essential Books, 1992.

Lappe, Anna, and Bryant Terry. *Grub: Ideas for an Urban Organic Kitchen.* New York: Penguin, 2006.

Nabhan, Gary Paul. *Coming Home to Eat: The Pleasures and Politics of Local Foods.* New York and London: W. W. Norton, 2002.

Norberg-Hodge, Helena, Todd Merrifield, and Steven Gorelick. *Bringing the Food Economy Home: Local Alternatives to Global Agribusiness.* Bloomfield, CT: Kumarian Press, 2002.

Pirog, Rich, and Andrew Benjamin. *Checking the Food Odometer: Comparing Food Miles for Local versus Conventional Produce Sales to*

Iowa Institutions. Ames, IA: Leopold Center for Sustainable Agriculture, 2003.

Pollan, Michael. *The Omnivore's Dilemma: A Natural History of Four Meals*. New York: Penguin, 2006.

Sams, Craig. *The Little Food Book: You Are What You Eat*. New York: Disinformation, 2004.

Schumacher, E. F. *Small Is Beautiful: Economics As If People Mattered*. London: Blond & Briggs, 1973.

Solnit, David, ed. *Globalize Liberation: How to Uproot the System and Build a Better World*. San Francisco: City Lights Books, 2004.

Vinton, Sherri Brooks. *The Real Food Revival*. New York: Penguin Books, 2005.

Weed, Susun S. *Wise Woman Herbal: Healing Wise*. Woodstock, NY: Ash Tree, 1989.

Wimberley, Ronald C., Brenda J. Vander Mey, Betty Wells, Godfrey D. Ejimakor, Conner Bailey, Larry L. Burmeister, Craig K. Harris, et. al. *Food from Our Changing World: The Globalization of Food and How Americans Feel about It*. North Carolina State University, 2003. http://sasw.chass.ncsu.edu/global-food.

Woelfle-Erskine, Cleo, ed. *Urban Wilds: Gardeners' Stories of the Struggle for Land and Justice*. Oakland, CA: water/under/ground publications, 2002.

Periodicals

Acres USA (monthly)
PO Box 91299
Austin, TX 78709
(800) 355-5313
www.acresusa.com

The Community Farm (quarterly)
3480 Potter Road
Bear Lake, MI 49614
(231) 889-3216
csafarm@jackpine.com

Growing for Market (monthly)
PO Box 3747
Lawrence, KS 66046
(800) 307-8949
www.growingformarket.com

Permaculture Activist (quarterly)
PO Box 1209W
Black Mountain, NC 28711
www.permacultureactivist.net

Small Farmer's Journal (quarterly)
PO Box 1627
Sisters, OR 97759
(541) 549-2064
www.smallfarmersjournal.com

Films

Global Banquet: The Politics of Food. Woodstock, VT: Old Dog Documentaries, 2001; www.olddog-documentaries.com.

Life in Debt. Directed by Stephanie Black. Tuff Gong Pictures, 2001; www.lifeanddebt.org.

Wal-Mart: The High Cost of Low Price. Directed by Robert Greenwald. Culver City, CA: Brave New Films, 2005; www.walmartmovie.com.

Organizations and Other Resources

Added Value
305 Van Brunt Street
Brooklyn, NY 11231
(718) 855-5531
www.added-value.org

Appalachian Sustainable Agriculture
   Project
729 Haywood Road
Asheville, NC 28806
(828) 236-1282
www.asapconnections.org

Bio-Dynamic Farming and Gardening
   Association
25844 Butler Road
Junction City, OR 97448
(888) 516-7797
www.biodynamics.com

Carolina Farm Stewardship Association
PO Box 448
Pittsboro, NC 27312
(919) 542-2402
www.carolinafarmstewards.org

Center for Ecoliteracy
2528 San Pablo Avenue
Berkeley, CA 94702
www.ecoliteracy.org
*Creator of the Rethinking School Lunch
program.*

Center for Food Safety
660 Pennsylvania Avenue SE, #302
Washington, DC 20003
(202) 547-9359
www.centerforfoodsafety.org

Chef's Collaborative
262 Beacon Street
Boston, MA 02116
(617) 236-5200
www.chefscollaborative.org

Community Food Security Coalition
PO Box 209
Venice, CA 90294
(310) 822-5410
www.foodsecurity.org

Ecological Farming Association
406 Main Street, Suite 313
Watsonville, CA 95076
(831) 763-2111
www.eco-farm.org

The Edible Schoolyard
Martin Luther King Jr. Middle School
1781 Rose Street
Berkeley, CA 94703
(510) 558-1335
www.edibleschoolyard.org

Food First/Institute for Food and
   Development Policy
398 60th Street
Oakland, CA 94618
(510) 654-4400
www.foodfirst.org

FoodRoutes Network
37 East Durham Street
Philadelphia, PA 19119
(814) 349-6000
www.foodroutes.org

Food Security Learning Center
World Hunger Year
505 Eighth Avenue, Suite 2100
New York, NY 10018-6582
(212) 629-8850
www.worldhungeryear.org/fslc

The Food Trust
1201 Chestnut Street, 4th Floor
Philadelphia, PA 19107
(215) 568-0830
www.thefoodtrust.org

Hartford Food System
191 Franklin Avenue
Hartford, CT 06114
(860) 296-9325
www.hartfordfood.org

International Forum on Globalization
1009 General Kennedy Avenue #2
San Francisco, CA 94129
(415) 561-7650
www.ifg.org

International Society for Ecology
   and Culture USA
PO Box 9475
Berkeley, CA 94709
(510) 548 4915
www.isec.org.uk

Journey to Forever Small Farms
     Online Library
www.journeytoforever.org/farm_
library.html

Just Food
208 East 51st Street, 4th Floor
New York, NY 10022
(212) 645-9880
www.justfood.org

Leopold Center for Sustainable
     Agriculture
209 Curtiss Hall
Iowa State University
Ames, IA 50011-1050
(515) 294-3711
www.leopold.iastate.edu

Local Harvest
220 21st Avenue
Santa Cruz, CA 95062
(831) 475-8150
www.localharvest.org
*Nationwide online searchable directory
of small farms, farmers' markets, and
other local food sources.*

Long Hungry Creek Farm CSA
Jeff Poppen
PO Box 163
Red Boiling Springs, TN 37150
www.barefootfarmer.com

Maine Organic Farmers and Gardeners
     Association
PO Box 170
Unity, ME 04988
(207) 568-4142
www.mofga.org

National Farm to School Program
Center for Food and Justice
Urban and Environmental Policy
     Institute
Occidental College
1600 Campus Road
Mail Stop M1
Los Angeles, CA 90041
(323) 341-5095
www.farmtoschool.org

Native Seeds/SEARCH
526 North 4th Avenue
Tucson, AZ 85705-8450
(866) 622-5561
www.nativeseeds.org

New Farm
www.newfarm.org
*A Rodale Institute–sponsored web portal
including CSA resources, farm journals,
student farm directory, and more.*

Northeast Organic Farming Association
411 Sheldon Road
Barre, MA 01005
(978) 355-2853
www.nofa.org

Ohio Ecological Food and Farm
     Association
PO Box 82234
Columbus, OH 43202
(614) 421-2022
www.oeffa.org

Organic Consumers Association
6101 Cliff Estate Road
Little Marais, MN 55614
(218) 226-4164
www.organicconsumers.org

Organic Volunteers
www.organicvolunteers.org

Oxfam
26 West Street
Boston, MA 02111
(800) 776-9326
www.oxfam.org

Pennsylvania Association for Sustainable
     Agriculture
PO Box 419
Millheim, PA 16854
(814) 349-9856
www.pasafarming.org

People's Grocery
3265 Market Street
Oakland, CA 94608
(510) 652-7607
www.peoplesgrocery.org

Pesticide Action Network
49 Powell Street, Suite 500
San Francisco, CA 94102
(415) 981-1771
www.panna.org

Plants For A Future
1 Lerryn View
Lerryn, Lostwithiel
Cornwall PL22 0QJ
United Kingdom
+44 1208 872936
www.pfaf.org

Robin Van En Center for CSA
c/o Center for Sustainable Living
Wilson College
1015 Philadelphia Avenue
Chambersburg, PA 17201
(717) 261-4141
www.csacenter.org

Rural Advancement Foundation
　　International (RAFI)
PO Box 640
Pittsboro, NC 27312
(919) 542-1396
www.rafiusa.org

Slow Food USA
20 Jay Street, Suite 313
Brooklyn, NY 11201
(718) 260-8000
www.slowfoodusa.org
*Creator of the Slow Food in Schools
program.*

Soil and Health Library
www.soilandhealth.org

Sustain: The Alliance for Better Farming
　　and Food
94 White Lion Street
London N1 9PF
United Kingdom
www.sustainweb.org

Sustainable Table
215 Lexington Avenue, Suite 1001
New York, NY 10016
(212) 726-9161
www.sustainabletable.org

Virginia Association for Biological
　　Farming
PO Box 1003
Lexington, VA 24450
www.vabf.org

Weston A. Price Foundation
4200 Wisconsin Avenue NW
Washington, DC 20016
(202) 363-4394
www.westonaprice.org
www.realmilk.com
*The Weston A. Price Foundation has
more than 300 grassroots local chapters
connecting consumers with local food
producers.*

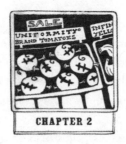

CHAPTER 2

Seed Saving as a Political Act

O ne January morning I sat at the kitchen table—the heart of our community and most others—with two of the people I live with, Daz'l and Laurel, figuring out which seeds we wanted to order for the coming growing season. This annual session of pouring over the catalogs together is something I have often dreaded, because it is the most consumeristic moment of the gardening experience. Glossy photos and seductive descriptions can whip folks into a buying frenzy, ordering more seeds than they'll ever get around to planting. In the past we've attempted to be systematic, comparison-shopping from a dozen different catalogs.

Somehow this year was lower-key. Daz'l had sorted through our seed stash, cleaned it up, and inventoried what we had. We put aside the stack of glossy catalogs and mostly ordered from a single supplier, Fedco, a worker-cooperative seed company in Waterville, Maine, whose catalog is black and white on simple newsprint. We decided which varieties to order largely based on the catalog's notations of which were raised by small-scale seed growers versus those supplied by large corporations.

When our seeds arrived a few weeks later, the package contained a letter from Fedco staff member CR Lawn, dated January 25, 2005:

Dear Seed Lover,

The day of reckoning was bound to come. We watched the increasing consolidation of the seed industry for years, wondering when it would next adversely affect us. This morning we heard that Monsanto, the *bête noire* of multinational genetic engineers, is buying out Seminis, the world's largest vegetable seed company with annual sales of over a half billion dollars. This creates a real ethical dilemma for us. We, and you who buy from us, are heavily dependent upon Seminis, particularly for top-notch hybrids. We carry sixty Seminis varieties, most available from no one else, including top sellers. . . . We have long opposed Monsanto because of their aggressive advocacy of genetic engineering. . . . Now we have to decide whether to drop the Seminis varieties. . . . If we drop them, our selection, particularly of hybrid melons, summer squash, peppers, and tomatoes, will be devastated. If we keep them, some of us may have trouble living with ourselves. . . .

Dependence upon ever-growing corporate entities for something as basic as seed is not pretty. Alfonso Romo Garza, the billionaire who masterminded the consolidation of Seminis prior to its sale to Monsanto, bragged to the *Wall Street Journal*: "Seeds are software. And we have the seeds."[1] That would now make Monsanto the Microsoft of food. Do we really want to be that dependent on a single corporation for our "operating system"?

Monsanto and the nine next largest seed corporations control more than half of the world's commercial seed supply.[2] "What you are seeing is not just a consolidation of seed companies," explains Robb Fraley, Monsanto's executive vice president and chief technology officer, "it's really a consolidation of the entire food chain."[3] Fedco decided to drop Monsanto's seeds and announced in its 2006 catalog that the company was "getting off the seed grid. . . .We do so because Monsanto epitomizes the road down which we no longer choose to go . . . the road that leads to our complete surrender of control of our seed and therefore of control of our food system."

Intellectual Property Laws.
Genetic Pollution, and Biodiversity

Expansion of the legal concept of intellectual property underlies corporate control of seeds. Intellectual property law deals with proprietary interests in innovations such as inventions, as well as abstractions such as words, ideas, sounds, and images. Over the past few decades, laws around the world have been rewritten to protect the intellectual property rights of plant breeders, allowing breeds to be patented and constraining ways in which farmers may sell, trade, give away, and even plant saved seeds. "Quite clearly a monopolistic patent regime cannot be established as long as farmers have the alternative of their own zero cost, reliable, time-tested, high-value seeds of their traditional varieties of indigenous agro-biodiversity," points out Vandana Shiva.[4] What has traditionally been viewed as a natural right—saving seed as an integral element of local agricultural practice—is being transformed by globalizing corporate interests into a legally granted (or denied) privilege.

In order to prevent farmers from "cheating" the patent holders by saving and replanting seed, the seed industry, in cooperation with the U.S. Department of Agriculture (USDA), has developed what is known as "terminator" technology, seeds that generate self-sterilizing plants. The disclosure of this technology in 1998 created an international furor. For now, the United Nations Convention on Biological Diversity has imposed an international moratorium on terminator technology, but it has been repeatedly challenged.[5] The technology exists, and those who stand to profit from it are likely to persist.

"Biotechnology essentially aims to eliminate sexuality as a means of passing on genetic material," contends Peter Lamborn Wilson. "Capital has now reached the theoretical stage of commodifying the life process itself. The principle of intellectual ownership of nature—the *final* enclosure—seems to have become the basis for the global world order and its economy."[6]

Increasingly, national governments and other, even less accountable, international regulatory institutions have been imposing plant-breed protection laws that deny the traditional right to perpetuate seed. "Farmers can't believe this is happening," says Terry Pugh, executive secretary of Canada's National Farmer's Union. "There are no benefits for farmers."[7] Profit-driven laws written to favor monopoly control, globalized markets, and economies of scale are attempting to supplant the ancient practice of saving seed, one of the foundations of agriculture and a tradition more central to culture and survival than even the rule of law. What choice does a life- and freedom-loving person have but to assert this natural right, even at the risk of violating the law?

The earliest legal expression of plant-breed ownership came into existence in the 1960s with the formation of the International Union for the Protection of New Plant Varieties. The rationale was to offer greater financial incentives for creative plant breeding. This international agreement created a registry of certified plant varieties, with registration criteria being qualities of distinctness, uniformity, stability, and novelty. In the United States, the 1970 Plant Variety Protection Act established specific ownership rights over seeds. In the original law, farmers were permitted to save enough of patent-protected seeds to plant their own land or to sell that amount of seed to a neighbor. A 1994 amendment prohibited the sale of any farmer-saved seed unless the variety owner granted permission. In addition, many jurisdictions around the world now prohibit any sale of seeds lacking government certification.

Increasingly in recent decades, farmers have been prosecuted for illegally exchanging seed they have saved. German organic farmer Josef Albrecht bred his own adapted variety of wheat, which he grew and sold to neighbors, until he was fined by the German government for the crime of selling seed that had not been certified for sale. Similarly, the exchange of seed potatoes among farmers was outlawed in the United Kingdom in 1995 by a court decision in which a Scottish farmer was fined £30,000 to cover royalties lost to the seed industry by direct farmer-to-farmer exchange.[8] In Canada, the Supreme Court affirmed the guilt of canola farmer Percy Schmeiser, prosecuted not for illegally exchanging seed but rather for saving and using his own seed, just as he had for the previous fifty years and as his father had before him. (We'll talk more about Percy's story later in this chapter.)

Understandings of what can be patented have grown rapidly with recent advances in genome sequencing. Genes and cell lines have been patented, as have even theoretical genetic crosses. Many biological creations, commonly held and freely shared up until now, are being claimed as private property. Activists have coined a descriptive term to describe this practice: biopiracy. The Coalition Against Biopiracy defines biopiracy as "the monopolization (usually through intellectual property) of genetic resources and traditional knowledge or culture taken from peoples or farming communities who have developed and nurtured those resources. Biopiracy includes bioprospecting, patents on nature (genes and molecules) and the trademarking of cultural knowledge."[9]

The Enola bean provides a clear example of biopiracy. In 1999 a U.S. patent was issued for this bean, which was later proven to be genetically identical to a preexisting Mexican yellow bean variety, one that had been previously known and grown in the United States. But meanwhile, yellow beans were stopped at the border, and the patent owner filed lawsuits against seed companies providing this seed and farmers growing this bean in the United States, charging patent infringement.

Following intervention from international agricultural institutions, the U.S. Patent and Trademark Office reviewed the patent, and after years of study, in 2005 the patent was rejected. "The real crime is that, despite the legal challenge, the U.S. patent system has allowed the patent owner to use bureaucratic delays and diversion to legally extend his exclusive monopoly on a bean variety of Mexican origin for over six years (and potentially more)—that's nearly one-third of the twenty-year patent term," says ETC Group. "In essence, the system enables holders of unjust patents to monopolize markets and destroy competition."[10] And despite its rejection, the Enola patent remains in force pending further appeal.

Plant and seed patents are no longer an issue of sovereign preroga-tive. The Uruguay Round of the General Agreement on Tariffs and Trades (1986–1994), in which the World Trade Organization (WTO) was created, "set a milestone on the road towards the privatization of living matter," observed the *Biotechnology and Development Monitor*. "It puts developing countries under the obligation to protect plant vari-eties by patents or by an alternative . . . system."[11] "The State is under siege," says Vandana Shiva.[12] Seed patent laws are being forced on people everywhere by the WTO. The WTO's 1994 Trade-Related Aspects of Intellectual Property Rights (TRIPS) treaty requires new intellectual property rights in the area of plant genetic resources. "Free trade" demands it.

Vandana Shiva has written about recent legislative efforts to bring India's laws into compliance with TRIPS by allowing for the first time there the patenting of seeds, plants, and other life forms. "Patents on seeds transform seed saving into an 'intellectual property crime,'" she observes. "This shift is associated with a transformation of farmers as breeders and reproducers of their own seed supply to farmers as consumers of proprietary seed from the seed industry. It is also a shift from a food economy based on millions of farmers as autonomous producers to a food system controlled by a handful of transnational corporations which control both inputs and outputs."[13]

All the nations of the world, like India, face pressure to conform to the new intellectual property regime, but Iraq's patent laws hold the distinction of having been revised by edict early in the U.S. occupation, evidently as an important step toward "democratic self-rule." In the spring of 2004, Paul Bremer, at the time the top U.S. administrator in Iraq, issued Order 81, "Patent, Industrial Design, Integrated Circuits and Plant Variety Law." The law extends patent protections to seeds and plants, legalizes genetically modified (GM) crops in Iraq, and prohibits farmers from saving seed from protected varieties. The order's introduction explains that it is necessary for Iraq's "transition from a non-transparent centrally planned economy to a free market economy."[14] Isn't the free market so free!

Investigative journalist Greg Palast obtained an internal State Department document from February 2003, a month *before* the U.S. invasion, that included seed and plant patents as part of the U.S. economic agenda in Iraq. "This is likely history's first military assault plan appended to a program for toughening the target nation's copyright laws," wrote Palast.[15] The plot gets thicker. The war devastated most Iraqi agricultural research centers and seed stocks, according to the United Nations Food and Agriculture Organization (FAO).[16] The now notorious Abu Ghraib prison, where U.S. soldiers tortured and sexually humiliated Iraqi prisoners, was previously home to Iraq's national seed bank and research facilities.[17] War-related damage and looting "has resulted in the loss of almost all generations of seeds of all crops," reports the FAO. "Moreover, much seed expertise was lost during the conflict." In Afghanistan, too, seed storage facilities were destroyed during the U.S. invasion. It appears from these facts that an element of the U.S. military agenda is to disrupt agricultural self-sufficiency and create dependency on the high-tech global seed market, while imposing the legal framework to permanently disempower local farmers.

As a practical matter, for plant patents to be meaningful, patented varieties must be consistent and uniform. Cary Fowler and Pat Mooney observe that "this kind of uniformity and the ongoing quest for greater and greater uniformity pleases both lawyers and pests, and is yet another factor contributing to the narrowing of the genetic base of our crops."[18] Crop uniformity leads to vulnerability to pests and diseases and now, when it involves genetically engineered traits, to genetic pollution.

Genetic pollution is fundamentally different from our more familiar notion of chemical pollution in that it is not a fixed quantity that is unleashed; instead, GM seeds self-replicate, and their genetic material spreads and proliferates. "A single molecule of DDT remains a single molecule or degrades," explains plant geneticist Norman C. Ellstrand. "But a single crop [gene] has the opportunity to multiply itself repeatedly through reproduction, which can frustrate attempts at containment."[19] The insidious engineered genes are spread easily, by pollinating bees and by the wind, and by commingling in huge processing and storage facilities, as well as by human error and manipulations.

Herbicide resistance is the most widespread GM trait so far. The biggest GM crops to date are those, like canola, that Monsanto has manufactured as "Roundup Ready," augmented with a gene enabling it to tolerate the herbicide Roundup, also marketed by Monsanto. But genetic drift is a pervasive reality. Whatever diversity existed among regional heirloom canola varieties in Canada is being rapidly homogenized by the Roundup Ready gene. Rene Van Acker of the University of Manitoba has found canola with Roundup Ready genes in ditches, schoolyards, and city lots; she found that even the purest, certified non-genetically engineered canola now contains up to 4.9 percent Roundup Ready material.[20] And researchers have identified weeds that have acquired the engineered genes for herbicide resistance, thereby undermining the effectiveness of the herbicide used to treat the herbicide-resistant crops.[21]

The very recombinant nature of genetic modification makes some scientists worry that the engineered genes are very likely to spread. "If you design genetically modified DNA to jump into genomes and to overcome species barriers," says geneticist Dr. Mae-Wan Ho, "then there is a chance that this DNA can . . . get into other unrelated species . . . to make new combinations."[22]

This process of widespread genetic contamination is happening to the wild teosinte of Mexico, the progenitor of corn in the place where corn was first domesticated. In Iraq, it's likely to happen to the wild precursors of wheat and barley indigenous to the Fertile Crescent, another of several places where civilizations built upon grain agriculture emerged. The contamination of wild progenitor plant populations leaves the crops humans have bred from these wild plants with a huge vulnerability to diseases. When diseases have ravaged cultivated varieties—as they have with increasing regularity as monoculture food production has replaced integrated subsistence farming—the solutions have repeatedly been found in the genetic diversity of the wild ancestors of the cultivars. Contamination of the ancestor populations by bioengineered genes contributes to their uniformity and diminishes their genetic diversity, reducing the gene pool from which to draw characteristics such as disease resistance.

Contamination of indigenous corn varieties in Mexico with GM genes was first documented by Ignacio Chapela, a Mexican-born professor of environmental science at the University of California at Berkeley. The Mexican government subsequently identified contaminated corn in many different locations—but not before Chapela's research had been attacked. The prestigious journal *Nature*, which published his report, came under enormous pressure and took the unprecedented step of publishing a partial retraction—the first retraction in its history—to distance itself from Chapela's controversial findings. Chapela was also denied tenure at Berkeley, despite enthusiastic campus support (though as a result of protests and lawsuits, the administration ultimately granted him tenure). His experience suggests that the institutions of science are not hospitable environments these days for a scientist willing to let the facts contradict a corporate funding agenda.

In the growing field of "biopharming," bioengineers are genetically modifying plants to be vehicles for the production of proteins for pharmaceutical use, hoping to produce antibodies to HIV, SARS, and tuberculosis and many other proteins with potentially promising medical applications.

The risk of genetic contamination carries especially high stakes in bio-pharming, because the genes used to produce these biopharmaceuticals, some active at mere billionths of a gram,[23] could be very dangerous if they were to accidentally enter the food supply or the seed supply. This almost happened in 2002 when experimental GM corn plants containing a pig vaccine were accidentally mixed with 30 million pounds of soybeans. All the soybeans had to be destroyed, and the company responsible for the mishap, ProdiGene, required a government bailout to pay $3 million in cleanup costs and fines.

Ventria Biosciences is gearing up for the largest commercial pharmaceutical planting to date: two hundred acres of GM pharmaceutical-producing rice crops in Missouri, with plans for twenty-eight thousand acres in the future. Widespread opposition from Missouri's conventional rice farmers (and their largest single customer, beer maker Anheuser-Busch) stopped Ventria from planting in 2005, but it persists in seeking the required permits. "There will be drugs in breakfast cereals sooner or later," predicts Craig Winters of the Campaign to Label Genetically Engineered Foods. "Those genes can't be recalled and they would be nearly impossible to clean up."[24] Even though engineering nonfood plants to produce biopharmaceuticals would be much safer, simply because they are further removed from the food supply, the industry prefers corn and rice and other food plants because they are ideal for producing high volumes of proteins.

No one really has any idea of just how pervasive genetic contamination really is. Besides the GM food crops already approved for commercial production (in the United States, that's soy, corn, cotton, canola, Hawaiian papaya, zucchini, and crookneck squash), there are more than one hundred other GM species, not yet approved for human consumption, that have been in field trials since 1987. "About forty-thousand test sites covering approximately half a million acres are virtually unregulated," writes Jeffrey M. Smith, the author of *Seeds of Deception* and *Genetic Roulette*. "Several are reported to have contaminated non-GM crops, but the overall extent of contamination is unknown and potentially widespread."[25]

Among the many exotic GM crops in development is rice with human liver genes, which are intended to enable the plants to digest pesticides, so that more pesticides can be "safely" used. This and other experimental GM crops contain genes that are considered confidential and proprietary, so there is little information available about which genes are being tested. "Because of the secrecy behind experiments in the United States, no one—not food companies, not even governments—will be able to test food products or food imports for contamination because they won't know what to test for," warned Adrian Bebb of Friends of the Earth Europe when the United States proposed safety regulations for experimental GM crops—regulations that failed to include testing of neighboring crops for contamination or any threshold limit for contamination.[26]

Genetic pollution makes it hard for *anyone* to be sure exactly what they are growing. Percy Schmeiser, a seventy-five-year-old Saskatchewan canola farmer, was saving seed just as he had for more than fifty years and just as his father had done before him. He wasn't an organic farmer or an ideologue. His farming practice was in every way conventional. All he did was continue doing things the way he always had, saving seed from the crop he produced every year, which cost nothing, rather than buying seed.

The Monsanto corporation manufactures a GM type of canola seed designated Roundup Ready, meaning that it is designed to tolerate the herbicide Roundup, which Monsanto also manufactures. Before it entered into the GM seed business, Monsanto was known primarily as a chemical manufacturer. The company was looking to diversify into something wholesome, such as feeding people, after hugely damaging scandals over two of its products—the defoliant Agent Orange and polychlorinated biphenyls, better known as PCBs, which are used in electrical equipment; both had been found to be environmental toxins linked to epidemics of cancer and many other health problems.

Some of Percy Schmeiser's Saskatchewan neighbors planted the Roundup Ready seeds. Wind carried pollen from the Monsanto canola into Schmeiser's crop. When Monsanto's private investigators—whom Schmeiser calls "the gene police"—came and took samples of his seeds, their tests verified the predictable drift of genetic material from the GM patent-protected seeds.

Monsanto sued Schmeiser for infringement of its patent, demanding monetary damages. The court ruled for Monsanto. Schmeiser appealed the case all the way to the Canadian Supreme Court, which ruled on May

21, 2004, in favor of Monsanto. The court's decision was nuanced, though, in that it recognized that Schmeiser did not profit from the copyright infringement and did not award Monsanto monetary damages.

Percy Schmeiser is not the only farmer whom Monsanto has attempted to force to pay for the privilege of having his seeds contaminated. The Center for Food Safety (CFS) reported in 2005 that Monsanto, which devotes an annual budget of $10 million and a staff of seventy-five solely to investigating and prosecuting farmers, had filed ninety lawsuits against farmers in twenty-five states. "These lawsuits and settlements are nothing less than corporate extortion of American farmers," says Andrew Kimbrell, executive director of CFS. "Monsanto is polluting American farms with its genetically engineered crops, not properly informing farmers about these altered seeds, and then profiting from its own irresponsibility and negligence by suing innocent farmers." The report tallied the total recorded judgments that farmers have been ordered to pay to Monsanto at over $15 million. "It's hard enough to farm as it is," says prosecuted North Dakota farmer Rodney Nelson. "You don't need a big seed supplier trying to trip you up and chase you down with lawyers."

The contamination of agricultural crops with GM traits that is occurring is an acceleration of a trend that began earlier as seed saving shifted from the realm of community-based generalists to that of seed breeder specialists. "The seeds came with the genetic code of the society that produced them," write Fowler and Mooney. "They produced not just crops, but replicas of the agricultural systems that produced them. They came as a package deal and part of the package was a major change in traditional cultures, values, and power relationships."[27] Subsistence-scale and community-based agricultural practices are being replaced by "improved" seeds, chemicals, and mechanization, just as global market economics displace traditional local food systems.

People on the ground everywhere are resisting this process—or trying to. "It is not that farmers are against new technologies," says Moses Shaha, chairman of the Kenya Small-Scale Farmers Forum, "so long as these technologies will not destroy our indigenous seed varieties, will not change our native farming systems knowledge, and will not render us helpless and at the mercy of the transnational companies to monopolize even on what we eat."[28]

Amateurism Breeds Diversity

Patent laws may have ceded ownership of seeds, but the mass of humanity cannot afford to abandon the seed-saving cycle so casually. Multinational seed corporations rely on reproduction engineers with PhDs, but historically, plant breeding and seed saving have been the work of generalists, not specialists. Amateurism doesn't necessarily mean incompetence; it can be general competence, which involves a process of demystification: learning important skills and spreading them.

Corporate control of seeds places us all in an exceedingly vulnerable position, for it means that the source of our food is centralized behind proprietary doors. Seed stocks have traditionally been decentralized, with control widely dispersed. Seed saving has always been a vital part of the agricultural cycle. Without saved seed there is nothing to sow and nothing to harvest. This is a fundamental law of annual plant cultivation.

Since the dawn of agriculture thousands of years ago, people have saved seeds. Over time people saved and replanted the seeds from the fleshiest fruits, from the sweetest- or the strongest- or the mildest-tasting plants, from the most storable, biggest, most prolific, most drought-resistant or heat-tolerant or cold-hardy individual plants. These gradually evolved into improved varieties, adapted to local conditions, whose seeds were traded and dispersed.

Seed selection and dispersal over many years and generations has led to tremendous local adaptation of varieties, as the characteristics of the plants most successful in a particular ecological niche were selected over time. "When traits people wanted appeared, they were not allowed to be lost but were encouraged, maintained, and perpetuated by the acts of the first farmers," write Cary Fowler and Pat Mooney. "This process of selecting certain plants and sowing their seeds, repeated every year for thousands of years, can have effects which are a marvel to contemplate."[29]

Seeds "got here in a dance of people and earth that will only go on if both partners are honored," writes British Columbia seed activist Dan Jason.[30] Not only have plant species evolved in this process, but human cultures have coevolved with the plants they have cultivated. For example, wild grass seeds were transformed over time into grains, which require human intervention for effective dispersal. In the process, civilizations were built around the grains and their cultivation, storage, distribution, and consumption. Our domesticated crops depend upon us for their continued existence in their current form just as surely as we depend upon them.

Traditional plant breeding, which has yielded uncountable varieties of cultivated plants around the world—often called heirlooms—is the work of amateurs. Like any other aspect of growing food, seed saving is best learned experientially; there's a learning curve. Certain crops need to be planted far from other members of their families so their seeds are true to type and they do not cross with genetically similar relatives. Tomato seeds need to be fermented in their pulp before being dried. Seed drying and storage practices influence seed viability. There is much to be learned, but for the most part, the process is simple enough.

In recent years gardeners and farmers have largely abdicated seed selection and saving, traditionally integrated elements of cultivating plants, to professionals. "For most gardeners, seed growing is a mysterious rite performed each year by gifted growers supervised by people with PhDs, the outcome of which is illustrated in bibles of various editions known as seed catalogues," writes Robert Johnston, Jr., in his informative pamphlet *Growing Garden Seeds*. "Certainly [it is] not a task to be undertaken by a mere gardener!"[31]

Government-funded breeding programs introduced farmers to "improved" hybrid varieties and induced them to stop saving their inherited heirloom seeds. The first hybrid seeds were produced in the 1920s. Hybridization involves crossing two inbred genetic lines, which requires greater technical know-how than traditional seed saving. The hybrid seeds produce uniform plants that often show increased vigor by virtue of cross-breeding (a phenomenon plant scientists call *heterosis* or "hybrid vigor"). However, when the hybrid plants generate seed, the genes that mixed in a predictable pattern in the first-generation (F1) hybrid reshuffle, producing highly variable progeny. Therefore, each year hybridization must be performed from the original two inbred parent lines to generate uniform F1 seeds. As farmers switched to buying hybrid seeds, most of them let go of the seed-saving tradition.

For decades plant breeding was undertaken primarily by scientists at state land-grant universities, whose work was funded by the government, in an effort to promote high yields. However, in recent years, as part of the overall trend toward privatization of resources and services, government research funding has shrunk, leaving corporate sponsorship as the driving force in seed development. For the seeds that are the basis of our sustenance, we have allowed ourselves to become utterly dependent on corporations whose motivations we all know are profit-driven. "Can we stop buying into processes and products that are designed only to make money before it becomes impossible not to?" asks Dan Jason.[32]

Another aspect of this dependence is that farmers are being reduced from creative generalists—whose concerns include seed saving and selective breeding—to "renters of proprietary germplasm from the Gene Giants or their subsidiaries," in the words of a 1999 communiqué from the Action Group on Erosion, Technology, and Concentration (ETC Group).[33] The results of this transformation have been disastrous. Achieving the high yields promised by hybrid varieties typically requires greater inputs, such as chemicals and water; these are expensive and degrade the environment, leading to the disintegration of farm communities and dizzying losses of both agricultural and natural biodiversity.

Much of the diversity of traditional, locally adapted crops has been replaced by a small handful of varieties. This increase in genetic uniformity gives rise to huge vulnerabilities to pests and diseases. Biodiversity is a key element of sustainability. "If diversity is to be saved," said plant geneticist Jack Harlan, "it may have to be saved by amateurs: people who love their seeds."[34]

I think I qualify as a seed-saving amateur. Every year that I have gardened I have saved some seeds, generally the ones that seem most straightforward. This year I saved okra seeds for the first time ever and there was nothing to it. I left some okra to dry on the stalks, then broke open the brittle pods and collected the seeds. Beans are also that easy, and it is my impression that they are the most widely saved seeds. Cilantro seeds are easy to harvest as well, whether to replant or to enjoy the distinctive flavor of coriander seeds. I've also been growing and replanting garlic bulbs and liver-regenerating milk thistle seeds for a number of years now. Other friends share with me the seeds they save.

One year I grew out corn and pole bean seeds gifted to me by Nance Klehm, a Chicago guerilla gardener and artist. I met Nance after I participated in a project of hers called *Cornography*, which was a sort of performance art installation featuring a few stalks of this corn growing in a shopping cart and many different people taking turns, over the course of more than a month, walking it across Chicago. "Folks volunteered to be pushers/farmers and traveled the streets and alleyways of Chicago with the corn and their own interpretations and agendas," says Nance. "The corn cart has visited community gardens, toured supermarkets, politicized a street fair, gone out for coffee, and rested in many backyards." Nance has also organized a neighborhood orchard of sorts, encouraging and assisting neighbors in planting fruit trees, grapevines, and garlic in their yards. "When you give someone a seed, it's such a small gift," observes Nance. "But it entails a responsibility to interact with the land."

At gardening-related gatherings, and even at political protest events, I've encountered other enthusiastic seed activists. These are folks sharing their seed abundances as a public service and a consciousness-raising exercise, asking for small donations or freely giving them away. It is such a generous and hopeful gesture to save the seeds of a few varieties to spread and swap and, more importantly, to inspire other potential amateur seed savers to reclaim this most basic of agricultural skills.

"Seeds, especially of food and other useful plants, should be taken care of *by the people*," insist Jude and Michel Fanton, the founders of Australia's Seed Savers' Network. "They are too precious for all of them to be placed under the exclusive control of the few. The more hands that hold them, the safer they will be."[35] It turns out that the Fantons enjoy not only saving seed but making good use of the many diverse plants they grow in their subtropical climate, and they are experienced fermentation enthusiasts. When my fermentation fervor tour took me to Australia, they invited me to their Seed Savers Center in Byron Bay, New South Wales. When I was inside their home and educational center, the Fantons kept pulling out jars of fermented vegetables and fruits for me to taste; outside as we toured their compact but richly diverse and productive gardens, Michel kept handing me seedpods, tubers, fibrous stalks, and bulbs. For the Fantons, fermentation and seed saving go together as forms of active engagement with the world of plants. "We can help ourselves to become independent again by saving seeds and passing on knowledge about propagation and plant usage," they write in their *Seed Savers' Handbook*.[36]

Over the past few decades, as it has become clear how rapidly seed resources are being lost (along with the amateur seed-saving skillbase required to maintain them), a number of organizations have emerged around the world to support and encourage seed saving. Diane and Kent Whealy started the Seed Savers Exchange in Iowa in 1975, after Diane's dying grandfather entrusted to their care the seeds of two garden heirlooms, Grandpa Ott's Morning Glory and German Pink Tomato, that his parents had brought from Bavaria when they immigrated to Iowa a hundred years earlier. "Seed Savers Exchange is a nonprofit organization that saves and shares the heirloom seeds of our garden heritage, forming a living legacy that can be passed down through generations," says the group's Web site. "Our organization is saving the world's diverse, but endangered, garden heritage for future generations by building a network of people committed to collecting, conserving, and sharing heirloom seeds and plants, while educating people about the value of genetic and cultural diversity."[37] The Seed Savers Exchange publishes an annual yearbook listing seed varieties cultivated by members. In the 2006 yearbook, 756 amateur seed savers offered 12,284 different seed varieties, more than the entire mail-order garden seed industry in the United States and Canada. Most seeds can be ordered directly from the listed members. Some rare varieties are available only on a "must reoffer" basis.

Because the nature of traditional seed varieties is dictated by adaptation to local conditions, the most practical level for seed exchange is local. In India, Navdanya, the seed-savers' organization started by Vandana Shiva, has helped establish eleven regional seed banks, which she describes as "spreading seeds of hope, helping farmers off the chemical treadmill and out of a vicious cycle of despair."[38] The Australian Seed Savers' Network, started in the mid-1980s, began devolving a decade later into local networks, of which there were sixty as of 2005. In my father's town of Gardiner, New York, Ken Greene, a local librarian who is also an aspiring farmer, has been teaching seed-saving workshops and has established a seed library with about fifty plant varieties. People "borrow" seeds from the library, grow them out, and then return fresh seeds at the end of the season.

Seed saving is a skill we can and must reclaim. "It's time for the rising up of a new generation of plant breeders out of the very soil of our farms and gardens," exhorts Carol Deppe, author of *Breed Your Own Vegetable Varieties*. "It is time for farmers and gardeners every-where to take back our seeds, to rediscover seed saving, and to prac-tice our own plant breeding. It is time to breed plants based upon an entirely different set of values."[39] For more information, see the list of excellent seed-saving books and other resources at the end of this chapter.

Biotech Food Safety: Corporate-Government Collusions and Delusions

Contrast the aggressive enforcement against individual farmers, such as Percy Schmeiser, found to have violated intellectual property laws, with the enforcement of the limited safety rules that apply to the biotech industry. Seminis (recently acquired by Monsanto) was fined a nominal $2,500 after it was discovered that the company had shipped unlabeled genetically engineered tomato seeds to the University of California at Davis, whose researchers distributed the seeds to scientists at other uni-versities who had ordered conventionally bred seeds. Scott's, a grass seed company, was fined only $3,125 when it failed to notify authorities that experimental, genetically engineered, herbicide-tolerant grass seed had escaped from a test field in Madras, Oregon.[40] The USDA and U.S. Environmental Protection Agency (EPA) covered up news that Swiss-based Syngenta had distributed around the world hundreds of tons of mislabeled experimental GM corn—not approved for commercial dis-tribution or consumption—from 2001 to 2004. The experimental corn was in the food supply for years before the story broke in the journal *Nature*, months after the U.S. government was notified by Syngenta and took no action to recall products containing the corn or to warn con-sumers.[41] The *Nature* editors later urged European regulators to inves-tigate how the error could have happened, since "their U.S. equivalents show little sign of rising to the challenge."[42] The USDA subsequently fined Syngenta $375,000, an inconsequential sum in light of the scale and length of the error.

These wrist-slapping enforcement actions are illustrative of the control biotech corporations have over the regulatory processes to which they are at least theoretically subject. Throughout the brief history of GM foods, corporations invested in the new technology have driven public policy. According to the *New York Times*, "It was an outcome that would be repeated, again and again, through three administrations. What Monsanto wished for from Washington, Monsanto—and, by extension, the biotechnology industry—got."[43]

The officials of federal regulatory agencies charged with evaluating Monsanto's applications are all too often once and future Monsanto employees, a classic revolving-door scenario that we find repeated in the stories of how control of our food supply has come to be so concentrated. For example, as a Washington-based attorney for the law firm of King and Spaulding, Michael Taylor worked for Monsanto drafting proposed regulations for GM crops for Monsanto's lobbyists to promote. When he was appointed deputy commissioner for policy at the U.S. Food and Drug Administration (FDA), Taylor was able to implement the regulations he had drafted. Taylor's good work at the FDA got him promoted to the position of administrator of the USDA's Food Safety and Inspection Service, where he continued to be involved in setting policy related to GM foods. He was later hired *back* by Monsanto as its vice president for public policy.

Attorney Steven Druker, a public-interest crusader whose organization, the Alliance for Bio-Integrity, filed a successful lawsuit under the Freedom of Information Act against the FDA, has had the opportunity to study the FDA's internal files. The lawsuit forced the FDA to release internal documents that are a fascinating study in politicized public policymaking. Certainly the agency had staff scientists who were raising safety questions. The FDA Task Group on Food Biotechnology: Progress Report 2, dated August 15, 1991, states: "Four broad concerns were identified: (1) New substances for which safety basis is not established; (2) Unexpected changes in food/feed composition that result from genetic modification; (3) Labeling; and (4) Environmental issues."[44] A few months later an FDA official wrote, "The process of genetic engineering and traditional breeding are different, and according to the technical experts in the agency, they lead to different risks."[45]

Nonetheless, FDA policy repeatedly stated that the GM foods were safe. "During Mr. Taylor's tenure as Deputy Commissioner," Druker writes, "references to the potential unintended negative effects of bio-engineering were progressively deleted from drafts of the policy statement (over the protests of agency scientists), and a final statement was issued claiming (a) that [GM] foods are no riskier than others and (b) that the agency has no information to the contrary."[46]

And so the official line is that these foods, radically altered on the genetic level, are "substantially equivalent" to traditional foods. The biotech food industry, the World Trade Organization, and the U.S. government all claim that there is no significant difference between foods that are genetically modified and those that are not, as if extensive research had definitively determined that truth. It is on the basis of this presumption of equivalence that these foods were released into the food supply—without any labeling to differentiate them.

The introduction of GM food has been devious and deceptive at every step. There *is* a huge experiment being conducted on the effects of GM food on human health and the environment. The experiment is completely uncontrolled, and its results have yet to be fully revealed or understood. We are all the subjects of this experiment. In the past decade, GM ingredients have saturated our diet in the United States through their widespread presence in processed foods. As of 2004, 85 percent of soy and 45 percent of corn grown in the United States was genetically modified.[47] Try finding processed foods without either corn or soy. Meanwhile, new GM foods keep being introduced every year. In 2005, for example, wine fermented with GM yeast entered the U.S. market.

Boosters of genetic modification point to the fact that we haven't all died or experienced dramatic illness after a decade of widespread consumption of GM foods. However, the causes of disease are not necessarily obvious, dramatic, or immediate. Often epidemiology (the study of disease transmission) takes decades to understand the impact of certain practices on health, such as smoking tobacco or eating trans fats.

Food-related illnesses doubled between 1994 and 2001, the period in which GM crops first entered the food supply.[48] "Unknown agents account for approximately 81 percent of foodborne illnesses and hospitalizations," reported the U.S. Centers for Disease Control and

Prevention in 1999.[49] In addition, obesity has become a national epidemic, the incidence of diabetes is rising sharply, and cancers and many other illnesses are becoming more and more prevalent. "Is there a connection to GM foods?" asks Jeffrey M. Smith. "We have no way of knowing because no one has looked for one."[50]

In fact, there has been very limited meaningful study of the effects of GM foods on human health. However, the few studies of the effects of GM foods on animals suggest problems. In 1995 biologist Arpad Pusztai received a grant from the Scottish Agriculture, Environment, and Fisheries Department to develop a model for testing the safety of GM foods. Pusztai studied the effects of a diet of GM potatoes on adolescent laboratory rats. After only ten days on a GM diet, the rats suffered immune system damage, white blood cell suppression, impaired organ development, and other problems. "I had facts that indicated to me there were serious problems with transgenic [GM] food," says Pusztai.[51]

After Pusztai went public with his findings, the institute that employed him would not permit him to speak further about his research, but a furor had already been unleashed, and he was invited to testify before Parliament, which superceded his contractually obliged silence. Sensational though Pusztai's revelations were, they have never been rigorously followed up. In 2005 Russian scientist Irina Ermakova conducted an experiment on the offspring of female rats, comparing three groups fed diets augmented by GM soy, non-GM soy, or no soy at all, beginning two weeks before conception and continuing through nursing. Within three weeks of birth, 56 percent of the rats born in the GM soy group died, compared to 9 percent in the non-GM soy group and 7 percent from the no-soy group. But then Ermakova's funding ran out, and she has not been able to perform detailed organ analysis or to repeat her experiment to confirm the results.[52]

"Those familiar with the body of GM safety studies are often astounded by their superficiality," reports Smith. With universities and research institutes increasingly dependent on corporate dollars, dissenting views are easily silenced by withdrawing funding. Research on GM food safety simply isn't happening, except under direct corporate sponsorship, which comes with strings attached. "When you have so many scientists . . . doing sponsored research, you start to wonder," says

Mildred Cho, a senior research scholar at Stanford University's Center for Biomedical Ethics. "How are these studies being designed? What kinds of research questions are being raised? What kinds aren't being raised?"[53]

One big concern about GM foods is the potential for unexpected allergic reactions. GM foods may contain greater concentrations of known allergens. Soy allergies increased 50 percent in the United Kingdom after GM soy was introduced to the country, and Russian scientists report that allergies in their country tripled in the three years when GM foods became widespread there.[54] GM foods can also produce new, unanticipated allergens. "No one knows if humans are allergic to [the GM foods'] proteins—they were never before part of the human food supply," observes Smith.[55]

GM StarLink corn, approved only for animal consumption, was discovered to be widespread in the human food supply in 2000. Although StarLink was planted on less than 1 percent of U.S. cornfields, it was widely mixed in silos with other corn and contaminated 22 percent of the corn tested by the USDA, thoroughly insinuated into all of corn's varied products. More than three hundred different products, totaling ten million individual food items, were eventually recalled from supermarket shelves, at a cost of about $1 billion, but not before hundreds of allergic reactions were reported, presumably triggered by Cry9C, a *Bacillus thuringiensis* (Bt) toxin unique to StarLink.[56]

"We all wish there was a test where you plug in a protein and out pops a 'yes' or 'no' answer," says Sue MacIntosh, a protein chemist with AgrEvo, a GM seed manufacturer. "But there is no such test . . . short of giving it to a lot of people and seeing what happens."[57] In 2006, more than a decade after GM foods entered the U.S. food supply, the EPA is for the first time offering grants, totaling $3 million, "to develop methods to assess the potential allergenicity of genetically engineered foods."[58] I wish that made me feel safer.

Worldwide Resistance to Genetically Modified Food

Most of the world is not accepting GM agriculture or food. More than half the acreage under GM cultivation globally is in the United States, and almost all of the rest is in four other nations: Argentina, Brazil, Canada, and China.[59] Most other nations have opposed GM (also referred to as GE, for genetically engineered) crops and products, either banning them outright or at least taking a more cautionary approach. In the United States, most people haven't so much embraced GM foods as remained oblivious to them, thanks to the lack of required labeling and the paucity of information about GM foods in the mainstream media. Despite the fact that GM ingredients are ubiquitous in processed foods in the United States, surveys consistently find that most people do not realize they are there.[60]

While the corporate forces of technological inevitability try desperately to impose GM crops and foods, people in most places are responding with an emphatic "No!" Zambia refused a donation of GM corn from the United States in 2002, and Angola, Lesotho, Malawi, Mozambique, and Zimbabwe have refused GM corn unless it is first milled to eliminate the risk of contaminating crops.[61] In 2006 a "farmers' jury" in Mali listened to arguments for and against GM crops for five days and then urged its government to reject them. Wangari Maathai, the Kenyan tree-planting environmental activist who was awarded the 2004 Nobel Peace Prize, warns that biotechnology "is the new frontier for conquest, and Africa ought to be wary because a history of colonialism and exploitation is repeating itself."[62]

In 2005 seventeen nongovernmental organizations from ten rice-growing nations across Asia came together in Bangkok to issue the GE-Free Rice Declaration, which concludes: "The future of our world's most important staple food crop will be secured through the protection and use of biodiversity rather than genetic engineering, and through ecological agriculture based on the traditional knowledge of farming communities."[63] When agricultural researchers met in Mexico City in 2004, "demonstrators tossed tortillas and ears of corn painted with fluorescent colors and skulls at a line of riot police guarding the hotel."[64]

Around the world many regions and localities have declared themselves "GE-free zones." In the United States, New England activists have brought the issue to town meetings, that venerable institution of direct democracy. In two days, March 4 and 5, 2002, thirty-one Vermont towns declared themselves "GE-free," and many more have since followed suit. By 2005 nearly one hundred New England localities, most in Vermont, had declared themselves GE-free zones, and the idea continues to spread.[65]

In California, citizen referendums have been a grassroots means of creating GE-free zones. Mendocino County passed the state's first ban in 2004, despite the fact that industry opponents of the ban outspent proponents seven to one in the campaign before the vote. Marin County voters passed a similar anti-GM referendum, and Trinity County joined the ban, not by referendum but by a simple vote of the county's board of supervisors. The group Californians for GE-Free Agriculture is offering trainings for teams of regional organizers in the hope of facilitating further local bans. "Perhaps the most important strategic tactic we have at the moment is passing local bans," says Ronnie Cummins of the Organic Consumers Association, "and then linking these local areas together so as to create regional GE-free zones, especially here in North America, the belly of the beast."

Of course, the biotech industry and the elected officials who answer to it are not submitting to grassroots democracy without a fight. As of 2005 Arizona, Florida, Georgia, Idaho, Indiana, Iowa, North Dakota, Ohio, Oklahoma, Pennsylvania, South Dakota, and West Virginia had passed preemptive laws prohibiting counties and municipalities from restricting crops. These laws are frequently referred to as "Monsanto laws," and similar measures are under consideration in more states, including California.

In the United States, some activists have focused on trying to get the government to require labeling of GM foods and ingredients. When asked in polls, Americans overwhelmingly (92 percent according to a 2003 ABC News poll) say they think GM foods should be required to be labeled as such. And yet they are not, and there has never been any serious national discussion of such a policy in the United States, though many other nations require GM foods to be labeled. In 2002 Oregon activists succeeded in getting a referendum on the ballot proposing to require labeling of GM foods. Industry opponents financed a $5 million media blitz to convince voters that passage would lead to higher grocery prices, and the referendum was defeated at the polls. A bill has been introduced in Congress to require GM labeling—the Genetically Engineered Food Right-to-Know Act—but it has gone nowhere. Congress is beholden to the biotech industry, which would be

destroyed by mandatory labeling. In 2005 Alaska became the first state
to require labeling of GM food, but only in the case of fish, as the FDA
considers approving fast-growing GM salmon.[66]

In response to the few states that have enacted or seriously considered their own food-labeling regulations, there has been a move toward
national policy prohibiting state food-labeling requirements beyond
existing FDA standards. In 2006 the U.S. House of Representatives
passed the National Uniformity for Food Act. If enacted into law, this
act will legally enforce ignorance and hide the truth.

The GM food industry has acted aggressively even against food
labeled as free of GM ingredients. Monsanto sued Oakhurst Dairy in
Maine because its label stated, "Our Farmers' Pledge: No Artificial
Growth Hormones," informing consumers that their milk is free of
genetically engineered recombinant bovine growth hormone (rBGH),
which is commonly used in milk production. The dairy settled the suit
by agreeing to add to its label the caveat "FDA states: no significant difference in milk from cows treated with artificial growth hormone."

In Europe, resistance to GM foods has been strong and largely
effective. Although GM food imports to the European Union are permitted, most retailers and manufacturers market their food products as
GM-free, and the European Union requires that any food containing
GM ingredients be explicitly labeled as such. The popular movement
against GM foods in Europe was sparked by direct action. In the fall of
1996, as the first ships bearing GM food arrived from the United States
in European ports, Greenpeace activists confronted the ships out in the
harbors. In Hamburg the first shipment of GM soy arrived in a ship
aptly named *Ideal Progress*, and activists drew attention to it by pro-
jecting onto the ship the words "We are not your guinea pigs!"[67] Two
weeks later activists confronted ships bearing GM soy in Amsterdam,
Liverpool, and Barcelona as well. Though these actions failed to prevent the GM soy from entering Europe, they were tremendously effective at alerting people to the issues.

Strong public opposition to GM food has prompted some European
governments to adopt bans or moratoria on GM crops. When GM
seeds have been imported to Europe or GM crops planted there, they
have often been destroyed by activists. In 1998 a group of two hundred
French farmers broke into a Novartis warehouse, opened sacks of GM

corn, and doused their contents with water. One of the organizers of the Novartis action, René Riesel, delivered an eloquent defense in court, asking, "Is it still possible to make the truth heard when so many political and economic powers are in league to cover it up? . . . My comrades and I felt it was urgent to act before it was too late."[68]

In 2005 a French court actually dismissed criminal charges against forty-nine activists who had uprooted a field of GM corn. "The defendants have shown proof that they committed an infraction of voluntary vandalism in a group to respond to a situation of necessity," said the court, affirming that genetic modification "constitutes a clear and present danger for the well-being of others, in the sense that it could be the source of contamination and unwanted pollution."[69] The same year another French court sentenced sheep farmer and activist José Bové to four months in jail for his role in destroying a field of GM corn. "They hope that by sending me to jail they can stop the movement," said Bové. "Our fight is more legitimate than ever, and it will go on."[70]

When Bové was invited to speak in the United States in 2006 at a conference at a university, he was denied entry into the country. Though direct action against GM crops has been common in Europe, and quite effective, in the United States, in this time of the so-called war on terror, these acts are defined as *agroterrorism*. "Agroterrorism is the willful, unlawful threatened or actual destruction of property or people through the agricultural and food industry to achieve the perpetrator's ends, usually political," writes agricultural economist Luther Tweeten. "It is not possible to dismiss the varied activity of agroterrorists as mere pranks because those who intend only to destroy property and science end up destroying lives both literally and figuratively. . . . Eternal vigilance is in order."[71]

In the United States most anti-GM direct action has been symbolic, such as in the 1998 action when members of the Biotic Baking Brigade threw a pie in the face of Monsanto CEO Robert Shapiro as he spoke at San Francisco's posh Fairmont Hotel. "Agent Apple" provided an eyewitness account:

> I could barely contain myself, the tension was so great. Shapiro waxed grandiloquently about Monsanto's crucial role in saving the Earth from soil erosion, pollution, overpopulation, famine,

and the destructiveness of industrial society. I kid you not. He described the inherent wastefulness of cars and other industrial products, especially agricultural. His solution: more technology. . . .

Finally, he finished his speech and left the podium in a hurry. I perceived Agents Custard and Lemon Meringue approaching him directly, so I prepared for a delicious case of culinary comeuppance. As Caesar said from the banks of the wide river Rubicon, while gazing across at Rome, "The pie is cast."

A young man at a table near the stage stopped Shapiro cold in his tracks with cries of "Shame, shame!" A dialogue ensued, then from Shapiro's three o'clock angle two pies originating from suited figures went airborne. The first made delightful contact with his upper left facial quadrant and left eyeglass piece, while the second sailed past harmlessly. Our victim directed some verbal unpleasantries toward the rapidly departing flan-ers, then barely stopped to wipe his glasses and face before returning to the argument, exclaiming loudly: "Roundup is perfectly safe!"[72]

The End of Sexuality and Other Apocalyptic Scenarios

Can any action avert humanity's technological downfall? I try to remain hopeful and cast my lot with the possibility of change, but our situation and prospects both appear rather bleak. So many nightmare scenarios have been imagined for us. Science fiction anticipated genetic tinkering generations before the technology existed to actually do it. The dangers I have just briefly described are very real. Yet I find that every new revelation seems strangely familiar, as if we had been expecting it. Each sensational news report seems like it must have come from science fiction.

For instance, on October 6, 2005, the *Washington Post* reported, "It has recently become clear that a few offspring of cloned pigs and cows are already trickling into the food supply."[73] Though the meat and milk industries have mostly observed a voluntary moratorium on producing food from cloned animals while the FDA formulates rules, some cloned animal products have entered the supply chain. The FDA is expected to rule that milk from cloned animals and meat from their offspring are safe to eat. "The FDA has made clear it won't require labels on clone products," wrote the *Post*, "which may leave meat-eaters who want to avoid them little practical way to do so."

This is surreal and scary. Our food supply is increasingly divorced from natural processes. Reproducing flocks of animals, like selected, saved, and replanted seeds, generate diversity in decentralized processes. Biotechnology creates uniformity. It seeks to control nature. But as we are seeing in the world around us, efforts to control nature typically have unpredictable repercussions, making us exceedingly vulnerable. The best protection of our food supply against disease and crop failures lies in the diversity of traditional decentralized agricultural practices. Unfortunately, decentralized systems of community food sovereignty are not high on the agendas of the multinational corporations vying for control of our food.

Toward what cataclysmic climax the path of biotechnology may eventually lead us, we can only speculate. The futuristic dystopian image I often think of comes from the 1973 film *Soylent Green*. Set only a couple of decades beyond our own time, the film envisions massive environmental collapse. The only foods available are processed food bars of undisclosed origin. One day a week people receive special green high-protein bars. "Tuesday is Soylent Green Day." The character of the cranky old man, Sol Roth (played by Edward G. Robinson), refuses when a young friend offers him a bar of Soylent Green:

> Tasteless, odorless crud. . . . You don't know any better. When I was a kid food was food. Before our scientific magicians polluted the water and soil and decimated plant and animal life. . . . Why in my day you could buy meat anywhere, eggs they had, real butter, fresh lettuce in the stores. . . .

Soylent Green turns out to be made of people, a not unreasonable source of nutrients in the absence of any others. But what generally conjures up this image in my mind is the fact that so much of what we consume already consists of mystery ingredients that the law requires *not* to be included on labels. These include not only actual GM ingredients but also many ingredients manufactured through processes that utilize enzymes produced by GM microbes.

My personal paranoid fantasy of where biotechnology industries are headed involves human reproduction. Isn't that the next frontier after plant reproduction and animal reproduction have been fully commercialized? There are already plenty of signs that human reproductive abilities are on the wane: decreasing fertility rates; reduced levels of sperm vitality and viability; the massive use of drugs by women to increase fertility and by men to overcome erectile dysfunction; and diminishing penis size linked to exposure to chemicals called phthalates, which are commonly found in plastics, cosmetics, and perfumes. It's not just us. "Animals throughout the world are undergoing unnatural sexual changes in response to environmental pollution," reports *National Geographic.*[74]

The biotech industry, composed of many of the same corporations that gave us the endocrine-disrupting chemicals in the first place, are well positioned to take over the complex mechanics of human reproduction. The flaw with life processes, from the point of view of capital, is that by their self-regenerating qualities they resist commodification. "If life is to be commodified," writes Vandana Shiva, "its renewability must be interrupted and arrested."[75] Biotechnology corporations profit by halting the continuous, endlessly cycling and regenerating spiral of life and requiring corporate products to accomplish various biological reproductive processes—from plant seeds to babies.

Already human reproductive processes have become medicalized, drawn into the realm of experts with an ever-expanding array of specialized technology. Will we come to accept that human reproduction requires technological intervention, as we seem to be accepting for the food we eat? If we do not reclaim natural reproductive processes for the food we eat, we risk our disconnection growing to encompass the remaining natural processes—such as human sexual reproduction—that are still considered the province of generalists. Retaining our biological power to share and exchange our own seeds (and related pleasures) may depend upon the outcome of political struggles happening now, upon farmers and gardeners asserting their inalienable natural rights by continuing the ancient tradition of saving and replanting seeds.

Recipe: Soaking and Sprouting Seeds

Seed germination is a miracle to behold. In its dry form, a seed is life in suspended animation, dormant, a bundle of potential. Once it is wet, a seed drinks in the water of life and begins to transform and become alive. A seed can remain in suspended animation for quite some time without losing its spark of life; in fact, scientists recently germinated a two-thousand-year-old seed they had unearthed in an archeological dig.

Dry seeds are nutritionally dense and protected by a skin and various chemical mechanisms that discourage critters (ourselves included) from eating them. Soaking seeds causes them to swell and sets in motion enyzmatic transformations that neutralize the protective toxins and digest proteins, carbohydrates, and fats into simpler forms. "The nutritional energy of the food is repatterned," writes Renée Loux Underkoffler. "The seed begins to transform its stored energy into the active, growing energy of the plant."[76] The process of germination produces vitamins and other nutrients.

Soaking seeds begins the process. Seeds include all the foods we know as nuts, grains, and beans, as well as sesame, pumpkin, flax, sunflower, and others that we generally refer to as seeds. Each seed is unique in its particulars, but generally this soaking improves digestibility and neutralizes toxic protective compounds. After just a few hours of soaking most seeds will be visibly swollen. Soaking overnight (six to twelve hours) is ideal for most seeds; for especially oily nuts, such as cashews, macadamias, and pine nuts, an hour or two of soaking is plenty, as they lack skins containing enzyme inhibitors, and longer soaking will leach out their rich oils. Drain off the soaking water and your seeds are ready for eating raw, cooking, sprouting, or making seed cheeses or pâtés (see page 183).

One seed toxin that has received much attention, thanks to the crusading work of Sally Fallon and the Weston A. Price Foundation (for more on them, see page 169), is phytic acid. Phytic acid is a phosphorous compound found in the bran (outer layer) of grains that can bind with minerals (calcium, magnesium, copper, iron, and especially zinc) in the digestive tract and prevent their absorption. Regular consumption of untreated whole grains can lead to depletion of these vital nutrients. Sprouting grains neutralizes the phytic acid. If the grains are not

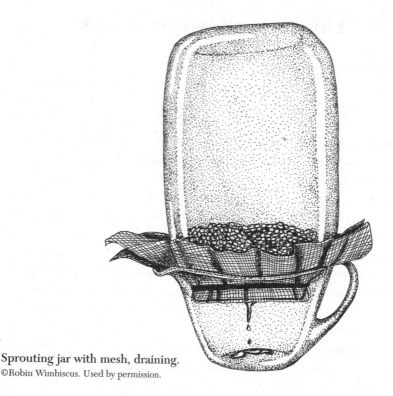

Sprouting jar with mesh, draining.
©Robin Wimbiscus. Used by permission.

to be sprouted but simply soaked, the addition of a small amount of an acidic liquid, such as vinegar, whey, sauerkraut juice, buttermilk, or sourdough starter, activates the enzyme phytase to break down the phytic acid.

To sprout, the swollen seed must be kept moist while also having access to air. This requires rinsing the seeds regularly, but not letting them sit in water, because they also need air. Think of a seed germinating in moist soil, wicking in moisture while also being exposed to air. The easiest way to create this condition is in a jar with window-screen mesh over the top, held in place with a rubber band or the circular screw-on band of a Mason jar top. Soak the seeds overnight right in the jar (leave space for them to swell), drain, then rinse the sprouts in the jar at least a few times a day. The more frequently you rinse, the better, especially in hot weather, when unrinsed sprouts can get funky and start to rot quickly. Leave the jar upside down while it is draining, supported up above the surface it is draining onto, so that the none of seeds will be sitting in a puddle of the drained water. Another good sprouting container is a bag made of fine-mesh fabric, which you can hang up to drip after each rinsing.

Radish sprouts are my favorites for a little fresh zing on a sandwich or salad. Mung bean sprouts are big, crunchy, sweet, and very versatile; I love them as elements in spring rolls, stir-fries, and kimchis. They may be rinsed for days to sprout longer tails. If the mung sprouts are protected from light, the tails will be white; exposed to light they will be green and more bitter. Once the sprouts are ready, refrigerate them and use them while fresh. They deteriorate after a few days, though continued rinsing can extend their life.

Only seeds with intact skins can be sprouted. Certain very small seeds, like millet, can be tricky to sprout, and flax is even more so because it is mucilaginous and impossible to rinse. Larger seeds are easier. The length of time required for sprouting will vary with the type of seed and the temperature. Seeds can also be sprouted to a greater or a lesser degree. Typically grains are sprouted just until their tails emerge. That's when they are sweetest, and as the tail grows the sweetness is consumed. Sprouted whole grains can be enjoyed raw; used in breads, beers, and delicious porridges; or further soaked into a fermented tonic drink called rejuvelac (find the recipe in my book *Wild Fermentation*).

Recipe: Roasting Squash or Pumpkin Seeds

I hate to see people throwing away the seeds of squashes and pumpkins. The seed is where the plant directs its greatest potency. It contains important nutrients—protein, fats, and minerals—that the plant is investing in its future generations. It seems like an extravagant insult to discard the most nutrient-dense part of the plant.

As we assert our natural right to save seeds and reclaim the seed as a missing link of continuity in the food chain, it behooves us to use rather than discard seeds. Making use of these precious resources honors them, recognizes their tremendous importance, and reintegrates them into our lives. And roasted seeds are so delicious!

Roasting seeds is easy. The slightly tedious part is separating the seeds from the pulp. Generally I collect the scraped-out seeds in a bowl of water and use both hands to pull chunks of pulp and fiber from the seeds. Eventually I decide the seeds are clean enough, and I drain off the excess water. Since these seeds are fresh, they lack the protective toxins that develop in dried seeds and so do not require soaking.

Sometimes I season seeds with salt and perhaps cayenne, and other times I toss them in a little tamari and/or liquid hot sauce. Then I roast them. You can roast seeds either in a pan on a stovetop or in the oven. The challenge is to not burn them, so it is important to stir the roasting seeds often. Stovetop roasting requires constant attention for ten to fifteen minutes. Roasting in the oven is somewhat more forgiving. Roast seeds at a moderate heat (325°F/160°C) for twenty to thirty minutes, until they're not only dry on the outside but crispy in the middle as well. As an alternative to roasting, if you wish to keep the seeds raw with enzymes intact (see chapter 5), you can also dry the seeds more slowly using a dehydrator.

Action and Information Resources

Books

Ashworth, Suzanne. *Seed to Seed: Seed Saving and Growing Techniques for Vegetable Gardeners*. 2nd ed. Decorah, IA: Seed Savers Exchange, 2002.

Cooper, David, Renee Vellve, and Henk Hobbelink, eds. *Growing Diversity: Genetic Resources and Local Food Security*. Warwickshire, UK: Intermediate Technology Development Group, 1992.

Deppe, Carol. *Breed Your Own Vegetable Varieties: The Gardener's and Farmer's Guide to Plant Breeding and Seed Saving*. White River Junction, VT: Chelsea Green, 2000.

Fanton, Michel and Jude. *The Seed Savers' Handbook for Australia and New Zealand*. Byron Bay, New South Wales, Australia: The Seed Savers' Network, 1993.

Fowler, Cary, and Pat Mooney. *Shattering: Food, Politics, and the Loss of Genetic Diversity*. Tucson: University of Arizona Press, 1990.

Fox, Michael W. *Beyond Evolution: The Genetically Altered Future of Plants, Animals, the Earth . . . and Humans*. New York: Lyons Press, 1999.

Jason, Dan. *Save Our Seeds, Save Ourselves: Means and Methods of Embracing Our Seed Heritage*. Ganges, Salt Spring Island, BC: self-published, circa 2000.

Johnston, Robert, Jr. *Growing Garden Seeds: A Manual for Gardeners and Small Farmers*. Winslow, ME: Johnny's Selected Seeds, 1983.

Lambrecht, Bill. *Dinner at the New Gene Cafe: How Genetic Engineering is Changing What We Eat, How We Live, and the Global Politics of Food*. New York: St. Martin's, 2001.

Lappé, Marc, and Britt Bailey. *Against the Grain: Biotechnology and the Corporate Takeover of Your Food*. Monroe, ME: Common Courage Press, 1998.

Nestle, Marion. *Safe Food: Bacteria, Biotechnology, and Bioterrorism*. Berkeley: University of California Press, 2003.

Shiva, Vandana. *Stolen Harvest: The Hijacking of the Global Food Supply*. Cambridge, MA: South End Press, 2000.

———. *Tomorrow's Biodiversity*. New York: Thames and Hudson, 2000.

Smith, Jeffrey M. *Genetic Roulette: The Documented Health Risks of Genetically Engineered Foods*. Fairfield, IA: Yes! Books, 2006.

———. *Seeds of Deception: Exposing Industry and Government Lies about the Safety of the Genetically Engineered Foods You're Eating*. Fairfield, IA: Yes! Books, 2003.

Tokar, Brian, ed. *Gene Traders: Biotechnology, World Trade, and the Globalization of Hunger*. Burlington, VT: Toward Freedom, 2004.

———. *Redesigning Life? The Worldwide Challenge to Genetic Engineering*. New York: Zed Books, 2001.

Weaver, William Woys. *Heirloom Vegetable Gardening: A Master Gardener's Guide to Planting, Seed Saving, and Cultural History*. New York: Henry Holt, 1997.

Films

Bullshit. Directed by PeÅ Holmquist and Suzanne Khardalian. Sweden: HB PeÅ Holmquist Film, 2005; www.peaholmquist.com.

Fed Up! Genetic Engineering, Industrial Agriculture and Sustainable Alternatives. San Francisco: Wholesome Goodness Productions, 2002; www.wholesomegoodness.org.

The Future of Food. Directed by Deborah Coons Garcia. Mill Valley, CA: Lily Films, 2004; www.thefutureoffood.com.

Life Running Out of Control. Directed by Bertram Verhaag. Reading, PA: Bullfrog Films, 2005; www.bullfrogfilms.com.

Organizations and Other Resources

Alliance for Bio-Integrity
2040 Pearl Lane #2
Fairfield, IA 52556
(206) 888-4852
www.biointegrity.org

Ban Terminator Campaign
431 Gilmour Street, Second Floor
Ottawa, ON K2P 0R5
Canada
(613) 241-2267
www.banterminator.org

Californians for GE-Free Agriculture
15290 Coleman Valley Road
Occidental, CA 95465
(510) 647-3733
www.calgefree.org

Campaign to Label Genetically Engineered Foods
PO Box 55699
Seattle, WA 98155
(425) 771-4049
www.thecampaign.org

Center for Food Safety
660 Pennsylvania Avenue SE, #302
Washington, DC 20003
(202) 547-9359
www.centerforfoodsafety.org

CorpWatch
1611 Telegraph Avenue, #702
Oakland, CA 94612
(510) 271-8080

Council for Responsible Genetics
5 Upland Road, Suite 3
Cambridge, MA 02140
(617) 868-0870
www.gene-watch.org

ETC Group: Action Group on Erosion, Technology, and Concentration
431 Gilmour Street, 2nd Floor
Ottawa, ON K2P 0R5
Canada
(613) 241-2267
www.etcgroup.org

Fedco Seeds
PO Box 520
Waterville, ME 04903-0520
(207) 873-7333
www.fedcoseeds.com

Garden State Heirloom Seed Society
PO Box 15
Delaware, NJ 07833
www.historyyoucaneat.org

GE Free Maine
PO Box 7805
Portland, ME 04112
(207) 244-0908
www.gefreemaine.org

Genetically Engineered Food Alert
1200 18th Street NW, 5th Floor
Washington, DC 20036
(800) 390-3373
www.gefoodalert.org

Genetic Resources Action International
Girona 25, pral., E-08010
Barcelona
Spain
34 93301 1381
www.grain.org

Greenpeace USA
702 H Street NW, Suite 300
Washington, DC 20001
(800) 326-0959
www.greenpeace.org

Indigenous Peoples Council on
    Biocolonialism
PO Box 72
Nixon, NV 89424
(775) 574-0248
www.ipcb.org

Institute for Responsible Technology
PO Box 469
Fairfield, IA 52556
www.responsibletechnology.org

Institute of Science in Society
PO Box 32097
London NW1 0XR
United Kingdom
44 20 8452 2729
www.i-sis.org.uk

Monsanto Watch
www.monsantowatch.org

National Farmers Union Seed Saver
    Campaign
2717 Wentz Avenue
Saskatoon, SK S7K 4B6
Canada
(306) 652-9465
www.nfu.ca/seedsaver.html

Native Seeds/SEARCH
526 North 4th Avenue
Tucson, AZ 85705-8450
(866) 622-5561
www.nativeseeds.org

Navdanya
A-60, Hauz Khas
New Delhi 110016
India
www.vshiva.net

Organic Seed Alliance
PO Box 772
Port Townsend, WA 98368
(360) 385-7192
www.seedalliance.org

Peoples' Global Action
www.agp.org

Primal Seeds
www.primalseeds.org

The Ram's Horn
S6, C27, RR#1
Sorrento, BC V0E 2W0
Canada
(250) 675-4866
www.ramshorn.ca

Restoring Our Seed
PO Box 520
Waterville, ME 04903
(207) 872-9093
www.growseed.org

Rural Advancement Foundation
    International USA
PO Box 640
Pittsboro, NC 27312
(919) 542-1396
www.rafiusa.org

Saving Our Seed
286 Dixie Hollow
Louisa, VA 23093
(706) 788-0017
www.savingourseed.org

Scatterseed Project
Khadighar Farm
PO Box 1167
Farmington, ME 04938

Seed Savers Exchange
3094 North Winn Road
Decorah, IA 52101
(563) 382-5990
www.seedsavers.org

Seeds of Diversity Canada
PO Box 36, Station Q
Toronto, ON M4T 2L7
Canada
(905) 623-0353
www.seeds.ca

True Food Network
2921 Chapman Street, Suite 2
Oakland, CA 94601
www.truefoodnow.org

UK Agricultural Biodiversity Coalition
www.ukabc.org

Union of Concerned Scientists
2 Brattle Square
Cambridge, MA 02238
(617) 547-5552
www.ucsusa.org

United Plant Savers
PO Box 400
East Barre, VT 05649
(802) 479-9825
unitedplantsavers.org

World Social Forum
Rua General Jardim, 660, 8th Floor
São Paulo, SP 01223-010
Brazil
www.worldsocialforum.org

CHAPTER 3

Holding Our Ground: Land and Labor Struggles

Without access to land, people cannot possibly create or otherwise obtain food. Security and survival depend upon access to physical, outdoor space: farmland, grazing meadows, foraging and hunting ranges, and shorelines for fishing. Unfortunately, getting such access is very often a struggle in itself. The histories of patriarchy, capitalism, racism, colonialism, and many other forms of oppression are long sagas in which people have been systematically torn from the specific ecological niches that previously sustained them, the unique places that are the basis of culture and its glorious diversity.

The earth is our mother. We all come from the mother, and to her we shall return. We are of the earth; it is absurd to imagine that we can "own" it, even in small pieces. And yet the earth has been divvied up as private property. Property is a legal concept, a cultural production, not an intrinsic quality of land. Notions of what can be privatized as "property" seem to be infinitely expansive: land is privatized; seeds and genes are privatized; and even water is privatized (see chapter 10).

My old friend Bill Dobbs used to say, "Real estate determines culture." He was generally describing urban phenomena and offering a materialist analysis for cultural trends, but I think of his words often in relation to our food system. Real estate determines culture when indigenous peoples, carrying on age-old subsistence lifestyles connected to the land where they live, are supplanted by land ownership. Real estate determines culture when productive small farms are forced to sell their land because their modest agricultural earnings simply cannot keep pace with rising property-tax rates and competing demands for golf courses, malls, and subdivisions. Real estate determines culture when urban community gardens, which brought vitality and activity to their neighborhoods, are doomed by their successes and auctioned off to the highest bidder.

The social construct we revere as "the logic of the market" doesn't do a very good job of taking care of the land or of meeting most peoples' needs. When real estate is allowed to determine culture, that culture is an expression of domination. Culture needs to be liberated from real estate, and liberation movements everywhere have the reclamation of land as a central goal. "Revolution is based on land," wrote Malcolm X in his 1963 "Message to the Grassroots" speech. "Land is the basis of all independence. Land is the basis of freedom, justice, and equality."[1]

The "commons" is an ancient tradition of land shared as a community resource, and what few commons remain are shrinking fast. In Britain the commons were privatized beginning in the mid-1600s, in four thousand individual "Acts of Enclosure," culminating in the Great Enclosure Act of 1845. The enclosures literally starved many people, peasant farmers who historically had depended on common land for their food. This harsh reality rapidly transformed the formerly landbound peasantry into cheap factory labor and facilitated the Industrial Revolution. The Diggers and the Levellers were two resistance movements that took down the enclosure fences as the landlords erected them. A Leveller tract of 1649 declared:

> The Work we are going about is this, To dig up Georges-Hill and the waste Ground thereabouts, and to Sow Corn, and to eat our bread together by the sweat of our brows. And the First Reason is this, That we may work in righteousness, and lay the Foundation of making the Earth a Common Treasury for All, both Rich and Poor, That every one that is born in the land, may be fed by the Earth his Mother that brought him forth, according to the Reason that rules in the Creation.[2]

This process of land privatization has been repeated around the world, as have movements of resistance to it. "This continual struggle shows that the current inequitable distribution of land and housing, though widely accepted by elected governments and even public opinion worldwide, is strongly disputed on an operational level by people with the short end of the stick," writes Anders Corr in *No Trespassing: Squatting, Rent Strikes and Land Struggles Worldwide.*[3]

This chapter looks at movements struggling to retain and reclaim land for growing food. These activists include small-scale farmers searching for strategies that will enable them to hold onto their land, urban community gardeners reclaiming abandoned lots in their neighborhoods, and liberation movements taking land redistribution into their own hands, such as Brazil's Landless Workers Movement (MST), settling hundreds of thousands of people on unused large agricultural holdings. This chapter also looks at some activist movements defined by their separation from land, such as landless farm workers organizing for living wages and safe working conditions.

Land Movements across Space and Time

Virtually everywhere on the earth indigenous peoples have been displaced, and conflicts over land rights, as well other questions of survival and self-determination, are ongoing. Certainly this is true in North America. "Struggles by native peoples to retain use and occupancy rights over our traditional territories, and Euroamerican efforts to supplant us, comprise the virtual entirety of U.S./Indian relations since the inception of the republic," observes writer, teacher, and activist Ward Churchill.[4] "All across this continent," according to Anishinaabeg activist (and former Green Party vice presidential candidate) Winona LaDuke, "there are native peoples—in small communities with populations of one hundred, five hundred, even five thousand—who are trying to regain control of their community and their territory."[5]

LaDuke is the founder of the White Earth Land Recovery Project (WELRP). She lives on the White Earth Reservation, an area thirty-six miles square, or about 837,000 acres, located in Minnesota. "A treaty reserved it for our people in 1867 in return for relinquishing a much larger area of northern Minnesota" says LaDuke. "Of all our territory we chose this land for its richness and diversity."[6] The Anishinaabeg have traditionally held land collectively. "In our language the words *Anishinaabeg akiing* describe the concept of land ownership. They translate as 'the land of the people,' which doesn't infer that we own our land but that we belong on it."

In 1887, in accordance with the federal General Allotment Act, the White Earth Reservation was divided into eighty-acre parcels, one of which was granted to each individual residing on the reservation. Previously, the Anishinaabeg had shared the land on a communal basis. "The allotment system had no connection to our traditional land tenure patterns," says LaDuke.

> In our society a person harvested rice in one place, trapped in another place, got medicines in a third place, and picked berries in a fourth. These locations depended on the ecosystem; they were not necessarily contiguous. But the government said to each Indian, "Here are your eighty acres; this is where you'll live." Then, after each Indian had received an allotment, the rest of the land was declared "surplus" and given to white people to homestead. . . . What happened to my reservation happened to reservations all across the country.

"Real estate determines culture." When the property owners couldn't pay their taxes, the state confiscated their property. The vast majority of the White Earth lands were taken in this manner, along with about two-thirds of all reservation land in the United States, according to LaDuke. "Our struggle is to get our land back," she explains. "That's what we've been trying to do for a hundred years. By 1980, 93 percent of our reservation was still held by non-Indians." Today most of the Anishinaabeg live off the reservation. "We're refugees, not unlike other people in this society."

As most of the Anishinaabeg have been forced off their ancestral lands, the state has replaced them by designating those lands as hunting and fishing areas and timber lots. Forests are being clear-cut, and most of the deer and fish taken from the land are by people from off the reservation. "We are watching the destruction of our ecosystem and the theft of our resources," laments LaDuke. She refers to *minobimaatisi-iwin*, an Anishinaabeg word meaning the practice of living in harmony with natural law. "*Minobimaatisiiwin* is our cultural practice; it is what you strive toward as an individual as well as collectively as a society. We have tried to retain this way of living and this way of thinking in spite of all that has happened to us over the centuries."

To continue this practice, WELRP is seeking to reclaim its land one parcel at a time.

> We bought some land as a site for a roundhouse, a building that holds one of our ceremonial drums. We bought back our burial grounds, which were on private land, because we believe that we should hold the land our ancestors lived on. These are all small parcels of land. . . . It is a very slow process, but our strategy is based on this recovery of the land and also on the recovery of our cultural and economic practices. . . . Our work is about strengthening and restoring our traditional economy.[7]

Unfortunately the Anishinaabeg have had to contend with the breeding of "improved" cultivated varieties of "wild" rice and the development of an industry in California able to produce cheap paddy-raised "wild" rice that diminishes the price the Anishinaabeg can get for the real thing. (For more information on Anishinaabeg wild rice activism, see chapter 4.)

Continuing on the subject of native land struggles, LaDuke states, "It is absolutely crucial . . . that our struggle for territorial integrity and economic and political control of our lands not be regarded as a threat by this society." She emphasizes that there is plenty of land for us all, and that existing native claims amount to less than one-third of the U.S. landmass. For those of us more recently transplanted to this land and seeking to develop deeper connection to it, our actions must respect the lives and lands of the earlier inhabitants. How can we value native foods without supporting the land claims of native people? Ward Churchill exhorts nonnative progressives and activists, "The land rights of 'First Americans' should serve as a first priority for attainment of everyone seriously committed to accomplishing positive change in North America."[8]

The struggles of many different people for survival and decent lives are struggles for land. "In every period of known history and in nearly every society touched by forms of inequitable property, people have struggled for a more equitable distribution of land and shelter," writes Anders Corr.[9] In Brazil, where land and wealth are distributed even more inequitably than in the United States, the Landless Workers Movement (MST) has mobilized more than a million people over the past twenty years to create settlements on unused land owned by large agricultural holders and forced the government to make good on its long-time promises of land reform. MST has succeeded in obtaining legal ownership of twenty million acres for 350,000 families in three thousand settlements.[10] "In every settlement we visited," report Angus Wright and Wendy Wolford, North American authors of a book on the MST, "people were enjoying a level of comfort, security, nutrition, education, health care, and sense of community participation that is remarkable among the Brazilian rural poor."[11] When people have access to land, their opportunities to meet the rest of their needs are vastly increased.

Land reform as a political agenda has had many different expressions and has been motivated by different forces. The United States supported post–World War II land redistribution as part of occupation reconstruction in Japan and Germany—modeling it on the traditional American farming model, just then beginning to erode—and justified land expropriations with the theory that the rise of fascism was due in part to the concentration of land and political power in the wrong hands. Nevertheless, the United States has frequently supported the concentration of land and political power in the hands of large holders, most notably in Latin America, where large landowners in many cases have been U.S. citizens and corporations. For if one thing is worse than a fascist concentration of land, according to the capitalist mindset, it's a communist expropriation of private property and redistribution of land.

In 1945 more than half of Guatemala's farmland consisted of plantations larger than one thousand acres, yet less than a fourth of the acreage of these plantation holdings was under cultivation.[12] One U.S. corporation, United Fruit (now known as Chiquita), was the largest employer, landowner, and exporter in Guatemala, growing and exporting bananas, primarily to the United States. United Fruit prospered in Guatemala largely because it was able to secure the support of government officials there.

In 1950 Guatemalans elected a new president, Jacobo Arbenz Guzmán, who initiated a land reform policy of expropriating uncultivated portions of large plantations and redistributing the land in small plots. Around 1.5 million acres were taken and divided among one hundred thousand families.[13] Some of the expropriated land belonged to United Fruit, which undertook a propaganda campaign in the United States to promote the idea that this represented the spread of communism to the Western Hemisphere.

Newly elected President Dwight Eisenhower was a Cold War warrior eager to combat the perceived communist threat. In addition, various members of his administration had direct ties to United Fruit. The U.S. Central Intelligence Agency (CIA) hatched a secret plot, codenamed Operation Success, that overthrew Arbenz in 1954, aborting the political process there and throwing Guatemala into a state of repression and violent civil unrest that has persisted ever since.

Chile is another Latin American nation in which a U.S.-backed military coup followed attempts at land reform. On September 11, 1973, its popular socialist president Salvador Allende was murdered and a military dictator named Augusto Pinochet took power. Pinochet dismantled Allende's land reforms and shifted Chilean agricultural policy toward export markets and foreign investment. Thanks in large part to this intervention, Chilean grapes are plentiful on U.S. supermarket shelves in wintertime. Aren't we lucky!

In 2005 Venezuela granted more than three hundred thousand acres of land to indigenous groups, returning to them control of their ancestral lands. "What we're recognizing is the original ownership of these lands," said President Hugo Chavez. "Now no one will be able to come and trample over you in the future."[14] A coup was attempted against Chavez in 2002 but failed, and prominent American broadcast commentators have freely suggested that the U.S. government assassinate him, but so far he remains in power.

Like Venezuela, Chile, Guatemala, and Brazil, Mexico has had some government-sponsored land reform. Traditional communal indigenous land holdings were guaranteed in Mexico's 1917 constitution, which remains in force to this day; however, these land provisions, contained in

Article 27, were revised in 1992, to bring Mexico's land into the private ownership system in accordance with the terms of the North American Free Trade Agreement (NAFTA). This abandonment of indigenous land rights propelled the Zapatista movement, composed of mostly indigenous people in the state of Chiapas, to take up arms. "We and our families have been sold down the river, or you could say that they stole our pants and sold them," explained Zapatista spokesperson Sub-Comandante Marcos in an interview at the time. "What can we do? We did everything legal that we could do so far as elections and organizations were concerned, and to no avail."[15] On January 1, 1994, the day NAFTA went into effect, armed Zapatista rebels seized towns in eastern and central Chiapas, declaring their intention to claim sovereignty on behalf of Mexico's people and to overthrow the Mexican government.

The Mexican army responded militarily, but support for the Zapatistas—both within Mexico and abroad—was so strong that the president ordered a cease-fire on January 12 and created a Commission for Peace and Reconciliation to negotiate with the rebels. The agreement the commission finally reached in 1996, known as the San Andrés Accords, recognized the autonomous rights of indigenous *pueblos*. However, Mexican president Ernesto Zedillo rejected the agreement.

The Zapatista rebels continue, a decade later, to hold a portion of Chiapas, hemmed in by Mexican troops. They have established thirty-seven autonomous *municipios* that have provided people with land, education, health care, and other services and continue to demand autonomy for indigenous communities. The Zapatistas have inspired people around the world. The word *zapatismo* has become an expression to describe any bold assertion of indigenous rights. Zapatismo involves both a love of the land and respect for its people.

Farmers Resisting Real-Estate Pressures

The United States is losing farmland, especially small farms, at a staggering rate. In most of the United States, people of all ages can recall farms that were around in their youth but have since been developed as real estate. Every ten seconds another acre of U.S. farmland is taken out of food production, according to the USDA. That's more than six acres each minute, three-hundred-seventy-six acres each hour, nine thousand acres each day, and three million acres per year. In the five years from 1997 to 2002 more than sixteen million acres of farmland were lost. The same rate of loss has been sustained all the way back to 1974, for a total loss of seventy-nine million acres.[16] Some of this acreage is paved over for expanding cities and suburbs; some of it becomes vacation getaways and second homes; and some of it lies fallow, because no one considers the potential agricultural earnings worth the effort.

In the first half of the twentieth century there were more than six million farms in the United States.[17] Today only a third of them, or two million farms, remain. Half the remaining farms are tiny, part-time operations with annual sales below $5,000. Around 177,000 of them are over one thousand acres. The only group of farms that has consistently grown is farms over two thousand acres. The globalized food commodity system rewards economies of scale, and the U.S. program of agricultural subsidies reinforces this by providing cash incentives—corporate welfare—for large-scale, industrial-style production. The largest farms are receiving more subsidies than ever. The largest 2 percent of farms received nearly 30 percent of U.S. agricultural subsidies in 2002, while the largest 30 percent received more than 80 percent of total subsidies.[18] According to the *Des Moines Register*, "The countryside is being divvied up among Wal-Mart-like mega-farms, which profit most from federal farm payments, and thousands of farmettes, comprising niche, part-time or hobby farmers who almost always require off-farm income to stay afloat."[19]

Factory-style farming does great harm to the communities where it is practiced. Large-scale agriculture concentrates polluting chemicals, antibiotics, and manure and can rapidly transform thriving ecosystems into toxic wastelands. Factory farms are noxious neighbors, polluting groundwater, creating unbearable odors, and diminishing property values. And economies of scale, which ignore externalized costs such as these yet are reinforced by government subsidies, enable factory farms to undersell smaller-scale farms. Small farms can't compete; economic opportunities shrink; and communities disintegrate. All over the country we've watched small farms disappear, and with them agrarian lifestyles and culture.

As small farms become more marginalized, selling the land for nonagricultural uses can be very alluring. The sad fact of our profit-driven property system is that housing and retailing provide a greater return on a land investment than the modest earnings yielded by small-scale agricultural use. "We can all survive without another condominium, Taco Bell, or shopping center," observes farmer Michael Ableman, who documented the survival of his farm, Fairview Gardens, in Goleta, California, in the book *On Good Land: The Autobiography of an Urban Farm.* "Can we really survive without fertile soils, without fresh and unpoisoned food, without a place to teach our children about interconnections and context, or a place to gather on the land?"[20]

An aerial photo from 1954 shows Fairview Gardens as one of many farms in a rural landscape of cultivated fields. Today it stands alone in a densely developed suburb of Santa Barbara. When the last other neighboring farm was being sold to developers, Ableman went to testify against the proposed zoning changes.

> I fought the demise of that land, feeling feeble standing in the city council chambers with a few other locals facing off against the highly paid lawyers for the developers. The story is always the same. Land is a mere commodity to be bought and sold, something to build on, pave over, mine, or drill. We protested the sacrifice of the richest topsoil on the entire West Coast. We cited the agricultural history of this valley, our perfect Mediterranean growing climate, the loss of farmland everywhere, and the importance of small farms and local food for our children. Our voices were drowned out by housing statistics, traffic studies, and promises for parks and tennis courts, all supported by sophisticated maps and graphs.[21]

After the plan went through, the farmer who had sold his land was quoted in the newspaper as saying, "Farming is a dying profession," to which Ableman reacted: "I had to wonder where *his* food came from."[22]

Once Fairview Gardens was the only farm in the area, its farming activities were increasingly viewed as a nuisance. Ableman received complaints about his roosters crowing early in the morning and the stink of his compost. "We spent an inordinate amount of time

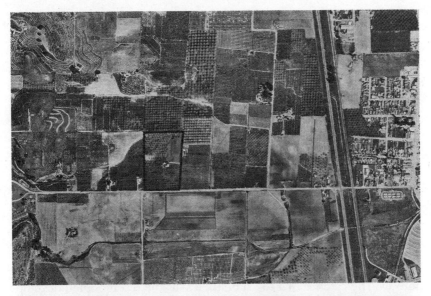

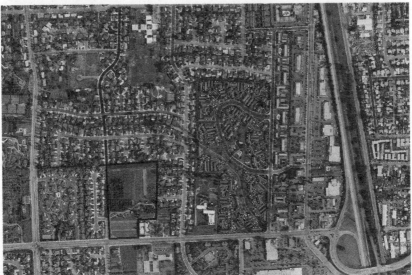

Fairview Gardens: 1954 and 1998. ©Michael Ableman. Used by permission.

defending our right to be," he recalls.[23] A few years later the owners of Ableman's farm (he rented it from them) decided to sell their land, no longer willing to sacrifice the potential income that their land could bring. Ableman didn't have the resources to buy the farm himself, but he and a group of devoted customers were able to organize a land trust and educational nonprofit, the Center for Urban Agriculture, which was able to raise enough money to purchase the farm. "If we could preserve this land in one of the most expensive real estate markets in the world, then our example could be used anywhere," he reflects.[24]

Land trusts can be organized at many different scales. The state of New Jersey—the "Garden State" despite the fact that it has lost most of its farmland to development over the past fifty years—formed the Garden State Preservation Trust in 1999 to help maintain agricultural land in the state. Financed by bonds and a portion of sales taxes, the trust has spent more than $500 million to protect 132,000 acres of farmland. The state accomplishes this by using a legal mechanism known as development easements. The state purchases the development easement for the farmland, thereby stripping the farmland of development potential and restricting its use to farming, theoretically forever. The catch is that the state then sells the disembodied development rights stripped from the farmland to developers to transfer them for use on other properties.

A related strategy for farmland preservation is the conservation easement, another legal agreement restricting use of the land "in perpetuity." An outside entity, such as a land trust, conservation organization, or government agency, monitors and enforces the limits spelled out in the easement. Easement terms are attached to the land, even if it is sold, and the owner of the restricted-use land is eligible for tax breaks. The American Farmland Trust is a clearinghouse for information related to farmland conservation strategies.

Another question related to farmland conservation is, who will run the farm after I'm gone? The average age of the remaining farmers in the United States was fifty-five as of 2002, and rising; fewer than 6 percent of "principal operators" of farms were under thirty-five.[25] In Iowa, the state with the greatest proportion of its land devoted to farms, half the state's farmland is owned by people over the age of sixty-five, and a quarter by people over the age of seventy-four.[26] To the extent that there remains an American farming legacy, who stands to receive it? Rural youth for the most part want out. They feel that their lives will be better off the farm. And who can blame them? The system of uniform globalized agricultural commodities has reduced most farmers to cogs in a machine—no longer independent creative entrepreneurs or

the stewards of diverse and productive farms, but rather monocultur-
alist debt-slaves to chemical and seed manufacturers and commodity
speculators.

Meanwhile, some young people—many from the cities and the suburbs—want to try their hand at farming. Many different organizations
link people interested in farm experience with farm opportunities. One
popular international network is World-wide Opportunities on Organic
Farms (WWOOF; known in many places as Willing Workers on
Organic Farms). Many varied farming associations help people find volunteer opportunities and apprenticeships on farms. For those with
experience who are looking for farms to run, programs have been
established in at least nineteen states to help link prospective farmers
with farmland. These groups match farmers seeking land with farmers
who have land, want it to remain in agricultural use, want to retire, and
have no heirs wishing to farm. There are plenty of folks in this situation!
State and regional organizations making these links have come together
as the National Farm Transition Network.

Of course, the best way to keep the next generation on the farm is to
make farming a viable way of earning a living. When the farm is prosperous, some of the next generation might stick around, reversing the
usual trend. At a recent Acres USA conference I met Daniel Salatin,
the twenty-something son of Virginia farmer and author Joel Salatin,
who runs many of the operations on the family's Polyface Farm, which
has become a model for the direct marketing of farm products. Daniel
is an enthusiastic and capable promoter of his family's farm. He is not
trapped in any dead end; he sees a bright future for the community-
supported farm he is set to inherit.

The explosion in community-supported agriculture (see page 11) has
enabled some small farmers to structure their farms in financially viable
ways. Many programs are trying to help small farmers find more profitable niches. In 2005 Woodbury County in Iowa became the first governmental entity in the United States to offer tax incentives to farmers
to transition to organic practices; then, in 2006, it adopted a policy of
purchasing foods for county services from local sources as much as possible. In the Southeast, several programs use tobacco settlement funds
paid to the states by cigarette manufacturers to help tobacco farmers
convert to organic crops. John Mullins, a Virginia farmer who made the

switch, reports earning $20,000 from an acre of organic grape tomatoes; his best acre of tobacco, he says, had netted only about $2,500. "Growing tobacco is like riding a dead horse," he has concluded.[27]

Other farms have sought to augment income with value-added products. These are foods such as preserves, pickles, cheeses, wines, breads, and cured meats (in many cases ferments), in which the raw agricultural product is transformed in some way that gives it greater value. I once spent an afternoon visiting L., a young Amish farmer in Pennsylvania. L. grew up dairy-farming the standard American way, selling the milk to the local dairy processor for a rate set by the government, eking out a small living. When his wife developed a health problem and was exploring ways to address it, she learned about the healing power of raw (unpasteurized) milk from grazing animals and its fermented products (see chapter 5).

As L.'s wife's health improved and she met others interested in obtaining the health benefits of real milk, their farm shifted. They went from grain-feeding to pasture-feeding; they reduced the size of their herd to what their limited pasture acreage could realistically accommodate; and they sold their milk directly to consumers, for a far better price than the mass processors ever paid. They also started making and selling raw cream, butter, sour cream, cottage cheese, yogurt, kefir, whey, and buttermilk, all value-added milk products. Selling raw milk is legal in their state, but selling other raw dairy products technically is not, though they have discovered that demand for them is great. Their farm has become prosperous enough that other Amish farmers are taking note and making similar changes, plugging into different forms of direct-marketing to health-conscious consumers.

Another strategy for increasing farm income is through farm tourism or farm education. Italy uses the designation *agriturismo* to denote farms that offer rooms for rent or meals, and many farms supplement their income by hosting tourists and feeding them home-grown food. I've heard that the Quillisascut Farm in Washington State has augmented its earnings through farm-based culinary education. The Quillisascut Farm School of the Domestic Arts offers week-long farm immersion programs in which students learn hands-on skills such as milking by hand, butchering a lamb, making cheese and sausage, canning, and vegetable gardening and have the experience of preparing meals using exclusively fresh, seasonal ingredients. There is a little bit of this happening in the United States, but there could be much more. Many people are hungry for the experience of a little time on a farm.

Fear and Loathing in Rural America

Before we get too nostalgic about reviving the disappearing agrarian culture of rural America, let's recall how entrenched and insular small-town culture can be, how inhospitable to outsiders, meaning both people from elsewhere and people who, by reason of race, religion, or other qualities, fail to conform to dominant local norms. This is an important issue for the movement for local food. "Praise of the local, the small, the self-contained can sound terrifying to people whose history includes being drummed out of small, local, and homogenous communities," notes food philosopher Lisa Heldke. "An expanded bioregionalist vision must include a deep, well-integrated commitment to ethnic diversity—and must regard this diversity not simply as a thing to be 'dealt with' but as a fundamental feature of the environment that is every bit as important to it as is the diversity of its plant life."[28]

Who owns farms, and who doesn't? Fully 97 percent of "farm operators" in the United States are white, according to the Census Bureau. Just 1 percent are African-American,[29] despite the fact that African-Americans comprise more than 12 percent of the U.S. population and until the past century mostly lived an agrarian rural life. "Real estate determines culture." And culture determines real estate, too. The initial promise of reparations to freed slaves after emancipation was "forty acres and a mule," a promise that was broken quickly, and no reparations have been offered since. "Landless people are but refugees in a strange land," says Gary Grant of the Black Farmers and Agriculturalists Association.[30]

A freed slave, Thomas Hall, recalled many years later when he was interviewed by the Federal Writers' Project that after emancipation "we still had to depend on the southern white man for work, food, and clothing, and he held us out of necessity and want in a state of servitude but little better than slavery."[31] Black farm laborers were often paid not in money but in "orders," which could be used only at a store controlled by the landowner. According to historian Howard Zinn, "The Negro farmer, to get the wherewithal to plant his crop, had to promise it to the store, and when everything was added up at the end of the year he was in debt, so his crop was constantly owed to someone.[32] Emancipation led to sharecropping and other forms of indentured servitude.

Across the South, the Ku Klux Klan rose as a powerful institution, using violence to enforce white supremacy. Lynching was a common form of terrorism and intimidation. From 1882, when the first attempt was begun to systematically tally newspaper reports of lynchings, through 1964, 3,445 lynchings of African-Americans were reported.[33] Given these circumstances, it's hardly surprising that the decades from the late nineteenth century through the mid-twentieth century saw a steady migration of African-Americans from the rural South to cities, North and South. From a 1920 peak of nearly a million African-American "farm operators," one in seven U.S. farmers,[34] the number of African-American farmers has steadily declined. By the latest count, in 1997, only eighteen thousand remained.

One important factor in the decline of African-American farmers has been lack of access to USDA credit and other programs that help small farmers buy land and equipment and survive lean years. These programs are administered by a system of "county committees," which are composed of local, generally white elites. Historically the USDA has mostly ignored complaints about racial discrimination by these committees and other USDA programs. In the 1980s the Reagan administration even closed the USDA's Office of Civil Rights. In 1996 the agency made a feeble attempt to address racial discrimination by reopening the Office of Civil Rights and forming a Civil Rights Action Team, which issued a report concluding that "minority farmers have lost significant amounts of land and potential farm income as a result of discrimination by [the USDA]"[35] and recommending actions to remedy the problem, few of which were ever implemented.

In 1997 a group of African-American farmers (and former farmers and their heirs) sued the USDA, alleging that they had lost their farms or farm income due to USDA discrimination. In 1999 the lawsuit was settled with a "consent decree," acknowledging a history of USDA discrimination. The agreement called for financial restitution to African-American farmers who had suffered discrimination, and their descendants, and created a process for settling claims.

Unfortunately, that process has become yet another denial of justice. The Environmental Working Group, which has monitored the settlement process, reports that "of the nearly one hundred thousand farmers who came forward with racial discrimination complaints, nine out of ten were denied any recovery from the settlement"[36] Government lawyers have strenuously fought the majority of the claims and have denied lawyers for the farmers access to documents that could substantiate claims of discrimination. "The lawsuit itself has turned out to be just as discriminatory as the past actions," says Thomas Burrell of the Black Farmers and Agriculturalists Association. "This is a double act of betrayal. The Black farmers got the barnyard version of jurisprudence."[37]

This case, and the history which gives rise to it, is a vivid illustration of the harsh realities of discrimination, and the continuing resistance to reconciliation. It's also a reminder of how closed rural communities can be—and closed-minded. It's not hard to imagine those good old boys on the county committee channeling those USDA resources to their own kind, wishing the others would disappear.

Rural communities can be inhospitable to people on many different counts. Where I live, membership in a church confers legitimacy. I am not a churchgoer, and being a Jew, I am far outside the mainstream here. I am not only a Jew but a queer Jew, living in a community of queer folks in this unlikely location. Before you conclude that a random Bible Belt rural area must import its queers, let me assure you that I have met many of the homegrown variety. In many and varied manifestations, we *are* everywhere.

A lot of the rhetoric around saving small farms and reviving agrarian culture revolves around the romantic ideal of the "family farm." This expression tends to suggest a heterosexual nuclear family—dad and mom, united in holy "one man and one woman" matrimony, and their willing-to-work offspring who will inherit the farm and carry on—as the ideal farm tenders. Queers have often been the first in the family to escape the farm, and the countryside, in search of other queers and queer culture in cities. The countryside can be isolating and lonely for people whose identities fall outside social norms. As a long-urbanized gay man who grew up on a farm said when I started to tell him about the place I live, "If I never see another tree it will be too soon."

It seems clear to me that any postmodern rural renaissance in the
United States needs to be expansive, embracing multiculturalism and
evolving identities. If we want to get real about community-based food
production, we have to encourage more folks to get involved in it—all
kinds of people—and embrace whomever chooses to follow that calling
and that path.

Urban Food Production and Cultural Change

As I walk the streets of the concrete jungle in my beloved hometown of
New York City, I ponder how people who live here can reclaim a sense
of connection to growing food. My father's garden was not here in the
city where he and my mother worked and we went to school, but rather
in "the country," an hour and a half from our apartment, where we
spent most weekends. Many affluent urbanites maintain two homes
and feel that their weekend getaways keep them grounded. I suspect
that many urban dwellers without the luxury of a country home may
imagine that participating in community food production is not a possibility for them, unless it is part of a fantasy of leaving the city one day.
In fact, there are many inspiring food production projects happening in
cities everywhere.

Wandering in Central Park, I notice along the fence lines burdock
and lamb's-quarters, two irrepressible weeds that make delicious and
extremely nutritious food, surviving in the margins between concrete
paths and mowed meadows. It is here in this park that I first harvested
burdock fifteen years ago. Though my developing interest in plants
back then led me out of the city and into the woods, these weeds are
potent symbols of the unstoppability of green power, of natural
processes, even in a densely populated, concrete-covered megalopolis.
The marginal spaces of cities are full of edible plants and offer tremendous possibilities for cultivation, especially if we can gain the support
and cooperation of authorities. Creating more gardens in cities makes
them more livable for everyone.

One question that often arises in relation to growing food in cities is
soil contamination. Heavy metals and other toxic pollutants in the soil
can contaminate vegetables. For this reason is important to test poten-

tial garden soil, especially on former building sites and in industrial areas. Activists in many places have been using techniques of an emerging field called bioremediation to improve the soil. Bioremediation employs certain plants, fungi, and bacteria to draw heavy metals and other toxins out of the soil and into their tissue or to digest them into harmless forms. Bioremediation activists have been applying these techniques in post-Katrina New Orleans, where chemical spills during the 2005 flood have contaminated soil in much of the city.

In some cities the scale of urban gardening is very impressive. A survey commissioned by the Canadian group City Farmer in 2002 found that 44 percent of people in Greater Vancouver and 40 percent of people in Greater Toronto live in households that grow some of their own food.[38] According to the Resource Centre on Urban Agriculture and Forestry,

> The scale of urban food production is generally underestimated. According to the most widely accepted estimate, [worldwide] about two hundred million urban dwellers now participate in urban farming, providing eight hundred million people with at least some of their food. Conservative estimates suggest that, in 1993, between 15 and 20 percent of the world's food was produced in urban areas. Although numbers are difficult to come by, it is further estimated that as much as 40 percent of the population in African cities and up to 50 percent in Latin America are involved in urban agriculture.[39]

Often spurred by circumstances of necessity, urban land and people can effectively produce food. This happened in the United States during the "victory garden" movements of World Wars I and II and the relief gardens of the Depression era, and it's been happening in Cuba's cities for the past fifteen years (see page 30). In Venezuela the government of President Hugo Chavez has set a target of supplying 20 percent of Venezuela's vegetable production from urban gardens.[40] According to a 2000 United Nations Food and Agriculture Organization report titled *Urban and Periurban[41] Agriculture (UPA) on the Policy Agenda,* "Numerous examples in recent years have shown the potential for UPA to ameliorate emergency food shortage situations: cities in Indonesia,

Kosovo, Russia and other war-torn and economic-crisis zones have turned to UPA."[42]

We are all inherently capable of growing food. We don't require the threat of starvation or dire emergency to motivate urban food production. Fresh food tastes better and is more nutritious; and the interaction with the land in the city is healing all around. We do not have to be dependent on a global corporate system that is neither stable nor sustainable. "I've got this land reclamation thing in my head," says Bernadette Cozart of the organization Greening of Harlem.

> When I look at Harlem, I see a community ready to burst forth. I see vacant lots as sources of jobs. I can see growing vegetables and herbs as going all the way from seed to shelf. . . . I envision watermelon rind jelly, tomato preserve, and "cha cha" with labels that say "grown and made in Harlem." . . . I can see making dyes and potpourris, raising herbs for healing and culinary uses. I can see a vineyard right here in Harlem. . . . Why not? . . . And grapes, fermented and bottled into Harlem Champagne.[43]

Urban dwellers everywhere are manifesting their gardening and food-production visions, usually just to create and share access to good fresh produce, but sometimes to generate income. If the market value of land is factored in, it's the rare urban farm that can generate enough income for land payments. But by partnering with nonprofit organizations, public agencies, generous benefactors, land trusts, or land outside the city, some urban farms have been able to generate income to fairly compensate the farmers.

One impressive example of urban farming is the Food Project in Boston, Massachusetts. With two gardens in the Roxbury neighborhood of Boston and a twenty-seven acre farm in the suburb of Lincoln, about fifteen miles away, the Food Project produces 130,000 pounds of vegetables each year. This produce is distributed widely. In addition to the produce for the one hundred CSA shareholders, food is sold at farmers' markets, served at large community meals, and delivered to "collaborators," including churches, organic shops, and chefs, as well as fifteen homeless shelters. The food is grown, marketed, and distributed primarily by teenagers, who are paid a weekly stipend.

Many of the most successful urban gardens are successful because they have plugged into existing neighborhood social networks and institutions. Schools usually have land they can devote to gardening or relationships they can use to find nearby land. School gardens not only produce food but also teach students useful skills and give them a connection to the earth that has become quite rare. "Once the seeds germinate, I've got the kids," reports Bernadette Cozart. "Kids here are so removed from nature they don't know that just about everything comes from nature—their clothes, their houses, their food."[44] Every school could have a garden.

When I visited Detroit I was amazed to see the extent of land being reclaimed by plants, and a scale of urban vegetable production beyond what I have witnessed anywhere else. I had the pleasure of visiting a visionary school-farm there, the Catherine Ferguson Academy, a public alternative high school for pregnant teens and young moms that has integrated farming into its curriculum. The small farm outside the school, taking up the rest of the city block, has milking goats and is also home to horses, sheep, angora rabbits, turkeys, chickens, ducks, and bees, as well as vegetable gardens and fruit trees. I was there in the summer, when school was out of session, but summer-camp kids, visitors, and young volunteers were plentiful and highly engaged. Some were trying to catch chickens to move them into a different grazing area, and it was very exciting to watch the drama and awe of kids interacting in the flesh with farm animals for the first time. Jesse, the farm manager at the school, reports that the young mothers and mothers-to-be learn important caretaking and nurturance skills by working with the animals.

Housing developments are another type of landed urban institution that can host gardens. In many cases housing is pitted against gardening, but the reality is that housing and quality of life are improved by the presence of gardens. When I visited Toledo, Ohio, Michael Szuberla of Toledo GROWs showed off thriving community garden plots at a public housing project. Organizations devoted to feeding hungry people are also potential partners for food-production projects. The Earth Works gardens I visited in Detroit, which were producing literally tons of vegetables, were cosponsored by a food bank and a soup kitchen.

Some urban park systems have dedicated space to edible fruit trees or community gardens. Nursing homes, drug rehabilitation centers, and other healing and care institutions sometimes incorporate gardens as part of their therapeutic programs. In a 1996 survey by the American Community Gardening Association, of 6,021 gardens reported, nearly 1,000 were public housing gardens, 500 were school gardens, 87 were "mental health or rehab gardens," and 85 were affiliated with senior centers.[45] Community activists can be catalysts for getting local institutions to initiate garden programs.

Activists can also be instrumental in making institutional change at a municipal level. In Tucson, Arizona, I visited with Brad Lancaster, an enthusiastic permaculture activist. *Permaculture* is a word coined by Australians Bill Mollison and David Holmgren, a fusion of *permanent* and *agriculture* (then later *permanent* and *culture*). Permaculture is a way of thinking about design for human needs in relation to natural forces such as sun, water, and wind. Of course, these considerations have always driven human settlement patterns, but such "common sense" grows more and more elusive as rectangular grids, property rights, and large-scale infrastructures dictate development patterns. "Permaculture gives us a vocabulary," says my permaculturalist friend Ashley Ironwood.

Tucson is a very dry place, and Brad is an explorer of water-harvesting strategies. In his densely planted yard, Brad has a washing machine that neighbors are invited to use. The graywater (dirty water not fit for drinking but not contaminated with fecal matter) from the washing of clothes is channeled through a series of earth and plant filters and then to native food trees. One action Brad has been actively promoting is the simple idea of harvesting rainwater by channeling storm runoff to trees. He has worked hard to convince the city "that runoff is an asset rather than a liability" and thus to make curb cuts to direct rainwater to trees.

"The majority of public land—our commons—in the urban setting is our public streets and adjoining right-of-ways," observes Brad.[46] So he has focused his efforts on street plantings. Desert Harvesters, a project Brad started, organizes neighborhood tree-planting events. The group distributes native food trees (paid for by a grant from a local utility) and shows people how to plant them in the earth in ways that enable the plants to capture the most water.

One of the main trees Desert Harvesters distributes is mesquite. Since traditional grinding of the edible mesquite seed is extremely time-consuming, the group purchased a small industrial grinding mill and mounted it on a mobile trailer. Each year at harvest time members of the group take the mill around the city to the neighborhoods where planting events have been held in years past and mill mesquite for people. "By planting, harvesting, and sharing the produce of the native ecosystem and backyard gardens these foods become sustainable parts of our daily experience, community and cultural identity, and food security," says Brad.

Another exciting frontier of urban food activism involves farm animals. Certain farm animals can live well and beneficially in certain cities, large and small, and the presence of these animals in the urban environment can help establish some degree of connection between people and the sources of their food. The legal scenarios vary widely, with local laws ranging from prohibition to regulation, and much gray area in between.

In some cities, raising chickens has always been part of the urban fabric. Mobile, Alabama, for instance, has always allowed chickens in the city, with a limit of twenty-five birds and, in the event that a neighbor complains, no roosters. "I believe it's time for urban chicken raisers everywhere to come out of the closet and let the rest of the world know what they've been missing all these years," wrote Bill Finch in the *Mobile Register*. "I have chickens not only because it is the destiny and ambition of every Finch to have a small home flock, just like Grandma did so many years ago in Mobile, but also because I've discovered that home-raised chickens are an indispensable part of my garden, and their exceptionally rich eggs are an invaluable addition to my diet."[47] Finch notes that in Alabama most of the older cities permit chickens, whereas many newly settled suburban communities forbid them.

In other cities people raising small flocks of chickens have persuaded city officials to sanction the practice. Mad City Chickens, the "poultry underground" of Madison, Wisconsin, got the laws there changed in 2004 to allow up to four hens (no roosters) in a coop, no closer than twenty-five feet to the nearest neighbor's living quarters. Seattle passed a chicken law in 1982 permitting up to three hens per household. In both cities activist educators offer classes to help aspiring city farmers get started, and the organization Seattle Tilth organizes an annual tour of chicken coops, inspiring both whimsical and functional innovations.

Another farm animal enjoying growing popularity in U.S. cities is the honeybee. Bees can easily blend into the cityscape as they forage for flower nectars, and by pollinating flowers, they increase plant fertility and greenery. Honeybees exhibit an elaborate social organization and are quite magical to observe. And the honey they produce from the flower nectars is, of course, a nectar in its own right. Our Short Mountain beekeeping queen Hush organizes an annual honey extraction evening, coordinating about a dozen of us worker bees in the exciting task of harvesting this incredible nectar. Beekeeping can be done anywhere, and I've met folks in many cities, large and small, tending hives of bees.

Michael Thompson has been keeping honeybees in Chicago for decades. He tends hives on the roof of City Hall, teaches beekeeping classes, and, along with other beekeeper friends, started the Chicago Honey Cooperative in 2003. The co-op has seventy hives on a former Sears parking lot on the west side of town, which the owner is renting to them (until a more lucrative offer comes along) for one dollar per month. They also collaborate with a local social services agency on a job-training program for formerly incarcerated people. With the trainees, the co-op tends the hives, sells honey at two farmers' markets, and runs a community garden. In 2005 co-op members extracted two thousand pounds of honey, and their plan, as more trainees join the coop, is to quadruple in scale to three hundred hives.

Michael sees cities as perfect environments for bees. In the case of Chicago, he explains that its lakeside location gives it a succession of blooms especially well suited for them, offering a huge quantity of nectar. Beekeeping is not prohibited in Chicago, unless someone complains to the building department. Other animals are permitted too, depending on numbers, space, and neighbors. Michael knows of people raising chickens, goats, sheep, llamas, and tilapia (fish, kept in ponds) within the city limits.

Even on the roofs of Manhattan skyscrapers, people are keeping beehives. David Graves, a beekeeper from Massachusetts who sells his honey at New York City farmers' markets, displayed a hive at his stand in 1996 with a sign reading: "We need a home. We are very gentle. We like to share our New York City honey. Do you have a rooftop?" Invitations came rolling in, and Graves helped set up more than a dozen rooftop hives. New York City has no law specifically prohibiting or regulating beekeeping, but the health code does prohibit keeping animals that are "wild, ferocious, fierce, dangerous, or naturally inclined to do harm," which officials interpret as banning bees. However, enforcement of the ban is impractical: the bees' foraging is decentralized, their hives are hidden on rooftops, and their presence is virtually invisible.

For urban dwellers, producing any type food is a departure from the norm, creating powerful connections with the biological sources of food. There is no shortage of creative ideas for encouraging food production in and around cities. It's making those ideas happen that is the hard work. The image of bees as invisible but indispensable pollinators has inspired many activists in their work, plugging away at small projects, no one of which will change the world, but which collectively create fertility, and the fruits of today's activism are—we hope—the seeds of a better tomorrow. "We're city folk, not experts at feeding each other or solving these insidious problems," writes urban garden-activist Andrea del Moral. "But this is exactly the point."

> This is where we all start: willing to be beginners. Taking a chance, we can shape our own circumstance. So that when spring comes around, there's a piece of earth nearby where we can come together with other people, dig our hands in, and begin to plant another seed. Knowing that we are the only ones who can make the worlds we desire—and that we have the power to make seeds grow.[48]

Guerilla Gardeners Reclaiming Abandoned Lots

Many community gardens have been started by people who were not afraid to go onto abandoned property that they did not own and start cleaning and cultivating it. They are squatters, making use of unoccupied property—but property nonetheless. They are willing to break the letter of the law for the greater good of green space and community well-being, and potentially even food production. "Look around you," writes Cleo Woelfle-Erskine, who traveled around the United States visiting and documenting community gardens and self-published an inspirational book titled *Urban Wilds: Gardeners' Stories of the Struggles for Land and Justice.* "Land is everywhere. If not horizontal, it's vertical. Your imagination is the limit: railway embankments, back gardens, golf courses, roofs, car parks, overgrown bits, cracks in the pavement. . . ."[49]

For those cracks in the pavement, Cleo offers guerilla gardeners this simple "recipe for rhubarb crumble":

1. Take rhubarb seed and stuff it in cracks in concrete
2. Sit back and watch the crumble take shape![50]

One of the early (1973) groups of community gardeners on the Lower East Side in New York City called themselves the Green Guerillas. "Armed with bolt-cutters and pickaxes, they conceived of themselves as a strike force to liberate the crumbling landscape around them," writes Sarah Ferguson in her "Brief History of Grassroots Greening on the Lower East Side."[51] They also assembled "seed green-aids"—balloons stuffed with earth and wildflower seeds—and tossed them into vacant lots and onto street medians. Another variation on this concept is "seed balls," developed by Japanese farmer-philosopher Masanobu Fukuoka. Seed balls are simply a variety of seeds mixed with clay and compost and formed into balls, which can be dropped anywhere in need of greenery.

Guerilla gardening is not an activity confined to the United States and other affluent lands. Like squatting, it's happening, by necessity, in most of the sprawling cities of the "developing" world. In Zimbabwe's capital city of Harare, where food has been scarce and expensive, growing numbers of city residents are growing food anywhere they can, both to feed themselves and as a source of income. "They use any piece of land they can find," observes one South African media report.[52] "Farming in cemeteries has been a lifeline for many Harare residents struggling to cope with the ongoing economic crisis and spiraling prices," according to another.[53]

The crazy thing about this Harare example of guerilla gardening is that the Zimbabwean government is actually dealing with gardeners as guerillas. Zimbabwe President Robert Mugabe is implementing a policy he calls Operation Murambatsvina, which translates to "Drive Out Trash." The operation involves destroying makeshift shelters, street-vending kiosks, and garden plots. There have been thirty thousand arrests, mostly of "street vendors the government accuses of sabotaging the failing economy by selling black market goods."[54] Subsistence gardeners, microentrepreneurs, and squatters are jailed for sabotage.

In the vastly different context of North America, I have met many different people engaged in small acts of horticultural subversion who refer to what they do as guerilla gardening. Nance Klehm, the Chicago seed saver I wrote about in chapter 2, describes herself as a guerilla gardener because she likes to plant her seeds in public spaces and construction sites. In this way she spreads her seeds, grows food and flowers on more land, and brings life and greenery to her urban landscape. She describes guerilla gardening as an "open-ended gesture."

Cailen Campbell, the cider maker whose story I told in chapter 1, was a guerilla gardener in the city of Asheville, North Carolina, until he had a run-in with the law. The small urban homestead he shared with several friends—as well as goats, chickens, ducks, and bees—was planted to capacity, so he expanded into a series of what he called "satellite gardens," some in neighbors' yards with their permission, others in vacant lots with absentee owners. When I visited, I walked with him, his housemate Zev, and their two goats through wooded trails to a dense grove of bamboo on a neglected lot. Cailen and Zev harvested bamboo for a building project while the goats did their own guerilla foraging. Every day Cailen took the goats out for a walk to a different overgrown lot. Lack of land was not an impediment to his farming aspirations.

What was an impediment was the law. Through a friend from Asheville I heard that Cailen had been forced by the city to get rid of his goats. I e-mailed him to inquire, and this was his story:

> The truth of the gossip is that the city did indeed come down on our little urban livestock scene. Someone actually called in a formal complaint upon witnessing one of my urban guerilla goat-herding forays across a busy street. The city officials were obliged to respond, and as it was the second visit to our

homestead, they "threw the book at us." The ordinance states that (among other things) all animal enclosures must be at least 100 feet from the nearest household (the actual home, not property line), except for bees, which must be 150 feet away. After actually measuring, it was determined that there was really no way to make it fit. . . . You would have to have at least a 1-acre lot to make it work for even a couple animals in cramped confinement.

So Cailen moved with his animals to Earthaven Ecovillage in the Blue Ridge mountains, forty-five minutes from Asheville:

> [I'm] starting a new life for me and my goats with lots of room and support to realize all of my wildest agricultural dreams and aspirations (I had long since outgrown the limitations of the ever-shrinking urban agricultural potential). . . . So, I didn't get rid of my goats. We are still together, with room for the herd to grow. I'm planning some interesting crossbreeding experiments as I endeavor to come up with my own bioregional dairy goat breed, as well as working my way into the wild wonderful world of draft animals, training our soon-to-be-ox Dexter calf, and looking for some young donkeys to purchase.

It sounds like getting busted for his guerilla goat-foraging forays is spurring Cailen on to bigger visions. Guerilla food production is not necessarily a goal in itself; rather it is a strategy to create and hold space in order to nurture more sustainable arrangements.

Many long-established community gardens began as guerilla gardens on abandoned land. In the 1960s, as their neighborhood was crumbling, some South Bronx homeowners started reclaiming vacant lots for gardens. "I struggled hard for my house, and I wasn't going to leave that easy," recalls Cordelia Gilford. "I love this area. If I left, I'd be abandoning the area the same way as the landlords and the city government. This is where our community was." So in 1967 Gilford and some of her neighbors started a garden in an abandoned lot. "We just got out there and did what we had to do. It was city land, but they didn't seem to care what happened to it, and we did. So we took it over."[55]

Forty years later many of the gardens scattered around the South Bronx are clearly beloved sacred sites, centers of vibrant community activity and evidence that people—at least some people—connect passionately with the land here. Yet in the South Bronx, as is the case elsewhere, small community gardens like these are pitted against housing demands. Some long-established gardens have been cleared to develop as housing or auctioned off to private interests. The broad desire for adequate and affordable housing is assumed to be more urgent than the need for green open space.

In this neighborhood there remain many vacant lots and abandoned buildings. There would be plenty of room to create new housing without displacing gardens if gardens were valued more highly by city planners and officials. But developers like large, continuous areas to work with, and housing is a more tangible good than gardens and is more likely to bring financial gain to the owners of the properties (in most cases the city, the supposed guardian of the public interest). Housing and gardens are both legitimate needs. However, they are not intrinsically in conflict but rather historically have been integrated. Our cities would be healthier places if we could weave more gardens back into the fabric of urban living.

One sweltering summer day while I was visiting New York, I found spontaneous refuge from the sea of concrete radiating heat in the lush oasis of cool green of the Sixth and B Garden on the Lower East Side. I sat in the shade and inhaled sweet floral scents, then I grazed lamb's-quarters in an overgrown garden bed. I noticed a schedule of free activities: yoga and qi gong classes, jazz saxophone, classical Indian ragas, poetry, a flamenco performance for kids, interactive storytelling, movies, even bingo. Even tiny green spaces in cities can be enormous community assets.

Instead, gardens are regarded as an inefficient use of land once more lucrative opportunities develop. Often, even after decades of gardeners investing themselves in the land to improve their lives and their neighborhoods, the land is taken away. On the Lower East Side of Manhattan, there used to be an extraordinary garden called the Garden of Eden, which was so unusual that it was featured in the pages of *National Geographic*. The Garden of Eden was a beloved neighborhood landmark until it was demolished by the city in 1986 to make room for housing. I visited the Garden of Eden once, shortly before it was demolished, before I was specifically interested in gardening and food production. I was just an adventurer, and this place was a kooky adventure. My friends and I climbed six flights of stairs to the roof of the building next door, which was squatted by the possessed artist who had created the garden, an old hippy named Adam Purple. Looking down from above, the garden revealed itself as a yin-yang design. "The demolition of Eden became symbolic of the city's maddening refusal to incorporate community-held green space into its designs," writes Sarah Ferguson.[56] As usual, housing and gardens were pitted against one another as competing uses, a classic divide-and-conquer tactic.

In the 1990s Mayor Rudolph Giuliani implemented a wholesale transfer of hundreds of city-owned lots with gardens on them to the city's Department of Housing Preservation and Development (HPD), which arranged to put 112 of them up for auction at once in the spring of 1999. When asked why the city was auctioning the gardens, the mayor responded, "This is a free-market economy; welcome to the era after communism."[57] The idea that the city would encourage permanent community-based gardening on its unused land was regarded as absurd and contrary to the laws of the market. Privatization of all resources is the "free-market" creed. "We are trying to privatize as many city-owned properties as we can," confirmed an HPD official.[58]

Rather than gardens being threatened individually, as they had been for more than a decade, suddenly the whole community-gardening movement was under massive systematic attack. Community gardeners and their supporters responded to this threat with action. "Now, gardeners know every gardener is under threat," observed Haja Worley, a Harlem gardener who helped start two gardens. "We can respond at one time, rather than being picked off one by one."[59]

The More Gardens! Coalition was founded during this period when New York City gardens were being auctioned; one of its pamphlets stated, "What Giuliani and his real estate supporters haven't bargained for is the strong fight we'll put up to save our green havens."[60] In addition to the usual petitions, appeals to local officials, and lawsuits, the coalition organized rallies and direct action. After the first of several civil disobedience actions over the gardens, the *New York Times* reported vivid contrasts: "Thirty people were arrested in an odd encounter between protesters carrying kazoos and police officers wearing riot gear."[61]

Protests escalated as the auction date approached. There were many small actions, such as a lone man dressed like a sunflower high up in a ginkgo tree in City Hall Park, screaming, "The gardens must be saved!" and a group that locked down with Kryptonite bicycle locks in a city office. There were also rallies of hundreds of people and a protest in which sixty-two people were arrested in the streets. The director of Operation Green Thumb, the city agency that administered temporary leases to the gardens, quit her job after fourteen years, joined the protests, and got arrested. The New York State Attorney General sued the city to block the auction, saying the city had skipped state-required environmental review processes.

All this pressure forced the city to reconsider its position. "Faced with three lawsuits and the kind of bad publicity that comes when pro-testers are willing to risk arrest for the sake of lilacs and tomato plants, the Giuliani administration is trying to strike a settlement," reported the *New York Times* the day before the scheduled auction.[62] In an eleventh-hour deal, singer Bette Midler and her privately funded land trust supplemented an earlier offer by the Trust for Public Land to pur-chase all 112 gardens, and the gardens were saved. Thank you, Bette, for saving all those gardens! But what we really need is for public authorities to respect and support community gardening.

As this book went to press, one of the largest urban community gar-dens in the United States, South Central Community Farm in Los Angeles, was evicted and bulldozed. South Central's fourteen acres contained the garden plots of 350 families with incomes below the USDA poverty standard. Most were immigrants from Mexico or Central America. "These aren't tiny weekend projects with a few toma-toes and California poppies," wrote Dean Kuipers in the *LA City Beat*. The plots were "crammed with a tropical density of native Mesoamerican plants" that the gardeners used to feed their families. "These are survival gardens."[63]

South Central Community Farm came to be, like most community gardens, because the land it sits upon was otherwise unused. The vacant land had been owned by private investors when the city of Los Angeles seized it through eminent domain (for $4.7 million) in the 1980s to build

Third-Space Farmers

Imagine a space where families gather every day to work on the community farm. Imagine they have made this special place into a sustainable source of local food. They have created an edible landscape: a green mosaic with an endless variety of food crops, medicinal plants, fruit trees, creepers, crawlers, and cacti. Imagine the people plant seeds that are family heirlooms and have been saved over countless generations. Imagine the seeds contain genetic information that is at least five thousand years old from the native ancestral crops of the Americas. Imagine a space where indigenous women cultivate heirloom crops and weave visions and memories of their cultural identity and heritage into the landscape. They are making place; they are making home. Imagine the passing of this knowledge to the next generation in memories of the plant stories and the social and ecological skills of the farmer. Imagine the youth eagerly pursuing the cultivation of crops like maize, beans, calabaza, guayaba, chipilin, and chilacayote. Imagine they know the wild and cultivated varieties, their nutritional and medicinal properties, and what it takes to grow them naturally.

Now, imagine this space is located not in a rural area of Mexico but at the center of one of world's largest and most important global cities: Los Angeles, California. Imagine then, nothing less than the amazing fourteen-acre urban farm known as the South Central Community Garden, at 41st and Alameda in Los Angeles. South Central is the largest urban farm in California and one of the biggest in the United States. For thirteen years, the community has relied on this precious and rare space to grow food while becoming self-reliant and building a sense of community. South Central Farmers Feeding Families is a grassroots organization of 350 families who manage this mosaic landscape of native row crops, fruit-bearing trees and vines, and medicinal herbs in a democratic fashion. . . .

I have observed youth and the elderly tending and harvesting crops at South Central. I am always struck by the way these relationships represent the shared social life of the garden. Perhaps the most important crop cultivated here is conviviality. These loving acts transmit knowledge of plants and farming but also build an ethic of self-reliance. The farmers grow

By Devon G. Peña, PhD

food and social capital: the inter-generational cooperation farming provides gives youth meaningful alternatives to gangs and drugs.

Now imagine another space: a fourteen-acre block of hulking gray warehouses and bare concrete parking lots. Imagine why the City of Los Angeles would choose to evict the 350 farming families at South Central to make room for another block of lifeless urban redundancy. . . . This space has a long contested history. It was the site of a key episode in the decades-long struggle against environmental racism in LA. In the 1980s the Concerned Citizens of South Central, led by Juanita Tate, successfully resisted efforts by the City to use the site for trash incinerators. The activists instead created an alternative "third" space compatible with the needs of the community.

LA needs a dozen more urban farms like South Central. It does not need to destroy a singular natural and cultural treasure to replace it with more of the same: an impoverished, homogenous landscape, a result of enclosure by privatization. The third space of human and natural capital created at South Central over the past thirteen years must be valued as a model of grassroots new urbanism.

Inner cities across North America are being re-invented from the grassroots in creative and hopeful ways. There is a sustainable Latina/o urban ecology and the South Central farmers embody this heritage of environmental self-governance. The process of re-visioning a sustainable and just city must not be diminished by the encroachment of the heartless soul that is the post-industrial urban landscape of neoliberalism. Imagine LA as a city without people, without culture, without ecology. Imagine the empty warehouses and blank parking lots; the buried Zanja Madre and the paved-over containment of wild rivers and creeks. Imagine a light post in place of a sacred tree, South Central's fallen Pochote. Imagine the silence—a space devoid of laughter and the chatter of children and their grandmothers tending fields of ancient heirloom corn.

Excerpted from "Third-Space Farmers," *Visions Magazine*, November 2005. Used by permission. Dr. Peña is a professor of anthropology at the University of Washington in Seattle. Find out more about the South Central Farmers fight to save the garden at www.southcentralfarmers.com.

a trash incinerator. Residents opposed placing a smelly, polluting incinerator in their neighborhood and successfully organized to defeat it; the city eventually abandoned the plan. The lot sat there unused and strewn with trash for years. After the Rodney King rebellion of 1992, as a gesture of goodwill, the city designated the site as a community garden.

Meanwhile, the city, with state and federal support, was investing heavily in a plan to develop the Alameda Corridor, where the garden is located, into a warehousing and distribution hub to facilitate the movement of goods arriving and departing by ship from the ports of LA and Long Beach. As the neighborhood around it was developed, the South Central site became potentially lucrative. The original owners decided they wanted to develop the site as a warehouse, and through backroom political deals the city sold it back to them in 2003 with no consideration for the hundreds of gardeners who had invested themselves there for more than a decade. "The facilitation of global trade, then, receives the unquestioned backing of city, state, and federal authorities," observes farmer and writer Tom Philpott. "Urban farming, with its myriad environmental and social benefits, gets different treatment."[64]

The South Central farmers fought the deal in court but lost. In March 2006 they received a final eviction notice, but for three months they defied the order and refused to leave the land. The farmers took turns guarding the farm—asserting that their right to grow food for their families is as important as the rights of land speculators and global traders—and were joined by an encampment of supporters. They only left after hundreds of police officers in riot gear surrounded the farm on June 13 and arrested more than forty farmers and protestors (including actress Darryl Hannah).

The destruction of South Central epitomizes the struggle between land as a source of sustenance for the people working it, and land as property controlled by the highest bidder. The South Central farmers continue to struggle for their land. "We're Taking Back the Farm!," they declared as this book was in production in June, 2006. "Come to the Farm and stand in solidarity with us as we continue with the 24 hour vigil to take back the Farm," they invite supporters. "Small bulldozers have already torn through plots but it is far from lost." The farmers continue to fight, in court and on the streets. "This is not the end," they promise.[65]

Landless Farm Workers Challenging Exploitation

Access to land is a distant dream for many people struggling to survive in a harsh world. A job is often a more immediate and pressing need. Many people are desperate enough for work that they will migrate thousands of miles in search of jobs, often risking their lives to cross borders illegally. Hardly anybody who lives here in the United States is willing to do the repetitive grunt work of agricultural labor, so we rely on migrants, mostly from Mexico and Central America, to do it for shockingly low wages.

Working conditions in the chemical-laden fields of factory farms can be quite dangerous. In May 2005 twenty-three women working in a California vineyard had to be rushed to the hospital after chemicals being sprayed on a neighboring field drifted in their direction and engulfed them. First they smelled something odd, then they started feeling dizzy and nauseous. They tried to run away. Four of them fell into convulsions.

Gruesome scenes like this are everyday occurrences. The World Health Organization reports that three million cases of pesticide poisoning occur every year, resulting in more than 250,000 deaths.[66] In 2004 thousands of Costa Rican banana pickers filed a class action lawsuit in Los Angeles against two chemical corporations (Dow and Royal Dutch/Shell) and three fruit corporations (Chiquita, Del Monte, and Dole) over exposure to a toxic pesticide, dibromochloropropane, which was banned in the United States in 1979 but is still in use in Costa Rica. The chemical is suspected of causing sterility, testicular atrophy, miscarriages, birth defects, liver damage, and cancer when inhaled or absorbed by the skin.

In many places farm workers are organizing to demand safer working conditions and living wages. Two campaigns in the southeastern United States have recently experienced notable successes. A five-year national boycott of Mount Olive Pickles, a North Carolina company, ended in 2004 when the Farm Labor Organizing Committee reached an agreement for better wages and working conditions with the company.

Union president Baldemar Velasquez credited the boycott for their victory. "There was so much scrutiny, attention, shedding light on the abuses in agriculture," he said. "Eventually they had to do something to make it go away."[67] Corroborating this point, Mount Olive's president quipped, "I am one pickle packer who is glad to be out of a pickle."[68] The agreement, signed not only by Mount Olive but also by the North Carolina Growers' Association, covers as many as eight thousand farm workers at more than one thousand North Carolina farms growing cucumbers as well as tobacco and a variety of other agricultural products.

Another recent farm labor victory was a 2005 agreement between the Coalition of Immokalee Workers (CIW), representing Florida tomato pickers, and Yum Brands, the world's largest restaurant corporation, following that union's four-year boycott campaign against Taco Bell, one of Yum Brands' chains. Yum Brands exemplifies the concentration of the produce-buying market that is occurring at present. Fast-food and supermarket chains dictate terms to growers, demanding low prices that are guaranteed by contracts signed prior to planting. As a result, in 2005 tomato pickers were being paid less to work longer hours than they had twenty-five years earlier. Pickers were being paid as little as $50 for picking two tons of tomatoes in a twelve-hour day.

The Taco Bell boycott spread through campaigns at universities and churches and through the involvement of high-profile figures such as Jimmy Carter and Martin Sheen. The agreement, which effectively raises pickers' wages by 75 *percent*, calls for Taco Bell to pay an additional *penny* per pound of tomatoes.[69] What a difference a single penny can make! CIW claimed a precedent-setting victory: "This agreement represents the first time—ever—that a fast-food leader has agreed to address directly the sub-poverty wages paid to farm workers in its supply chain," announced the union. "With this agreement, farm workers from one of the country's poorest towns took on a corporate giant larger than McDonald's and won."[70]

A boycott is a consumer action against a practice you oppose. Another tactic being successfully employed in the realm of consumer action is the opposite of a boycott: rather than *not* buying a product because you disagree with some aspect of the methods used to produce it, you *do* buy a product because you approve of the methods used to produce it. Fair-trade merchants give consumers a positively defined product to buy, typically coffee or chocolate or other tropical treats,

produced and procured in accordance with benevolent fair-trade practices, which include paying living wages to growers and using ecologically sustainable growing methods.

Fair trade is definitely better than unfair trade. For the lucky
farmers who are able to market their coffee or cacao at fair-trade prices,
no doubt this is an important movement. However, in general there is
nothing either fair or free about the global system of commodity
exchange. It is a profitable game for the traders, generally at the
expense of the growers and workers. Though fair-trade projects create
on a limited scale a more benevolent model of trade, they do not really
alter or challenge a global trading system that favors big players and dis-
empowers small growers and farm workers. People anywhere could
survive better by growing food for themselves to eat first, and export
crops second, or not at all, rather than putting all their eggs in one
basket by growing a single crop for export.

Coffee provides a clear example: Coffee prices have been in a downward spiral in recent years due to global overproduction. Global traders
encourage overproduction, because it drives down their prices.
Between 1999 and 2002 alone, the price of coffee fell by half "in a race
to the bottom that has trampled many of the world's twenty-five million
small coffee farmers, throwing millions out of work and off their land,"
reports *Smithsonian*.[71] Global market forces far beyond the farmers'
control have "condemned the growers to poverty, exile, death, or
charity," writes Mexican journalist Luis Hernandez Navarro.
"Meanwhile transnational traders . . . accumulate huge fortunes."[72]

Our regular consumption of luxury imports—"fair trade" or not—
encourages dependency on global trade rather than food security and
food sovereignty in the places from which our tropical treats come. "If
the people of a country must depend for their next meal on the vagaries
of the global economy, on the goodwill of a superpower not to use food
as a weapon, or on the unpredictability and high cost of long-distance
shipping, that country is not secure in the sense of either national security or food security," writes Peter Rosset of Food First.[73]

Farmers' dependency on global markets for survival is intrinsically
not fair. Although the growth of the fair-trade consumer movement is a
positive step, we must acknowledge that "fair trade" is an upscale marketing niche, not unlike "organic." Folgers and Starbucks now offer

fair-trade coffees, and a campaign is under way to encourage Mars, the world's largest chocolate maker, to buy fair-trade cacao. For these corporations, fair trade is a public relations maneuver—not an ethical stance. My fear about fair trade is that—for coffee drinkers and chocolate lovers as a whole—it may simply pacify us and make us feel better about ourselves, while continuing to perpetuate the grotesque inequities of power that the affluent North American consumer has in relation to the tropical farm worker.

If the toil of human hands could be removed altogether from agricultural production, imagine how much better everyone could feel about gratifying their desires completely free of worker exploitation! The *Los Angeles Times* described a fruit-picking robot under development, with funding from the federal government:

> Part robot, part tractor, the contraption is an unusual combination of one internal-combustion engine, four rubber tires, eight digital cameras, eight electronic arms and an excruciating number of computer algorithms that choreograph every movement. Its metal arms maneuver among the branches, where "eyes" spot the fruit and suction-cup "hands" grasp them even more gently than human hands, which is what they are designed to replace. In fact, just one human finger is involved in this entire enterprise, for the thing also needs no driver. The robot sets its own course and speed, relying on a human only to push the on/off button on a remote control. . . . Many believe machines offer a better, cheaper, and possibly more humane way to harvest.[74]

. . . thus creating even more people without any way to earn money and severing humans even further from the earth, which provides us with its bounty.

Recipe: Eat Some Dirt

Try it. Choose a place that seems clean, away from chemical waste, lead paint, traffic, and fresh excrement. In a garden perhaps, or a forest.

Taste a little dirt. On its own, or what you find clinging to a fresh carrot or radish or burdock root. It may be gritty, so protect your teeth and don't bite down on it too hard. Savor the flavor. The earth is good for you. Pregnant and lactating women in many places routinely eat dirt to obtain minerals, a practice known as *geophagy*. And probiotic formulations marketed as soil-based organisms (SBO) are some of the most expensive nutritional supplements on the market. Don't buy a capsule; taste the earth to get your SBOs. This is another important aspect of eating locally: eating the local soil organisms further integrates us into the web of life of our environment and adapts us to the local microbial ecology. Be here now. Learn to love the flavor of the earth.

Recipe: Herbal Elixir Mead

Land struggles are not simply over ownership. They are about claiming a connection to the land. And one way to claim that connection is through plants. People use plants for their culinary, medicinal, nutritional, energetic, tonifying, mind-altering, and fibrous qualities. Virtually all plants have traditions of usage by the people (as well as other creatures) who interact with them. That people use plants seems to be a universal element of human culture (at least in subarctic zones) and how we live on the land. For me, an important aspect of connecting with the land, the particular land in the particular place where I find myself, is through the plants that are there. Getting to know the plants that thrive where you exist is a way of becoming more connected to that place. Using those plants as medicine and food and fiber connects you through both matter and spirit to the land. Using local honey similarly connects you to the land, through the magical nectar-collecting and pollinating activity of honeybees.

Herbal elixir meads (these words were joined together by my friend Frank Cook, who is a plant explorer and teacher) take plants, with all their flavors, nutrients, and medicine, and ferment them with honey to enhance and preserve their botanical potency. Fermented honey, or mead, is generally regarded as the original form of alcohol. Adding herbs to the mix is nothing new; practitioners in many herbal healing traditions incorporate herbs into fermented brews. In fact, a great variety of herbs

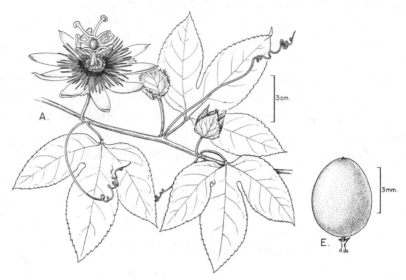

Passionflower. ©Bobbi Angell. Used by permission.

have been incorporated into not only meads but beers and wines as well. Through reclaiming mead as a medium for ritual, magic, and healing, we can reconnect to plant spirits and plant medicine, and also to the land, which produces all these elements and invites us to weave them together. An elixir mead can cast a spell upon the people gathered to enjoy it, as our friends are woven in with these other elements, as well as being woven together in community, fellowship, and solidarity.

When we walk the land, observe the land, and get to know the land, the plant spirits begin to reveal themselves to us. My herbal elixir meads are typically inspired by the abundant presence of some plant friend. For example, as I contemplated writing this section of the book, I kept stumbling upon wild passionflower vines around our land. I placed a small wire cage over one vine, to give it something to climb. Passionflowers are extraordinarily beautiful: with their delicate, curvy, undulating forms, they look like they're in a perpetual state of vibration. They got the name passionflower because a Jesuit missionary, inspired by this unique and gorgeous flower, sent one from Peru to the Pope in 1605, with a letter suggesting that it represented the passion of Christ.[75] Medicinally passionflower is used to calm and sedate. It should be avoided during pregnancy, however.

One day I collected more than a dozen flowers and started a passion-flower elixir. Flowers and fruits are typically host to wild yeasts, so I prepared it as a wild fermentation. Here's how:

The proportion of honey to water depends upon whether you intend to ferment the elixir fully, which takes a year or more, or enjoy it as a short term (one week to one month) ferment. For a long-term ferment, mix one part honey with four parts water. For a shorter-term ferment use less honey, about one part honey to seven parts water. Stir until the honey is thoroughly dissolved in the water. Then put the honey-water into a bowl or other vessel with the flowers. This method is not exclusively for use with passionflowers; you can substitute any edible flowers, aromatic herbs, or fruit. Stir, stir, stir. Agitation stimulates fermentation and introduces yeast from the surface into the elixir. Stir, stir, stir. I like to stir around the edge of the bowl to create a vortex in the center, first in one direction, then the other. (Biodynamic farmers make compost teas like this and say that the vortex heightens the life forces in the tea.) Between stirrings, keep the bowl covered to protect it from flies.

After a few days (usually somewhere between two and five days; it depends on the ingredients and the environment) of periodic stirring, the elixir will be bubbling. Add more flowers, fruit, or herbs if you wish to make it stronger. With this passionflower elixir, I added flowers a second time. Keep stirring every day while it's in an open vessel; if you forget, molds may start to develop on the surface. Let the elixir bubble in the bowl for about a week. Then strain out the plant material, squeezing any excess liquid from it into the elixir. You can drink it now for an immediate gratification treat, if you wish. Historically this is how most people have enjoyed ferments, as airlock technology and bottling have not always or universally been available. In many parts of the world, this is how alcoholic beverages are still routinely enjoyed.

Or, you may continue to ferment as follows. Transfer the elixir to a narrow-neck jug and add honey-water, mixed at the same 1:4 ratio, to fill the jug, not to the very top, but to the point at which the neck narrows all the way. Protect the elixir from oxygen, which encourages vinegar formation, by using a water-filled airlock or balloon. Plastic airlocks are inexpensive and available at beer- and wine-making supply shops; balloons are a decent alternative, though they require you to release built-up CO_2 pressure periodically. Bottling and aging can produce sublimely smooth meads but, unfortunately, are beyond the scope of this book. See my book *Wild Fermentation* or my Web site (www.wildfermentation.com) for the details of that.

Elixirs can be made many different ways. You can prepare the herbs as infusions (steeping flowers or leaves in hot water but not actually boiling them) or decoctions (boiling the more fibrous parts of plants, such as barks and roots), then mix the infusion or decoction with honey. Once the brew cools to body temperature, you can add an already bubbling starter, fresh fruit or flowers, or commercial yeast. Experiment and vary your methods. Be part of the herbal elixir mead plant medicine-making revival.

Action and Information Resources

Books

Ableman, Michael. *Fields of Plenty: A Farmer's Journey in Search of Real Food and the People Who Grow It.* San Francisco: Chronicle Books, 2005.

———. *On Good Land: The Autobiography of an Urban Farm.* San Francisco: Chronicle Books, 1998.

Berry, Wendell. *The Gift of Good Land: Further Essays Cultural and Agricultural.* San Francisco: North Point Press, 1981.

Bové, José, and François Dufour. *The World Is Not for Sale: Farmers against Junk Food.* Translated by Anna De Casparis. New York: Verso, 2001.

Buhner, Stephen Harrod. *Sacred and Healing Herbal Beers: The Secrets of Ancient Fermentation.* Boulder, CO: Brewers, 1998.

Churchill, Ward. *Acts of Rebellion: The Ward Churchill Reader.* New York: Routledge, 2003.

Collier, George A., with Elizabeth Lowery Quaratiello. *Basta!: Land and the Zapatista Rebellion in Chiapas.* Oakland, CA: Food First Books, 1999.

Corr, Anders. *No Trespassing: Squatting, Rent Strikes and Land Struggles Worldwide.* Cambridge, MA: South End Press, 1999.

Fussell, Betty. *The Story of Corn: The Myths and History, the Culture and Agriculture, the Art and Science of America's Quintessential Crop.* New York: North Point Press, 1992.

George-Warren, Holly, Dave Hoekstra, and the Founders of Farm Aid. *Farm Aid: A Song for America.* Emmaus, PA: Rodale Press, 2005.

Herman, Patrick. *Food for Thought: Towards a Future for Farming.* Translated, adapted, and updated by Richard Kuper. Sterling, VA: Pluto Press, 2003.

Hynes, H. Patricia. *A Patch of Eden: America's Inner-City Gardeners.* White River Junction, VT: Chelsea Green, 1996.

Kimbrell, Andrew, ed. *The Fatal Harvest Reader: The Tragedy of Industrial Agriculture.* Washington, DC: Island Press, 2002.

LaDuke, Winona. *All Our Relations: Native Struggles for Land and Life.* Cambridge, MA: South End Press, 1999.

Lancaster, Brad. *Rainwater Harvesting for Drylands.* Tucson, AZ: Rainsource Press, 2006.

Magdoff, Fred, John Bellamy Foster and Frederick H. Buttel, eds. *Hungry for Profit: The Agribusiness Threat to Farmers, Food, and the Environment.* New York: Monthly Review Press, 2000.

Schlesinger, Stephen, and Stephen Kinzer. *Bitter Fruit: The Untold Story of the American Coup in Guatemala.* New York: Anchor Books, 1983.

Stamets, Paul. *Mycelium Running: How Mushrooms Can Help Save the World.* Berkeley, CA: Ten Speed Press, 2005.

Wilson, Peter Lamborn, and Bill Weinberg, eds. *Avant Gardening: Ecological Struggle in the City and the World.* New York: Autonomedia, 1999.

Woelfle-Erskine, Cleo, ed. *Urban Wilds: Gardeners' Stories of the Struggle for Land and Justice.* Oakland, CA: water/under/ground publications, 2001.

Wright, Angus, and Wendy Wolford. *To Inherit the Earth: The Landless Movement and the Struggle for a New Brazil.* Oakland, CA: Food First Books, 2003.

Films

The Bitter Aftertaste. Directed by Philip Thompson. WORLDwrite, 2005; www.worldwrite.org.uk/bitter.

Black Gold. Directed by Marc and Nick Francis. Speakalt Productions, 2006; www.blackgoldmovie.com.

The Real Dirt on Farmer John. Directed by Taggart Siegel. Awakened Media, 2005; www.therealdirt.net.

Organizations and Other Resources

Added Value & Herban Solutions
305 Van Brunt Street
Brooklyn, NY 11231
(718) 855-5531
www.added-value.org

Agribusiness Accountability Initiative
www.agribusinessaccountability.org

American Community Gardening
   Association
c/o Council on the Environment
51 Chambers Street, Suite 228
New York, NY 10007
(877) 275-2242
www.communitygarden.org

American Farmland Trust
1200 18th Street NW
Washington, DC 20036
(202) 331-7300
www.farmland.org

Black Farmers and Agriculturalists
   Association
PO Box 61
Tillery, NC 27887
(252) 826-2800
www.bfaa-us.org

Center for Rural Affairs
PO Box 136
Lyons, NE 68038-0136
(402) 687.2100
www.cfra.org

Chicago Honey Cooperative
2000 West Carroll Street, Suite 301
Chicago, IL 60612
(773) 848-2246
honeycoop@gmail.com

City Farmer
Canada's Office of Urban Agriculture
Box 74561, Kitsilano RPO
Vancouver, BC V6K 4P4
Canada
(604) 685-5832
www.cityfarmer.org

City Repair Project
PO Box 42615
Portland, OR 97242
(503) 235-8946
www.cityrepair.org

Coalition of Immokalee Workers
PO Box 603
Immokalee, FL, 34143
(239) 657-8311
www.ciw-online.org

Community Farm Alliance
614 Shelby Street
Frankfort, KY 40601
(502) 223-3655
www.communityfarmalliance.org

The Cornucopia Institute
PO Box 126
Cornucopia, WI 54827
(608) 625-2042
www.cornucopia.org

Desert Harvesters
www.desertharvesters.org

Earth Works Gardens
1820 Mount Elliot
Detroit, MI 48207
(313) 579-2100 x211
www.earth-works.org

Environmental Working Group
1436 U Street NW, Suite 100
Washington, DC 20009
(202) 667-6982
www.ewg.org

Fair Trade Resource Network
PO Box 33772
Washington, DC 20033-3772
(202) 302.0976
www.fairtraderesource.org

Family Farm Defenders
PO Box 1772
Madison, WI 53701
(608) 260-0900
www.familyfarmdefenders.org

Farm Aid
11 Ward Street, Suite 200
Somerville, MA 02143
(800) FARM-AID
www.farmaid.org

Farmers' Legal Action Group
360 North Robert Street, Suite 500
St. Paul, MN 55101
(651) 223-5400
www.flaginc.org

Farm Labor Organizing Committee
1221 Broadway Street
Toledo, OH 43609
(419) 243-3456
www.floc.com

Farmworker Justice Fund
1010 Vermont Avenue NW, Suite 915
Washington, DC 20005
(202) 783-2628
www.fwjustice.org

Food First/Institute for Food and
    Development Policy
398 60th Street
Oakland, CA 94618
(510) 654-4400
www.foodfirst.org

Food for the Cities
Food and Agriculture Organization of
    the United Nations
www.fao.org/fcit

Food Not Lawns
31139 Lanes Turn Road
Coburg, OR 97408
www.foodnotlawns.com

The Food Project
PO Box 705
Lincoln, MA 01773
(781) 259-8621
www.thefoodproject.org

Global Exchange
2017 Mission Street, #303
San Francisco, CA 94110
(415) 255-7296
www.globalexchange.org

Green Guerillas
214 West 29th Street, 5th Floor
New York, NY 10001
(212) 402-1121
www.greenguerillas.org

Greening of Harlem Coalition
406 Lenox Avenue, #4N
New York, NY 10037
(212) 491-7926

Growing Gardens
2003 NE 42nd Avenue, #3
Portland, OR 97213
(503) 284-8420
www.growing-gardens.org

Growing Power
5500 West Silver Spring Road
Milwaukee, WI 53218
(414) 527-1546
www.growingpower.org

Heifer Project International
PO Box 8058
Little Rock, AR 72203
(800) 422-0474
www.heifer.org

Institute for Agriculture and Trade
    Policy
2105 First Avenue South
Minneapolis, MN 55404
(612) 870-0453
www.iatp.org

Institute for Community Economics
57 School Street
Springfield, MA 01105
(413) 746-8660
www.iceclt.org

International Confederation of
    Autonomous Chapters of the
    American Indian Movement
www.americanindianmovement.org

International Culinary Tourism
    Association
4110 SE Hawthorne Boulevard, #440
Portland, OR 97214
(503) 750-7200
www.culinarytourism.org

The Land Institute
2440 East Water Well Road
Salina, KS 67401
(785) 823-5376
www.landinstitute.org

Land Stewardship Project
2200 4th Street
White Bear Lake, MN 55110
(651) 653-0618
www.landstewardshipproject.org

Land Trust Alliance
1331 H Street NW, Suite 400
Washington, DC 20005
(202) 638-4725
www.lta.org

Mad City Chickens
madcitychickens.com

More Gardens! Coalition
376 East 162nd Street, #2
Bronx, NY 10451
(718) 585-2109
www.moregardens.org

Movimento dos Trabalhadores Rurais
    Sem Terra (MTS; Brazil's Landless
    Workers Movement)
www.mstbrazil.org

National Family Farm Coalition
110 Maryland Avenue NE, Suite 307
Washington, DC 20002
(202) 543-5675
www.nffc.net

National Farm Transition Network
www.farmtransition.org

National Immigrant Farming Initiative
88 Atlantic Avenue, #8
Brooklyn, NY 11201
(718) 875-2220
www.immigrantfarming.org

Native Web: Resources for Indigenous
    Cultures around the World
www.nativeweb.org

New England Small Farm Institute
275 Jackson Street
Belchertown, MA 01007
(413) 323-4531
www.smallfarm.org

Organic Volunteers
www.organicvolunteers.org

Pesticide Action Network North America
49 Powell Street, Suite 500
San Francisco, CA 94102
(415) 981-1771
www.panna.org

Program on Corporations, Law, and
    Democracy
PO Box 246
South Yarmouth, MA 02664-0246
(508) 398-1145
www.poclad.org

Quillisascut Farm School of the
Domestic Arts
2409 Pleasant Valley Road
Rice, WA 99167
(509) 738-2011
www.quillisascutcheese.com

Resource Centres on Urban Agriculture
and Food Security
www.ruaf.org

Rhizome Collective
300 Allen Street
Austin, TX 78702
(512) 385-3695
www.rhizomecollective.org

Root Activist Network of Trainers
(RANT) Collective
www.rantcollective.net

Seattle Tilth Association
4649 Sunnyside Avenue N, Room 120
Seattle, WA 98103
(206) 633-0451
www.seattletilth.org

South Central LA Farmers
7309 Clybourn Avenue, Suite 1
Sun Valley, CA 91352
(818) 255-1483
www.southcentralfarmers.com

Spiral Gardens Community Food
Security Project
2880 Sacramento Street
Berkeley, CA 94702
(510) 843-1307
www.spiralgardens.org

Toledo GROWS
(419) 936-2975
www.toledogarden.org

Trust for Public Land
116 New Montgomery Street, 4th Floor
San Francisco, CA 94105
(800) 714-LAND
www.tpl.org

Via Campesina (International Peasant
Movement)
www.viacampesina.org

Western Shoshone Defense Project
PO Box 211308
Crescent Valley, NV 89821
(775) 468-0230
www.wsdp.org

White Earth Land Recovery Project
32033 East Round Lake Road
Ponsford, MN 56575
(218) 573-3448
www.nativeharvest.com

Women, Food, and Agriculture Network
59624 Chicago Road
Atlantic, IA 50022
(712) 243-3264
wfan.org

World Social Forum
Rua General Jardim, 660, 8th Floor
São Paulo, SP 01223-010
Brazil
www.worldsocialforum.org

World-Wide Opportunities on Organic
Farms
www.wwoof.org

World-Wide Opportunities on Organic
Farms (WWOOF) USA
PO Box 510
Felton, CA 95060
(831) 425-3276
www.wwoofusa.org

Zapatista Network
www.zapatistas.org

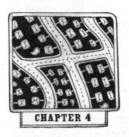

CHAPTER 4

Slow Food for Cultural Survival

Slow Food is a movement that began in Italy in 1986. It was sparked by the outrage of an Italian journalist, Carlo Petrini, at the opening of a McDonald's at Rome's landmark Spanish Steps. The movement originally defined itself by its opposition to fast food. "A firm defense of quiet material pleasure is the only way to oppose the universal folly of Fast Life," states the 1989 Slow Food Manifesto.[1]

Slow Food struck a chord and has since developed into a worldwide organization with eighty thousand members in 800 local "convivia" or chapters, 150 of them in the United States. I've made presentations to several of these groups; after all, food doesn't get any slower than fermentation. Many of these groups host regular tasting events. The Slow Food group that I spoke with in Atlanta had recently held a tasting of different salts from around the world. To a food geek like me, that sounds really interesting and fun.

"Taste is a part of knowledge," says Petrini,[2] and taste education is one of the goals of Slow Food. One manifestation of taste education, and the firm defense of quiet material pleasure, is connoisseurship. Unfortunately, too much emphasis on buying fancy foods becomes highbrow consumerism, a costly pursuit of the very finest foods and wines that is disconnected from questions of sustainable production and far beyond the means of ordinary people. Some critics have dismissed Slow Food as elitist. Indeed, that is a reasonable critique of any organization that charges a $60 annual membership fee and typically sponsors events at expensive restaurants. To be fair, some Slow Food convivia organize mostly free, potluck events. But then $500 is the going rate for attending a dinner with Petrini himself, "A Rare Opportunity to Talk (and Eat) with Slow Food's Founder."[3]

Yet Petrini's rhetoric and many of the projects that Slow Food has undertaken around the world suggest an agenda beyond fine dining. "Saving gastronomy is not possible if we cannot save the very context in which it is developed," Petrini says. "The challenge ahead is to reconnect the umbilical cord of traditional knowledge that once joined man and nature and has almost been severed by industrialization."[4]

Accordingly, Slow Food has championed traditional local food production. It has focused on issues of biodiversity, both at the level of preserving heirloom breeds of plants and animals in the face of homogenization and extinctions and in terms of the cultural diversity that homogenized agricultural practices threaten. Without an emphasis on supporting small-scale food producers, warns Petrini, "we all become top-class gourmets and connoisseurs of rare delicacies while ignoring the need to prevent the disappearance of those who actually work the land and supply the products."[5]

In 2004 Slow Food organized an unprecedented gathering of small-scale food producers from around the world. Of course these are people with limited budgets for international travel, so this coming together was facilitated by the largesse of the Italian government (promoting food tourism) and augmented by the fund-raising efforts of Slow Food convivia worldwide. The gathering, known as Terra Madre ("Mother Earth"), brought together more than five thousand small-scale food producers—farmers, bakers, brewers, and other food processors using traditional methods at a community-based scale—from 130 countries! These producers represent what Petrini calls "food communities," which "bind together the destinies of women and men pledged to defending their own traditions, cultures and crops."[6]

"Terra Madre changed the essence of Slow Food," reflects Petrini.[7] "It became evident that if we want to properly develop actions of defense, support and service, it is essential to start looking at food communities with a much broader and more complex perspective than we have to date."[8] Vandana Shiva, one of the Terra Madre keynote speakers, calls this Terra Madre perspective "earth democracy," which "implies having both a planetary consciousness and a local embeddedness of how we produce and consume, and how we experience our identity and sense of self."[9]

Shortly after Terra Madre, I attended a presentation at the Carolina Farm Stewardship Association given by several farmers who had gone to Italy for the gathering. They all had come home feeling inspired by people they had met at Terra Madre. "There are people all over the world doing what we're doing here," reported farmer Libby Outlaw. For people doing the most localized of work there is—working particular land to grow food—this is needed affirmation and encouragement. After experiencing the solidarity of food producers from all over the world, farmer Emile DeFelice saw "movement potential." The movement he envisions is a coming together of small-scale food producers and "food communities," empowered by numbers, unity, and solidarity, keeping traditions alive in the face of global homogenization and expanding corporate concentration of the food chain.

A huge sign on the wall at Terra Madre read, "Today thirty plants feed 95 percent of the world's population. In the past one hundred years, 250,000 plant varieties have gone extinct, and one plant variety disappears every six hours. Since the beginning of the twentieth century, Europe has lost more than 75 percent of its agricultural variety, while the United States has lost 93 percent of its crop diversity. One third of native cattle, sheep, and pig breeds have gone extinct or are on the road to extinction."

We've already touched upon this issue in chapter 2 in the discussion of the disappearance of heirloom vegetable varieties, ones that evolved over time through selection by farmers and are thereby adapted to local conditions. "Improved" varieties developed by scientists in university and corporate laboratories—not adapted to local conditions—have largely replaced traditional heirloom varieties, along with the habit and practice of seed saving. Most traditional varieties listed in seed catalogs a century ago are forever lost. The plant varieties, the seed-saving practices, the farmers themselves, and their roles in their communities—all of these are manifestations of the loss of diversity, with loss of biological diversity reflecting loss of cultural diversity, and vice versa. The globalization and homogenization of food diminishes diversity on all these levels, and only by reconnecting with traditions of food production can we reclaim and reestablish practices that support and rebuild both biological and cultural diversity.

One Slow Food project is the Ark of Taste, which lists foods—either from specific breeds or made through specific processes—that are perceived to be in some danger of extinction. In most cases potential food extinctions are due to disuse and neglect. For instance, the pawpaw (*Asimina triloba*), a custardlike fruit that grows on a tree of the same name native to the eastern United States, is the largest fruit indigenous to the United States. The thick, sweet flesh of the fruits is compellingly delicious, yet the pawpaw is bizarrely obscure today. Pawpaws and other native "first fruits" suffered as the indigenous tribes of the eastern United States were forced to move westward without their orchards.

Pawpaw trees are still part of the landscape in the Southeast and Midwest. We enjoy pawpaws here in Tennessee every fall. The ripest pawpaws are found on the ground and are intensely sweet, with a rich, complex flavor and a gorgeous, creamy texture that melts in your

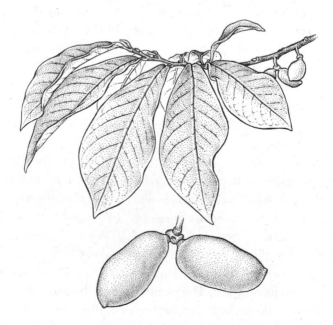

Pawpaw. ©Bobbi Angell. Used by permission.

mouth. My friend Hector Black sells some pawpaws at his stand at the Cookeville, Tennessee, farmers' market, but on an extremely small scale. *USA Today* reported on a California pawpaw grower who sells the fruits at one of San Francisco's premier farmers' markets:

> Even there, at a market known as a magnet for serious foodies and chefs who welcome the most obscure fruits and vegetables, customers puzzle over the mottled green-brown fruits the size of small mangos. When he can get them to actually taste the pawpaws, they're hooked. A quick cut to one end, a squeeze of the creamy, custardy flesh straight into the mouth and customers lap up the explosion of flavors that are reminiscent of banana, papaya, coconut, cream and even hints of caramel in the ripest. But five minutes of explanation for each sale isn't the way to move a harvest's worth of fruit.[10]

Slow Food's Washington, DC, convivium is spearheading a "Three Sweet Sisters" campaign to generate renewed interest in pawpaws, along with two other neglected indigenous fruits, native persimmons and wild strawberries. The Three Sweet Sisters project has sponsored tasting events, Three Sweet Sisters Gardens (including one at the National Arboretum), and Restaurant Dialogues, sessions that encourage chefs to incorporate these fruits into their menus.

It is not only plant varieties that face potential extinction. According to animal geneticist John Hodges, 45 percent of existing chicken breeds, 43 percent of horse breeds, 23 percent of pig breeds, and 23 percent of cattle breeds are at risk of extinction.[11] As one example, turkeys have been bred to be so grotesquely large-breasted that the single breed (Broad Breasted White) that constitutes more than 99 percent of the commercial market in the United States can no longer accomplish reproduction without human intervention.[12] Bigger is not always better!

An organization called the American Livestock Breed Conservancy (ALBC) is working to preserve traditional breeds of farm animals, which, like seeds, have historically been bred to adapt to varied local conditions. Heritage farm animals have largely been replaced by "improved" breeds with the generic appeal of producing more meat (or milk or eggs) more quickly, though the resulting animals are often less healthy, less fertile, and less able to thrive on pasture and thereby require more inputs (such as water, feed, reproductive assistance, or antibiotics). The ALBC has helped to bring back from the brink of extinction a number of heritage farm-animal breeds, most notably turkeys; traditional American breeds such as the Standard Bronze and Narragansett are making a comeback. The ALBC provides information and technical resources to breeders and farmers and works with Slow Food to develop markets for heritage breeds.

Slow Food is collaborating with the ALBC and several other organizations, including the Seed Savers Exchange and Native Seeds/SEARCH, in a project called Renewing America's Food Traditions (RAFT). RAFT has begun holding regional events to celebrate regional foods, to brainstorm lists of regionally distinctive foods, plants, and animals, and to determine which species are abundant, threatened, endangered, extinct, or recovering. The first workshop, in the "Salmon Nation" of the Pacific Northwest, came up with a list of 180 regional foods, two-thirds of which are at risk. Workshops in the other regions will be held over the next several years, contributing to the RAFT "Redlist" of endangered foods and creating "tangible tools of eco-gastronomic conservation."[13]

Traditional foods can be saved not by preaching ideology, insists Petrini, but only by reviving pleasure:

> The beginning of the organic movement had a mistaken attitude because it didn't place any emphasis on pleasure. It was an ideological, almost religious approach. It ignored pleasure. Pleasure is not antithetical to health, pleasure is not the enemy of sustainability. Pleasure is moderation and with moderation we can be sustainable. An environmentalist or an organic farmer that is not also cultivating pleasure is just out of this world. Throughout history, all of humanity has always wanted to produce food also to produce pleasure. . . . This idea is part of the complexity of a new gastronomy. We can't change the world by just preaching boring messages. We have to re-discover the value of taste and understand that at its root, taste is connected to pleasure. Taste is pleasure that reasons, or knowledge that enjoys. Nice, eh?[14]

Though his agenda is pleasure-based, Petrini maintains a sense of urgency: "Either we go back to local agriculture, and go back to giving pride to these farmers, having a human rapport with these farmers, or we might as well just blow our brains out."[15]

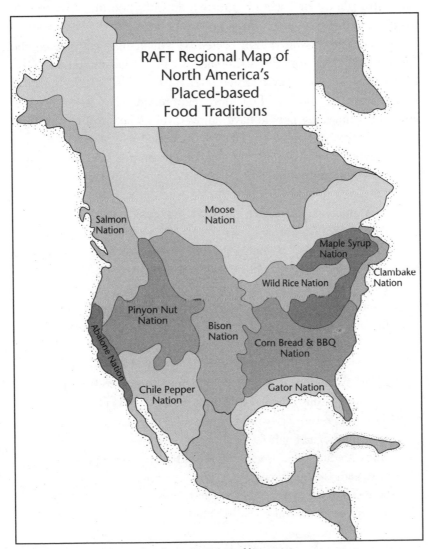

©2006 Renewing America's Food Traditions (RAFT). Used by permission.

Wild Rice and Other Indigenous-Food Culture Struggles

The previous chapter highlighted the land struggles of the Anishinaabeg people of northern Minnesota and southern Ontario. Their struggle for their land is intertwined with their ongoing struggle to continue their age-old cultural practice, specific to that very land, of harvesting, eating, and trading wild rice, which they call *manoomin*, "good berry." The story the Anishinaabeg tell of their migration to this land involves a prophecy instructing them to settle "where the good berry grows on water."[16] For more generations than anyone could count, Anishinaabeg people have enjoyed the delicious and nutritious good berries of the northern lakes. "Our rice tastes like a lake," says Anishinaabeg activist Winona LaDuke.[17] The annual harvest is a time-honored community ritual.

> It is *Manoominike-Giizis*, the wild rice moon, and the lakes teem with a harvest and a way of life. "Ever since I was bitty, I've been ricing," reminisces Spud Fineday, of Ice Cracking Lake. Spud rices at Cabin Point, and then moves to Big Flat Lake, lakes on Minnesota's White Earth Reservation. "Sometimes we can knock four to five hundred pounds a day," he says, explaining that he alternates the jobs of "poling and knocking" with his wife, Tater, a.k.a. Vanessa Fineday. The Finedays, like many other Anishinaabeg from White Earth, and other reservations in the region, continue to rice, to feed their families, to "buy school clothes and fix cars," and get ready for the ever returning winter. The wild rice harvest of the Anishinaabeg not only feeds the body; it feeds the soul, continuing a tradition that is generations old for these people of the lakes and rivers of the north. . . . It is a community event, a cultural event, which ties the community intergenerationally to all that is essentially Anishinaabeg, Ojibwe.[18]

Unfortunately the annual Anishinaabeg rice harvest is threatened by the pursuit of biotechnological innovation, without regard for the integrity of either indigenous plants' genetic identity or indigenous peoples' cultural identity.

Wild rice offers us another example of biopiracy. Early in the twentieth century anthropologists from the University of Minnesota studied the Anishinaabeg and determined that "wild rice, which has led to their advance thus far, held them back from further progress, unless, indeed, they left it behind them, for with them it was incapable of intensive cultivation."[19] Intensive cultivation—growing more on less space, so the land's productivity is intensified—is understood to be progress and traditional seasonal gathering as backward! So university plant breeders set out to improve wild rice, and in the 1950s and 1960s they developed a domesticated, paddy-grown "wild" rice.

The genetic material they started with and manipulated came from native wild rice, of course; the researchers felt free to avail themselves of this as a public resource, even though native peoples' rights to the rice have been repeatedly recognized by treaties. As a result of this breeding effort, a domesticated "wild" rice industry developed in Minnesota, and wild rice was officially declared the state grain. As the industry grew it shifted to California, where the damaging hail and winds common in Minnesota could be avoided. "Wild" rice prices plummeted, from $4.44 per pound in 1967 to $2.68 per pound in 1976.[20] The Anishinaabeg and other peoples of the northern waters, who until then had been the sole sources of wild rice, felt the impact of domestication.

Thirty years later public funds continue to be channeled into breeding for the domesticated "wild" rice industry. The University of Minnesota continues to fund studies with titles like "Molecular Cytogenics for Plant Improvement, Wild Rice Breeding/Germplasm, and Toward the Identification of Functional Genes in Wild Rice." The Anishinaabeg, who have always harvested wild rice from Minnesota's lakes—and whose livelihoods have already been diminished by the crop "improvements"—worry that new, genetically modified varieties will contaminate the indigenous wild rice. For them, the increasingly sophisticated genetic technology is not value-neutral science at all; it diminishes their culture. A coalition of northern Minnesota Anishinaabeg bands has demanded that the University of Minnesota declare a moratorium on genetic research on wild rice.

In addition to challenging the biopiracy of their resources and restoring their land base, LaDuke and her fellow Anishinaabeg activists are actively working to reintegrate traditional foods into the contemporary lives of their people. Their organization, the White Earth Land Recovery Project (WELRP), is promoting food sovereignty as a means of cultural survival through several related projects: encouraging rice harvesting as a source of both food and income; actively marketing wild rice online and through networks like Slow Food; encouraging other food production on the reservation; and combating an epidemic of diabetes by distributing traditional foods to diabetics and their families. In 2003 LaDuke and White Earth elder Margaret Smith were recognized for their efforts with an International Slow Food Award for the Defense of Biodiversity. More importantly, their work is taking hold and changing Anishinaabeg peoples' lives.

The program to bring traditional foods to diabetics is called Mino-Miijim ("Good Food"). Native Americans have the highest prevalence of type 2 diabetes in the world. A third of the residents of the White Earth Reservation are diabetic, as is an estimated 40 percent of Native Americans over the age of forty nationwide.[21] According to the WELRP Web site:

> The process of colonization effected a dramatic change in patterns of exercise and diet. The forced adaptation of a sedentary lifestyle and the subsequent increase in obesity rates facilitated the spread of diabetes, heart disease, and other related health complications. In addition, the switch from a traditional diet, which was high in dietary fiber and lean sources of protein (wild game), to a diet rich in sugars, refined carbohydrates, and fats has fueled the diabetes epidemic.[22]

Many of the Anishinaabeg rely upon highly processed government-issue commodity foods. "Ironically nearly all the foods the government issued to the tribes were less nutritious and more fattening than their native foods," says Gary Paul Nabhan, an Arizona ecologist, writer, and food activist who founded the organization Native Seeds/SEARCH.[23] "It seems as though it is the poorest among us who most desperately need such traditional foods to regain their health, for they are otherwise treated as the dumping grounds for the worst of junk foods."[24] In other words, everybody needs "slow food"—not just food adventurers with disposable income.

Margaret Smith, an elderly diabetic Anishinaabeg herself, decided to assemble monthly care packages of Anishinaabeg foods—foods such as wild rice, hominy corn, and buffalo meat (bought from other reservations)—and distribute them to other diabetic Anishinaabeg elders on the reservation. Smith visits with the elders and encourages them to share the native foods with young people. WELRP sends elders into schools to introduce native foods, advocates for native-food-based school lunch programs, and teaches people to grow the traditional American "three sisters" companions of corn, beans, and squash. WELRP recognizes food sovereignty as an integral element of land sovereignty and healthy lives and seeks, on many fronts simultaneously, to reintegrate traditional food production into the lives of the Anishinaabeg people.

In the Sonoran Desert of Arizona and Mexico, Gary Paul Nabhan organized the Desert Walk for Biodiversity, Heritage, and Health, a twelve-day, 220-mile, multicultural trek through the desert intended to create awareness of the relationship between diet and diabetes. Among the participants were more than twenty Native Americans with diabetes from the Seri, Pima, and O'odham peoples. According to Nabhan, the O'odham have the highest diabetes rate of any ethnic group in the world.[25] The walkers learned about indigenous foods from communities along the way, feasting on meals including venison, rabbit, birds, tomatillos, squash, pumpkins, tepary beans, mesquite, lamb's-quarters, purslane, mustards, cress, ocotillo blossoms, prickly pear and other cacti, mistletoe, pinole, chia seeds, and mescal.

One of the ways in which these traditional foods contrast with the high-fat, high-sugar, highly processed standard American diet is that their nutrients are metabolized much more slowly (which gives us another perspective on the concept of slow food). "Traditional diets of desert peoples formerly *protected* them from diabetes and other life-threatening afflictions," writes Nabhan.[26] He and the other walkers were able to dramatically experience the physiological differences that a diet of native foods can produce.

> These foods enabled us to hike across rugged terrain for ten hours a day, followed by another hour or two of celebratory dancing. Our collective effort made us more deeply aware that

our own energy levels could be sustained for hours by slow-release foods. . . . A return to a more traditional diet of their ancestral foods was not merely some trip to fantasy land for nostalgia's sake; it provided them with a deep motivation for improving their own health.[27]

Native Americans in many different places are organizing around traditional foods as a strategy for survival. Patricia Cochran, an Inupiat from northwestern Alaska near the Bering Strait, directs an organization called the Alaska Native Science Commission, which promotes cultural survival via environmental protection and health advocacy. Inupiat people eat mostly fish and sea mammals. Among their traditional delicacies are stinkfish, which are fish that are buried in the tundra to ferment, and *muktuk*, or whale blubber. *New York Times* critic Frank Bruni traveled to Alaska and wrote about sampling *muktuk*: "I did as told: grabbed the hide and bit into the blubber. It tasted like a wedge of solid rubber that had spent several months marinating in rancid fish oil. And it flew instantaneously from my mouth into a thicket of nearby birch trees."[28] Then the big-city critic watched a ten-month-old baby as he "gummed and licked that slimy whale fat as if it were Alaska's biggest, brightest lollipop," concluding that "a palate, like a mind, works better with exposure and education and is a product of its environment."[29]

Both the food itself and the taste for it are products of their environment. This is exactly why globalized food makes no sense. Each ecological niche has its own unique abundance to offer. Different regions offer different sources of abundance. Human beings have been remarkably adaptable in terms of diet. What we eat has historically been central to what defines our culture. Though their traditional diet made the Inupiat and other peoples of the Arctic among the healthiest on the earth, today atmospheric and oceanic currents are now known to carry chemicals and emissions from the rest of the world and concentrate them there. "The Arctic has been transformed into the planet's chemical trash can, the final destination for toxic waste that originates thousands of miles away," writes Marla Cone in *Mother Jones*.[30] PCBs, DDT, mercury, lead, and other dangerous chemicals are present in Arctic fish, and in the breast milk and umbilical cords of Arctic mothers, at alarming levels.

Some might conclude that the Inupiat people should abandon their traditional fish-based diet. But the food of any culture is more than a collection of nutrients; it is a central element of identity. Says Cochran:

> How we get our food is intrinsic to our culture. It's how we pass on our values and knowledge to our young. When you go out with your aunts and uncles to hunt or to gather, you learn to smell the air, watch the wind, understand the way ice moves, know the land. You get to know where to pick which plant and what animal to take. It's part, too, of your development as a person. You share food with your community. You show respect to your elders by offering them the first catch. You give thanks to the animal that gave up its life for your sustenance. So you get all the physical activity of harvesting your own food, all the social activity of sharing and preparing it, and all the spiritual aspects as well. You certainly don't get all that, do you, when you buy prepackaged food from a store.[31]

The Makah, a Washington State tribe that traditionally subsisted largely on the meat of the gray whale, made an attempt a few years ago to revive their food tradition. The gray whale is so central to their culture that in an 1855 treaty with the United States, the Makah traded 90 percent of their land for the right to continue whaling. As the commercial whaling industry grew, the Makah watched whale populations dwindle. In the 1920s they made the voluntary decision to stop whaling altogether, fifty years before the gray whale became legally protected as an endangered species. An international moratorium on commercial whaling, in place since 1986, has been effective enough that gray whale populations have rebounded, and in 1994 it was removed from the endangered species list. Because of that 1855 treaty, and the fact that they do not hunt for commercial purposes, the Makah are at least theoretically exempt from the commercial whaling ban. They decided to resume tradition, and after a rigorous training program, in 1999 a group of Makah went out hunting into the sea and brought home the first whale in nearly eighty years. "The biggest thrill of my life was to feed fresh whale to my grandson," said a Makah woman in the television documentary *The Meaning of Food*. Some misguided environmentalists and animal-rights activists protested the Makah whale hunt with slogans such as "Abolish the treaties!" and "Save a Whale—Hunt a Makah!" In 2000 a federal court ordered the Makah to stop whale hunting, treaty or no treaty, extinction threat or not, preventing them from practicing their ancient food traditions in a sustainable way.

Other cultures in the Pacific Northwest are connected to salmon. However, dams, irrigation projects, and development have ruined most rivers for salmon spawning, and in 2004 the Bush administration scaled back *by 80 percent* protected salmon habitats.[32] Cultures organized around salmon are struggling to survive. Susana Santos, one of the few remaining members of the Tygh band of the Lower Deschutes River in Oregon, has watched the demise of the salmon that have traditionally sustained and coexisted with her people.

> I wanted to dance the salmon, know the salmon, say goodbye to the salmon. Now I am looking at the completion of destruc- tion, from the *Exxon Valdez* to . . . those dams. . . . Seventeen fish came down the river last year. None this year. The people are the salmon, and the salmon are the people. How do you quantify that?"[33]

Food is an integral aspect of movements for environmental justice. The Karuk of the Klamath River Valley in northern California are another native people whose diet centered around wild salmon. Since the destruction of salmon spawning in the Klamath in the 1970s, the Karuk diet has become dominated by processed foods; as is the case for other native peoples abruptly cut off from their traditional foods, obe- sity and diabetes rates have steadily risen in the Karuk population. As the dams come up for relicensing by the Federal Energy Regulatory Commission, the Karuk are asserting that their health crises have been caused by the destruction of salmon habitat on the Klamath, and that at least three dams on the Klamath River should be knocked down.[34]

On the Pine Ridge Reservation in South Dakota, a group called Village Earth is helping Oglala Lakota people get their land back from the Bureau of Indian Affairs, which leases roughly 60 percent of the land allotted to the Oglala Lakota in the 1887 General Allotment Act to cattle ranchers for as little as $3 a year per acre. Village Earth is providing new Oglala Lakota settlers with various forms of assistance toward living sustainably on the land, among them "seed herds" of buffalo. The project is an effort to restore the buffalo and the people to their land, and to promote the interaction of the two. "Home, though, is a bit different than it used to be," reports the Village Earth Web site. "Despite the promising movement toward land restoration, Pine Ridge landowners still are required to fence in their land or it will be immediately revoked again."[35]

Two hundred years ago forty to fifty million buffalo roamed the northern plains. In the early nineteenth century buffalo extermination was federal policy, a means of wiping out one way of life and opening up space for the establishment of a new one—with profitable railroads and cattle ranching. "Forty-five and a half million cattle live in this same ecosystem now, but they lack the adaptability of the buffalo," writes Winona LaDuke. The cattle require extensive infrastructure to support them. "The prairies today are teeming with pumps, irrigation systems, combines, and chemical additives. Much of the original ecosystem has been destroyed."[36]

Many different projects that share the goal of restoring buffalo herds to the northern plains are under way. Forty-two tribes are collaborating on buffalo restoration and marketing efforts as the Intertribal Bison Cooperative, and the World Wildlife Fund and the American Prairie Foundation have started a buffalo restoration project on a 32,000-acre wildlife preserve in Montana. These projects are steps toward the larger goal of restoring the buffalo commons and, more broadly, healing the ecosystem and restoring the balance between people and buffalo on this land. "When we talk about restoring buffalo, we're not just talking about restoring animals to the land," says Fred Dubray of the Cheyenne River Nation, executive director of the Intertribal Bison Cooperative, "we're talking about restoring social structure, culture, and even our political structure."[37] As we discussed in chapter 3, the United States has a long tradition of ignoring tribal land claims. Supporting a revival of native food traditions means supporting a return of native lands.

People, communities, and cultures suffer when they are cut off from the sources that have always sustained them. People can change and adapt, certainly, but abrupt change is profoundly destabilizing and debilitating. Food and drink, and the methods of their production, are

integral elements of culture. For transplanted cultures as well as
indigenous peoples, strategies for cultural survival *must* incorporate
food, in both its consumption and its production. This does not mean
that we must all be slaves to tradition. Traditions change, slowly but
surely; they evolve, adapt, and influence other traditions. But even so,
traditions are vitally important, for they embody accumulated cultural
knowledge. "We've got to defend ancient wisdom," exhorts Carlo
Petrini. "It's not a retrograde battle, it's an avant-garde battle, because
we find for ourselves so much richness inside this traditional wisdom."[38]

Illegal Food: The War on Small-Scale Production

Many traditional foods and methods of food production have been prohibited by laws imposed in the name of hygiene. My current favorite
example of an outlawed food is the Italian cheese called *casu marzu*, a
traditional product of the island of Sardinia. *Casu marzu* is made from
pecorino, an Italian sheep's milk cheese, that is left out in the sun. Flies
land on the cheese and lay eggs, which hatch into maggots that digest
the hard, mild pecorino into *casu marzu*, "a viscous, pungent goo that
burns the tongue," according to the *Wall Street Journal*.[39] *Saveur* also
featured a vivid account of tasting *casu marzu*: "We happened to be in
a light-filled room as we prepared to taste it, and the maggots started
jumping around like crazy and landing everywhere, including on us."[40]
As you eat *casu marzu*, you must cover your eyes with a hand to protect
them from jumping maggots.

I've told many fermentation-enthused audiences about this sensational cheese, and it never fails to get people to cringe in horror. In my
fermentation practice I've periodically encountered maggots in foods
I've been aging. Anywhere flies can land and lay eggs, maggots will
develop. It's happened to me most often on cheeses I've tried to age in
summer. People worry about the bacteria that flies could potentially
spread, but the acids in an aging cheese make it inhospitable to pathogenic bacteria (see chapter 5 for more information about this).
Emboldened by reading about *casu marzu*, I've tasted a few accidentally maggoty cheeses. The cheese digested by the maggots is incredibly creamy and strong. In my observation, the maggots themselves

migrate from the creamy area to fresh cheese, so I've ended up with mostly viscous, gooey, pungent maggot-digested cheese and not much of the squirmy maggots themselves. No maggots jumping. And whatever maggots are there blend right in.

Really, people in this world eat all sorts of things, even insects, creepy-crawly things, and molds. People eat fish that has been buried for months until it decomposes into a cheesy paste; they eat years-old eggs and decades-old hams. My friend Alan Muskat presents me with crunchy dried ants for lunch, while the Wildroots Collective in western North Carolina serves me raccoon stew and other roadkill delicacies (see page 296). My friend Roman, when he was a little kid, used to eat worms, centipedes, and grasshoppers, without ill effect. The more grossed-out people were, the more encouraged he felt. Notions of what is appropriate to eat are largely subjective and culturally determined. There is no objective universal boundary between food fit to eat and food that is inappropriate or "spoiled."

People in Sardinia have been eating *casu marzu* for hundreds of years, apparently without ill effect. *Casu marzu* sells for twice the price of the maggot-free pecorino. Except that you can't buy it any more—at least not legally. "Selling it or serving it can be punished with a hefty fine," according to the *Wall Street Journal.* Evidently the E.U. bureaucrats in Brussels cringed at the thought of maggoty cheese, so they declared it illegal, not in compliance with E.U. hygienic standards. The cultural homogenization machine grinds on, saving us from corruption by eccentric cultural variations.

Of course, the tradition of *casu marzu* continues. People do not simply say, "Okay, we will end our inherited tradition because you say so." People resist any new order imposed upon their culture. And so *casu marzu* continues to be made and eaten, though now not sold, at least not openly. The tradition now holds a different place in the culture, as a symbol of resistance against an ever-more-distant, out-of-touch, centralized authority.

Most of the traditional foods that are being made illegal are less sensational than *casu marzu*. The typical story is simply that small-scale production methods have effectively been outlawed by hygiene regulations that are designed for mass production. The regulatory unification of Europe has rendered all sorts of small-scale food-processing operations illegal. "The laws and regulations are endless and forever changing," writes a German farmer I corresponded with, "but as always in favor of the ruling bunch." A dairy farmer and cheesemaker in a small town in central Italy reports that changes in Italian food-hygiene laws, in an attempt to make them "harmonize" with E.U. regulations, have made legal farmstead cheese production there difficult and expensive.

"In Italy," writes E., "if you want to sell 'transformed products,' you have to have an E.U. standard workshop *for each separate product*. The only thing we can legally sell is fruit and vegetables 'just as they are picked.' Even wine and oil are 'transformed' just by being bottled." Therefore a small-scale farm can no longer use a kitchen or other general work area to make cheese for sale; the cheese must be produced in a dedicated space, used solely for the production of cheese, that meets factory production standards. This means that legal cheese production in Italy now requires heavy capitalization, beyond the reach of the average small farmer.

So E. and other small-scale food producers in her area have started an underground market.

> Our market meets at a different farm each month, on a Saturday afternoon. We start at 3 p.m. in order to allow people who have animals to get back in time for milking/feeding. Most of the farms are small and "self-sufficient," all are organic, some are biodynamic. We started the market in 2001 after a big anti-G8 protest in Genoa during which many peaceful protesters were beaten by riot police. My companion and I, together with another local couple, were trying to think what we could do to change things since protesting in public seemed so fruitless, and we decided that we should start at home, on a very local level, and behave as if life were organized as we wish it were. So we called a meeting of all the local "alternative" people we thought might be interested in exchanging the food we produce.
>
> We sent out fifty invitations, but at the first meeting there were only eight people. Nevertheless, we decided to start a small monthly market, and at the first one we were twelve people, at the second, sixteen, at the third, twenty. Now we

have done these markets once a month for four full years and we have a list of about ninety people who participate. Out of these, about twenty are producers. At any given market, there are about fifty to seventy people. We refer to the market as *il mercatino*, the little market, or as "the clandestine market."

My companion, M., and I do the organizing: We send out a letter once a month to everyone on the list with a map showing how to get to the next farm. The letter also gives local news, and we include small notices and ads from participants who want to sell/buy/exchange/donate animals/land/equipment etc. Once a year, we ask everyone for money for stamps and photocopies (10 euros each). People are happy to host the market and one reason for moving it around is so that everyone can see how other people live and work. The host usually provides cake/wine/tea and the whole event has a useful and fun social side: people meet and talk and exchange advice and news. They also arrange the buying of big items like the year's supply of hay or wheat.

This clandestine market sounds strikingly similar to the bread club described in the introduction. E. also told me about other clandestine markets she knows of in the central Italian countryside. In many variations, all of them small and informal, such underground markets are widespread, and we need to create many more of them.

Similar regulatory changes are occurring elsewhere in the world. In 1998 India banned the sale of mustard oil and imposed new packaging requirements on other oils. This action was triggered by the death of fifty people in New Delhi, caused by contaminated mustard oil with suspicious details. The mustard oil was found to be tainted with petroleum products as well as an inedible seed oil (from an *Argemone* species) that contained toxic alkaloids. Contamination was found to be present in many different brands and at levels as high as 30 percent. A spokesperson for the government-owned brand of mustard oil charged, "There is a strong case for sabotage."[41] Vandana Shiva agrees: "There was no other way to explain why the contamination was so extensive."[42]

The Indian government announced the ban on mustard oil on the very same day that it lifted all restrictions on the importation of soy oil.

Its markets were quickly flooded with imported soy oil, most of it genetically modified. Vegetable oils in India have traditionally been quite diverse and their production small-scale, localized, and informal. People in communities all around India have always extracted oil from not only mustard seeds but also coconuts, peanuts, linseed, sunflower seeds, and sesame seeds, in small cottage industries. The contrast is stark: community-based self-sufficiency and economic democracy replaced by homogenized corporate consumerism, and in the name of hygiene and "free trade." Free trade of locally produced goods among people at the community level is outlawed, in favor of a global free trade among huge corporations. "Mustard oil and our indigenous oilseeds symbolize freedom for nature, for our farmers, our diverse food cultures and the rights of poor consumers," says Shiva. "Soyabean oil symbolizes concentration of power and the colonization of nature, cultures, farmers and consumers."[43]

It is ironic that a contamination scare led to further concentration of oil production and distribution, since centralized systems are most vulnerable to sabotage and manipulation. In the United States we have seen a growing fear of ways in which our food supply could be vulnerable to contamination as a form of terrorist attack. When Tommy Thompson, the secretary of the U.S. Department of Health and Human Services, resigned in 2004, he remarked upon his surprise that the food chain had not yet been attacked: "I, for the life of me, cannot understand why the terrorists have not attacked our food supply, because it is so easy to do."[44] And in 2005 the National Academy of Sciences published (in defiance of being asked not to by the government) an exploration of a scenario in which a single gram of botulinum toxin released into the U.S. milk supply could kill fifty thousand people.[45] Vulnerability exists at this scale only because the milk is processed at this scale! Decentralized local food systems provide security because they spread and dissipate the myriad food-safety risks— not only the terrorist variety, but also accidental contamination—so that even a worst-case scenario is contained and does not have as catastrophic an impact.

The scale of impact in the event of contamination is one of the reasons that it is appropriate to hold mass producers to more stringent safety standards than small-scale producers. Unfortunately, regulations justified in the name of safety often have the effect of forcing out small producers, thereby increasing reliance on centralized supplies. In 2005 India proposed a broad new food safety and standards law that Shiva calls "food fascism." She argues that the new law would impose upon all food production uniform standards appropriate for large-scale production, even though most of the food consumed in India (like oils until 1998) is still locally processed at a small scale and highly decentralized. "Clearly, the law has been designed to lubricate international trade and the expansion of the global agribusiness," says Shiva. "Consumer health, nutrition, and food culture are not even mentioned as objectives of the integrated food law. . . . [It] is a law to dismantle our diverse, decentralized food economy."[46]

The rhetoric of free trade is that the governments get out of the way and let market forces do their thing. Despite this rhetoric, observes Vandana Shiva,

> the government is a major player in the transfer of production from small scale decentralized systems to large scale, centralized systems under monopoly control. The state in fact is the backbone of the free trade order. The only difference is that instead of regulating big business, it leaves big business free, and declares small producers and diverse cultures illegal so that big business has monopoly control on the food system.[47]

This process—the transfer of production from small-scale decentralized systems to large-scale, centralized systems—is arguably the foundation of the state as an institution. It seems widely agreed that nation-states first emerged in those places where settled patterns of grain agriculture developed. The storability of grains created unprecedented potential for accumulation of resources and power. If food is all perishable and fleeting, it cannot be hoarded but must be eaten. Grains, in contrast, can be stored, hoarded, and amassed. With grain agriculture came larger-scale and more hierarchical social organization, and power has been concentrated more and more ever since. Each of us reclaims some of our power when we become small-scale producers or part of the informal sector that supports them, living the slow food ethic.

Street Food and the Importance of the Informal Economy

One way in which regulatory bureaucracies all around the world bear down upon informal, small-scale food production is through mass enforcement actions against street vendors. I receive online reports of crackdowns on street food vendors almost every week. It's happening on every continent, always in the name of safety and hygiene, as well as in defense of "legitimate" businesses that bear greater overhead costs. In many places, rules categorically exclude street vendors, without regard for the safety standards they practice. Carts and food are confiscated, and vendors are harassed, fined, or even arrested (as in Zimbabwe; see page 104).

Personally, I love street food. It's cheap, fast, and easy. I know the theme of this chapter is *slow* food, but I think that informal street food, even though it is fast, is an important part of the cultural context championed by Slow Food. "Fast food, street food, market food, is a part of the cultural idiom of nations; it can't be franchised out any more than oral history can be," writes cultural historian Katherine Dillon through the Listserv of the Association for the Study of Food and Society. "It's that local, that loved, that known."[48]

Some of the most delicious and memorable food I have ever eaten has been from street vendors. Wherever in the world I have traveled, I have enjoyed street food. I think of street food from my travels in Africa most vividly. *Harira* is a spicy tomato-based soup served in infinite variations by Moroccan street vendors. In West Africa, sticky, starchy *fufu* was a daily staple I frequently bought at street stalls; it's made from pounded cassava, usually sharp from fermentation, and served with stew for dipping.

Typically a street vendor is a small-scale operation. In its simplest manifestation it is simply food prepared in the home and then brought out to the street to sell. This is the informal economy, an easily accessible way to use culinary skills to earn some money without a wage job and without investing big bucks. In this informal realm many people support themselves and feed themselves. It seems like free trade to me. Expensive facilities do not guarantee good hygiene. Conscientious practices do.

When I was a kid, some of New York City's Upper West Side neighborhood food shops sold pastries that were prepared by old women, immigrants from Europe, in their home kitchens. This was considered acceptable practice and even something to boast about. Increasingly, though, such informal practices are not tolerated. In 2005 the Tennessee agriculture department cracked down on vendors at the Greeneville Farmers' Market in eastern Tennessee. Vendors were informed they could no longer sell jams, jellies, pickles, baked goods, or any other prepared foods unless they were prepared in a licensed, up-to-code kitchen. In most places in the United States, a home kitchen in which daily food preparation takes place cannot be licensed as a commercial kitchen. Period.

Some of the vendors challenged the enforcement officers, asking how selling baked goods at the farmers' market was any different from selling them at a charity bake sale. "We just physically can't get to all of them," replied an agriculture department official. "We don't actively seek out somebody having a charity fund-raising sale."[49] But legally, in more and more places, even bake sales—that venerable tradition of grassroots fund-raising—are illegal.

Food production in an unregulated home kitchen is considered a potential public health danger. Because the kitchen hasn't been inspected, something could be contaminated; people could get sick; someone could die. Therefore the only way to be safe is for all food to come from inspected facilities. A friend reports that her child's school prohibits parents from sending homemade food to school events with their children. They must send prepackaged food. Without state inspection and factory standards, we are all presumed to be at risk.

And yet, look at all the informal food-swapping that goes on in peoples' lives, from kids trading sandwiches at school to potluck dinners and the informal commerce of roadside garden stands and bake sales. "Without involving any advertising agencies, shipping firms, fancy packaging, or middlemen, millions of pounds of American foods have been bought with cash in hand, bartered for, or given away as gifts every summer of our lives," writes Gary Paul Nabhan.[50] Almost always, it's okay.

Occasionally there are freak incidents of contamination, both within and outside of the system of kitchen health inspections. Sure, there are people with disgusting kitchens you wouldn't want to eat from, just as there are inspected restaurants with disgusting kitchens you wouldn't want to eat from. Eating has its inherent dangers that no amount of policing can prevent, and enforcement is always subject to corruption and officials "looking the other way." Don't succumb to the paranoid fantasy that only licensed food is safe! The free trade of delicious home cooking is a neighborly tradition everywhere that must be practiced and safeguarded.

Fortunately, centralized control can never be complete. Informal-sector food economies thrive in many varied forms. In Italy a popular the latest underground movement is informal roving restaurants called *fai date* ("do-it-yourself"). Hosts publicize locations via cell-phone text messages and offer meals for around fifteen euros. "The authorities have taken a dim view of the practice . . . because the hosts avoid paying taxes and sidestep health and safety rules," according to a British news report.[51] A similar trend has been reported in the United States. "Restaurants of dubious legality, where food is cooked in apartments and backyards, abound across the United States," writes the *New York Times*.[52] The *San Francisco Chronicle* calls them "culinary speakeasies."[53] "Unlicensed restaurants tend to be very, very, very hidden, and reticent about admitting strangers," says New York food critic Jim Leff, who also reports that "home kitchen take-outs are fairly common in the African expatriate community."[54]

Legal action taken against these marginal microenterprises does not make people safer. It only outlaws amateurism in food production and makes us more dependent upon specialists and mass production. This erodes small-scale traditional practices and promotes cultural homogenization and centralized control. Freedom-loving people everywhere can resist this process by participating in informal-sector, community-based food production.

Rediscovering Traditional Food Processing

The skills needed for community-based production of many foods have become rare and require rediscovery. In fact, this is the reason that I have come to meet so many food activists working on so many different important projects: the skills of home fermentation, just like the skills of seed saving, are low-tech rituals that people have been practicing for literally thousands of years but that have become obscure in our time;

they are mystifying to most folks because they have disappeared into invisible faraway factories, leading people to believe that they are potentially dangerous or require great scientific expertise or technical precision. We need to revive traditional food-processing wisdom and skills, which have the potential to improve health and nutrition and to increase the potential for community food sovereignty.

The promise of industrialized food processing was liberation from drudgery. "However much I value elements of the old ways," explains Gary Paul Nabhan, "neither my political fervor for them, nor my intellectual curiosity about them, would be enough to convince my mother or my aunts and uncles that there was anything more than drudgery in all that daily food preparation." When he asks his mother to teach him how her mother cooked, she replies, "That was too much work. . . . I don't want to go back there." Nabhan reflects:

> Whenever I tell them I'd like to learn some of our family's traditions in order to integrate them into my life, they hear but one thing: *He wants to go back.* . . . What is curious is that while my elders see "back" as someplace that progress has allowed them to escape from—the wrong end of a linear trajectory—I imagine my life as looping and relooping, circling back to pick up something that we have forgotten, something that we desperately need for our health and our happiness, something precious we stoop down to cradle and carry along with us, as we curve out in a new direction.[55]

The daily grind of food production—shared by all members of the household rather than heaped upon one overburdened person—is actually an important rhythm that can structure our lives and create a context for social interaction and community building. In our "liberation" from the drudgery of these activities, much has been lost. Children have been deprived of opportunities for skill-building and meaningful contributions to family life; for stimulation they turn instead to television and computer games. Harvest and food processing have historically brought people together for purposeful and ritualistic activity. The loss of control over our food in the name of convenience and liberation has actually been a major factor in community disintegration.

Reviving traditional food-processing skills involves a learning curve. Even with a great teacher, discovery is experimental, because subjective judgment is acquired only through experience, and every food can be produced in a multiplicity of ways. It is an adventure to learn to make cheese, butcher and cure meat, and ferment vegetables and grains. In the summer, when the milk from our herd of goats is most abundant, the Short Mountain kitchen becomes a cheese workshop, where several of us amateur experimentalists learn cheesemaking techniques by observing one another's successes and failures. This summer I've discovered molds, not the kinds that can grow on cheese, but rather the kinds that express shapes and hold forms. I've learned that people are much more excited to eat a given cheese if it has a cute shape rather than the amorphous blob that is formed when cheese hangs in cheesecloth. Producing food well takes some learning, at any scale. When I visited an Amish dairy farmer in Pennsylvania, he was eagerly awaiting the arrival of a one-hundred-gallon cheese tank. Though he already was producing butter, yogurt, kefir, cottage cheese, and buttermilk, he had no experience making harder cheese and quizzed me about aspects of making cheese with rennet.

In many parts of the United States we are seeing a revival of local cheesemaking and brewing (in microbreweries). I'm also finding locally produced sauerkraut and other vegetable ferments in more areas. But butchers have mostly disappeared from American life, and all those cured meat products people love (bacon, ham, salami, and so on) are complete mysteries to most of us. But they don't have to be. They simply require that we be willing to learn.

My neighbor J. and his boyfriend S. have cured ham from pigs they raise. The first year, the hams were great. Then, the next year, they brought the first of the hams to S.'s family's Christmas dinner. The ham tasted awful, but the family pretended it was delicious to be polite. J. and S. were mortified, and they realized that the ham had gone off because the weather during the initial curing period had been unseasonably warm. They waited to slaughter their next pig until it was colder outside, so the meat could cure in a cooler environment. And that seemed to do the trick.

Bill Keener, another Tennessee farmer friend, showed me a ripening salami he and his daughter Ann had prepared using methods she learned from an Italian pork farmer whose family has been making it for generations. Techniques for curing meat without chemicals have become quite obscure. Bill was concerned about the film of green mold growing over the surface. I was able to reassure him that molds are very common on the surfaces of aged foods, because the surface is the place where a food comes into contact with the spore-rich air. When we scraped it with a knife, the mold came right off and the salami was beautiful and aromatic. The Keeners were not ready to go into salami production yet, but they're learning, and one day soon, they will.

The revival and dissemination of traditional food-production skills is at the core of a slow-food movement that seeks to be accessible and democratic, promoting community-based economies, indigenous foods, and diverse cultural practices. "I think it is important for those of us who appreciate slow food to also be doing slow food," writes Jessica Prentice. "This is the only way to keep alive the idea of real food as everyday food, accessible food, common food. . . . Let's get back into our kitchens and discover the magical things that happen when cabbage meets salt, or when honey meets yeast."[56] Rediscovering, reviving, and reinterpreting traditional food-production methods reinvigorates local food systems and helps diverse cultures survive the insidious erasure caused by the global thrust for homogenization.

Recipe: Gefilte Fish with Horseradish Sauce

Gefilte fish is a Jewish Passover tradition: fish is mixed with eggs, onions, and matzo meal, then formed into balls and cooked; the fish balls are usually eaten cold with carrots and horseradish sauce. *Gefilte* means "stuffed," though this recipe, like all the interpretations I have tried, makes simple fish balls.

I associate gefilte fish with my grandmother. Nobody learned how to make it from her. My mother and her sisters viewed my grandmother's hours in the kitchen as Old World drudgery. And so gefilte fish disappeared from our lives, at least as a homemade food, as my grandmother neared the end of her life. Her gefilte fish was an annual Passover tradition that I took for granted until it was over, and then I discovered how bad commercially available gefilte fish in jars is—bland and overly fine-textured.

My grandmother, Betty Ellix, was born in 1909 near Brest, in what she always referred to as Poland, though these days it is part of Belarus, near the Polish border. Pogroms and war forced her family to emigrate, and she arrived as a child in New York, where the family settled in Brooklyn. She met my grandfather, Sol Ellix, at Coney Island. How romantic is that? One of the ways Betty showered her family with love was through the elaborate preparation of food. She would come over to our house and spend hours making savory cheese blintzes to put in the freezer that we could heat up as a quick meal. The most quoted line of my childhood was when I told her, "Grandma, it's not that I don't like *your* chopped liver. I don't like *anybody's* chopped liver."

It is common for assimilated Jews who have lost many of our food traditions to bemoan the loss of gefilte fish and other traditional holiday feast foods, as if their preparation were so mysterious and elaborate that we could not possibly learn to master them. In fact, gefilte fish is quite straightforward. It's basically the "Hamburger Helper" of fish, a classic poor people's culinary tactic of stretching scarce fish (or meat) by mixing it with other more abundant, cheaper ingredients. I taught myself to make gefilte fish, rescuing this delicious ritual from extinction within my family. Every time I make it, the familiar smell of the boiling fish stock brings me back to my grandparents' apartment, and I feel uplifted by the presence of my grandmother, as if the fishy smell of revived tradition channels her spirit into my kitchen.

Ingredients (for about twenty-five gefilte fish balls, or 5 pounds)
$2^1/2$ pounds fish meat (a mix of carp, whitefish, and pike, or others), plus bones and a head
2 tablespoons vinegar
6 large onions
6 carrots
2 large eggs
$1^1/2$ cups matzo meal
1 tablespoon honey
1 tablespoon salt, plus more to taste
1 teaspoon freshly ground black pepper, plus more to taste

My grandmother made her gefilte fish out of a mix of three fresh-
water fish: carp, whitefish, and pike. Carp is very cheap, at around a
dollar a pound. It is also rather dense in texture, and adding other types
of fish lightens the gefilte mix. To begin, filet the fish, separating the
flesh from the bones as best you can. Leaving the flesh aside, make the
fish stock: gently simmer the bones and head, along with the vinegar,
half the onions, and half the carrots, in about 2 gallons of water, uncovered. Vinegar's acidity helps release minerals from the bones. The head
is full of important fat-soluble nutrients and also contains the thyroid
gland, which releases compounds that nourish our own thyroids. Fish
stock does not benefit from all-day cooking like other meat stocks.
According to Harold McGee's *On Food and Cooking: The Science and
Lore of the Kitchen*, fish collagen melts at lower temperatures and dis-
solves much more quickly than the collagen in mammal and bird bones,
and it can be damaged by overcooking.[57] For this reason, the stock
should simmer for only about an hour.

As the stock cooks, chop the fish. A meat grinder is ideal, or you can
finely mince it with a sharp knife. My friend Merril uses a rounded-
blade chopper, sometimes called a *mezzaluna* (half moon), in a wooden
bowl. Or you can use a food processor, though if you do, be sure not to
overprocess it into a paste or you will lose the texture of the fish. Finely
chop or process the remaining onions. Scramble the eggs, and mix
them together with the fish, onions, matzo meal, honey, salt, and
pepper. Traditionally matzo meal is used in gefilte fish, but any bread
crumbs will do. Mix these ingredients thoroughly. If the mixture is too
dry and fails to bind, add a little water to help it hold together.

Strain the stock and discard the spent solids. Add salt and pepper to
the stock to taste. Slice the remaining carrots (diagonally is how my
grandmother always sliced them). Form the fish mixture with a spoon
and your hands into oval fish balls. Drop the fish balls and carrot slices
into the hot stock, and gently simmer for twenty minutes. Remove the
gefilte fish and carrots from the stock. Cool the stock, which will thicken
into a somewhat gelatinous consistency. Pour the cooled gelatinous stock
over the gefilte fish and carrots, and refrigerate. The gelatinous stock
keeps the gefilte fish from drying out. The stock was my grandfather's
favorite part of gefilte fish, and we grandchildren would watch him slurp
that gelatin down in grossed-out disbelief. Now I've come to enjoy the

gelatin—concentrated nutrients from the whole fish—and appreciate its rich flavor and unusual consistency. I grew up eating gefilte fish cold, with a few carrot slices, and always with plenty of horseradish sauce.

Horseradish sauce is extremely simple to make: At least a few hours before serving, finely grate horseradish roots. Salt to taste and add just enough vinegar so that when you press down on the grated horseradish, it is submerged in liquid. Grate a little beet into the sauce too, for red color. Horseradish is an easy-to-grow perennial plant. Harvesting inevitably leaves root fragments that regenerate into new plants.

You can vary the gefilte fish recipe with whatever fish are available to you. I made delicious gefilte fish in Maine with hake, sole, and monk-fish tails my friend Ed brought home from the fish auction where he works. It was winter, and we enjoyed them not only cold, the way I grew up eating gefilte fish, but hot in the rich and soothing fish stock, like fish dumplings in a Vietnamese soup.

Recipe: Shav

Shav, a cold sorrel soup, is another compellingly delicious Old Country food that I associate with my grandparents. They kept a pitcher of it in the refrigerator in summer and drank it out of a glass. Sorrel is a sour green with cooling qualities, a perfect refreshing treat for a hot summer day. Sorrel is not commonly found in U.S. supermarkets, but it is among the easiest foods you can grow yourself, because in contrast to other greens, sorrel is perennial. This means that the plant lives for years, sending up fresh greens each year from the same roots. Sorrel also grows wild; the variety that grows as a weed in our gardens looks something like clover and is known as wood sorrel.

> **Ingredients** (for 1 gallon, or eight large or sixteen small servings)
> 1 pound potatoes (some recipes specify "mealy" potatoes)
> 1 pound sorrel
> 1 tablespoon butter or oil
> Salt to taste
> Sour cream

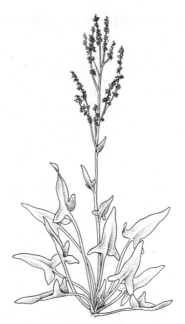

Sorrel. ©Bobbi Angell. Used by permission.

Peel and coarsely chop the potatoes. Clean the sorrel and separate the leaves from the fibrous stalks. Tie the stalks into a bundle with cheesecloth, and boil them with the chopped potatoes for about fifteen minutes in $3^1/2$ quarts of water (or a stock for a richer flavor). Meanwhile, chop the sorrel leaves and sauté them in butter or oil for just a moment, until they wilt. Remove the bundle of stalks from the stock, squeeze any excess water from them back into the stock, and then discard the stalks. Mash the potatoes in the stock to thicken it, add the sautéed sorrel, and simmer for five minutes. Add salt to taste. If you have pickle brine or sauerkraut juice on hand, you can use it instead of salt, adding it to the soup after it has cooled to body temperature; the brine or juice will contribute not only the salt it contains but also other flavors and live-culture goodness. Allow the soup to cool and store it in the refrigerator. Serve shav cold with a dollop of sour cream (see recipe, page 178).

The sour cream served in shav not only enhances the flavor but also plays an important protective role. Sorrel has high levels of oxalic acid, which can create problems, including kidney stones, when consumed in large quantities. Dairy calcium neutralizes the oxalic acid.

Action and Information Resources

Books

Alley, Lynn. *Lost Arts: A Celebration of Culinary Traditions*. Berkeley: Ten Speed Press, 2000.

Heldke, Lisa M. *Exotic Appetites: Ruminations of a Food Adventurer*. New York and London: Routledge, 2003.

LaDuke, Winona. *All Our Relations: Native Struggles for Land and Life*. Cambridge, MA: South End Press, 1999.

Nabhan, Gary Paul. *Why Some Like It Hot: Food, Genes, and Cultural Diversity*. Washington, DC: Island Press, 2004.

Nabhan, Gary Paul, and Ashley Rood, eds. *Renewing America's Food Traditions (RAFT): Bringing Cultural and Culinary Mainstays of the Past into the New Millennium*. Flagstaff, AZ: Center for Sustainable Environments at Northern Arizona University, 2004. Available online at www.environment.nau.edu/raft.

Petrini, Carlo, and Ben Watson, eds. *Slow Food: Collected Thoughts on Taste, Tradition, and the Honest Pleasures of Food*. White River Junction, VT: Chelsea Green, 2001.

Prentice, Jessica. *Full Moon Feast: Food and the Hunger for Connection*. White River Junction, VT: Chelsea Green, 2006.

Shiva, Vandana. *Biopiracy: The Plunder of Nature and Knowledge*. Cambridge, MA: South End Press, 1997.

————. *Tomorrow's Biodiversity*. New York: Thames and Hudson, 2000.

Periodicals

Cultural Survival (quarterly)
215 Prospect Street
Cambridge, MA 02139
(617) 441-5400
www.cs.org

Food, Culture & Society: An International Journal of Multidisciplinary Research (quarterly)
Association for the Study of Food and Society
www.food-culture.org

Slow: The International Herald of Good Taste (quarterly) and *The Snail: All the Food That's Fit to Print* (quarterly)
Available from Slow Food USA (see below)

Film

The Meaning of Food. Pie in the Sky Productions, 2005; www.pbs.org/opb/meaningoffood/.

Organizations and Other Resources

Alaska Native Science Commission
429 L Street
Anchorage, AK 99501
(907) 258-2672
www.nativescience.org

American Chestnut Foundation
PO Box 4044
Bennington, VT 05201
(802) 447-0110
www.acf.org

American Livestock Breeds Conservancy
PO Box 477
Pittsboro, NC 27312
(919) 542-5704
www.albc-usa.org

American Prairie Foundation
PO Box 908
Bozeman, MT 59771
(406) 585-4600
www.americanprairie.org

Bring the Salmon Home Campaign
Karuk Tribe of California
PO Box 1016
Happy Camp, CA 96039
(530) 493-5305
www.karuk.us

California Food & Nutrition Program
Northern California Indian
    Development Council
241 F Street
Eureka, CA 95501
(707) 445-8451
www.ncidc.org

Indigenous Environmental Network
PO Box 485
Bemidji, MN 56619
(218) 751-4967
www.ienearth.org

Indigenous Peoples Council on
    Biocolonialism
PO Box 72
Nixon, NV 89424
(775) 574-0248
www.ipcb.org

Intertribal Bison Cooperative
1560 Concourse Drive
Rapid City, SD 57703
(605) 394-9730
www.intertribalbison.org

Makah Tribe
PO Box 115
Neah Bay, WA 98357
(360) 645-2201
www.makah.com

Native Seeds/SEARCH
526 North 4th Avenue
Tucson, AZ 85705-8450
(866) 622-5561
www.nativeseeds.org

Native Web
Resources for Indigenous Cultures
    around the World
www.nativeweb.org

Navdanya
A-60, Hauz Khas
New Delhi 110016
India
www.vshiva.net

Pawpaw Foundation
The PawPaw Foundation
c/o Pawpaw Research
147 Atwood Research Facility
Kentucky State University
Frankfort, KY 40601-2355
www.pawpaw.kysu.edu

Renewing America's Food Traditions
    (RAFT) Coalition
Center for Sustainable Environments at
    Northern Arizona University
PO Box 5765
Flagstaff, AZ 86011
(928) 523-0637
www.environment.nau.edu/raft/index.htm

Seed Savers Exchange
3094 North Winn Road
Decorah, IA 52101
(563) 382-5990
www.seedsavers.org

Sequatchie Valley Institute/Moonshadow
1233 Cartwright Loop
Whitwell, TN 37397
(423) 949-5922
www.svionline.org

Slow Food International
Via Mendicità Istruita, 8
12042 Bra (CN)
Italy
(39) 0172 419 611
www.slowfood.com

Slow Food USA
20 Jay Street, Suite 313
Brooklyn, NY 11201
(718) 260-8000
www.slowfoodusa.org

Society for the Preservation of Poultry
    Antiquities
Route 4 Box 251
Middleburg, PA 17842
(570) 837-3157
www.feathersite.com/Poultry/SPPA/SPPA
.html

Village Earth
PO Box 797
Fort Collins, CO 80522
(970) 491-5754
www.villageearth.org

White Earth Land Recovery Project
32033 East Round Lake Road
Ponsford, MN 56575
(218) 573-3448
www.nativeharvest.com

CHAPTER 5

The Raw Underground

Everything we eat starts out raw. Cooking transmutes the raw products of agriculture into many wonderful forms, but in the application of heat, certain nutrients are diminished. Enzymes critical for digestion and nutrient assimilation are destroyed, as are bacteria that both protect the raw food from pathogenic bacteria and contribute to our intestinal microbial ecologies. Raw food is literally alive with these bacteria and enzymes. I love hot food, and I'm not promoting a raw-only dogma. However, most of us would do better to incorporate more raw foods into our diet. This chapter explores various movements promoting raw foods.

Unfortunately, raw foods are increasingly viewed as dangerous, and laws enacted in the name of public health and safety are requiring more and more foods to be sterilized prior to sale, by pasteurization or irradiation. Pasteurization, named for pioneering French microbiologist Louis Pasteur, involves heating the food to the point at which most bacteria die. Specifically, the food is heated to at least 161.5°F (72° Centigrade) and held at that temperature for at least fifteen seconds. Ultra-high-temperature pasteurization means heating the food to an even higher temperature (at least 280°F/138°C) for at least two seconds, for more thorough sterilization and longer shelf life.

Pasteurization has come to refer to a range of sterilizing processes. In 2002, as part of its massive "farm bill," the U.S. Congress explicitly granted the U.S. Food and Drug Administration (FDA) the power to approve any technology capable of killing pathogens as a form of "pasteurization," not requiring special labeling.[1] Irradiation, one such process, uses high doses of radiation—"seven million times more irradiation than a single chest X-ray," according to the Centers for Disease Control[2]—to kill pathogens and extend shelf life. This technology, developed in the 1970s by the U.S. Department of Energy as part of its Byproduct Utilization Program, uses cobalt 60 and cesium 137, both nuclear industry by-products. Irradiation, sometimes referred to as "cold pasteurization," is often applied to fruit juices, fruits, vegetables, spices, meats, and seafood. Yet irradiation has been shown to diminish the nutritional value of food. Irradiation also alters the molecular structure of the food and generates free radicals and radiolytic products, including benzene, formaldehyde, and other known mutagens and carcinogens, as well as "unique radiolytic products" for which no rigorous safety testing has ever been performed.[3] Nevertheless, Congress has prohibited the U.S. Department of Agriculture (USDA) from restricting distribution of irradiated foods through school lunch and child nutrition programs.[4]

Irradiation has been embraced by global food traders because it facilitates long-distance transport of their products. Irradiation plants are being constructed around the world and are considered an essential element of a food-exporting economy. As more foods are routinely irradiated—without being labeled as such—I wonder whether *all* commercial food will come to be irradiated over time, required to be devoid of life forces.

Is raw food dangerous? It certainly can be. Food can be a vector for the spread of a host of diseases, including bacterial food poisoning, such as from *Salmonella*, *Listeria*, and *E. coli*. But the reasons these pathogens are so prevalent in our food all have to do with the scandalous practices of factory farming and industrial food. Raw food is not inherently dangerous. Most often, food is contaminated in the course of its processing, handling, and storage or as a result of diseased animals. Healthy plants and animals produce safe food. Go outside of the factory-farming system and find (or help create) sources you can trust.

If we do not eat raw food, and every food we eat is cooked, pasteurized, or irradiated, then we fail to obtain important nutrients, and our health *will* suffer.

Challenging Milk Dogma

Many different foods are now routinely sterilized, but the food most strongly associated with pasteurization is milk. In most places milk cannot be legally sold unless it is pasteurized. In its raw, unprocessed form this most basic food is widely viewed as a threat to public safety. Nevertheless, a growing movement of people around the world are coming to the conclusion that milk as it is when it comes out of the udders, without being processed by pasteurization, irradiation, or homogenization, is superior to the processed product available legally. Raw milk enthusiasts are banding together to form distribution networks, and they are finding small-scale dairy farmers willing to join them in circumventing or defying mandatory pasteurization laws. The raw milk underground is one of the most widespread civil disobedience movements in the United States today.

Milk in its raw state, like any food in its raw state, is alive. It tastes better than pasteurized milk, is more nutritious because its vitamins haven't been degraded by heat, and is easier to digest because the naturally occurring enzymes and bacteria that break it down inside our bodies haven't been destroyed. The bacteria found in healthy milk also *protect* the milk from developing pathogenic bacteria, functioning as a built-in immune system.

Mark McAfee owns Organic Pastures, a 350-cow dairy that is the largest raw dairy in the United States, in California, one of the states where raw milk is legal for retail sales. "Twenty-four million servings and zero reported illnesses," states the crusading McAfee, describing his company's safety record. "Eleven thousand tests and no human pathogens!" McAfee has even inoculated pathogenic bacterial contaminants such as *E. coli* O157:H7, *Listeria*, and *Salmonella* into his raw milk and into pasteurized milk. In the raw milk, none of the pathogens were able to survive, because the naturally occurring bacteria and the acids they produce do not allow them to. However, in the pasteurized milk, which is devoid of bacterial and enzyme activity, the introduced pathogens easily proliferated. McAfee is so proud of his milk's testing record that he posts test results on his Web site.[5]

In addition to bacteria, milk naturally contains many enzymes, almost all of which are inactivated by pasteurization. One enzyme, lactase, digests lactose, the milk sugar that so many people cannot digest. Pasteurization is what *makes* milk indigestible for many people; among people who do not drink milk because they cannot tolerate lactose, many find that they *can* digest and enjoy milk raw, due to the presence of lactase. Another enzyme, phosphatase, is essential for the release and absorption of the minerals phosphorus and calcium. Calcium is a major nutrient people seek in milk, and pasteurization renders it largely unavailable. And still another enzyme, lactoperoxidase, produces hydrogen peroxide, another built-in system for protecting the milk from potentially pathogenic bacteria. Beyond destroying these and other enzymes and bacteria, pasteurization diminishes milk's content of heat-sensitive vitamins (including B_6, B_{12}, and C) and otherwise alters many other of its nutritional qualities. Real milk—from healthy animals and consumed raw—provides important nutrients.

Pasteurization is not the only problem with contemporary milk production. As has been the case in other food industries, control of our milk has been concentrated in a handful of corporations. Dean Foods is the largest milk corporation in the United States, processing more than two billion gallons of milk per year, and it owns many regional milk labels, including Alta Dena, Berkeley Farms, Borden, Brown's, Mayfield, Meadow Gold, Mountain High Yogurt, Purity, Shenandoah's Pride, and Horizon Organic Milk, as well as soy processors Silk, Sun Soy, and White Wave. According to the USDA, producers with sales of $800 million or more accounted for 69 percent of U.S. dairy sales in 1998.[6] Industry concentration continues to increase.

Much of this milk—nobody knows exactly how much, but then it all gets mixed together in bulk tanks anyway—is produced using the recombinant bovine growth hormone (rBGH), a genetically engineered drug that increases milk production in cows. This hormone is manufactured by Monsanto and is banned all around the world except in the United States, Mexico, and Brazil. Canada banned rBGH after a group of scientists convened by the government reviewed the rBGH studies that were the basis of the U.S. approval; their report concluded that the FDA approval process "was largely a theoretical review taking the manufacturer's conclusions at face value. No details of the studies nor a critical analysis of the quality of the data was provided."[7]

In overstimulating milk production, rBGH also causes udder infections. Milk from infected udders is really a mixture of milk and pus, the polite euphemism being "high somatic cell count." The drive to maximize production creates disease, and pasteurization makes the diseased product somewhat safer. To try to avoid infection, use of rBGH is usually accompanied by even heavier dosing of cows with antibiotics, leading to heightened risk of antibiotic-resistant diseases in both cows and humans. Milk from cows treated with rBGH also has elevated levels of insulin-like growth factor-1 (IGF-1), a compound found in all milk, but at higher concentrations in rBGH milk, that is linked to breast, prostate, lung, and colon cancer in humans.

Beyond all these health implications of contemporary methods of milk mass production, another compelling reason to seek out real milk—local raw milk—is taste. Milk from healthy animals, in its raw state, is much more satisfying and delicious than the processed product you can buy in the supermarket. As is the case with any other food, farm-fresh and unprocessed tastes best. Try some and see for yourself; chances are, there is a real milk distribution network near you.

A Brief History of Mandatory Pasteurization

Perhaps you are wondering how raw milk came to be illegal and associated with disease if all these virtues I'm singing are for real. The reality is that not all milk is created equal. Traditionally, cows have been pastured (not pasteurized), given plenty of space to graze on grass. This is how ruminants thrive. This practice makes for mostly healthy animals and safe, nutritious milk. Ruminants evolved grazing, and milk (as well as meat) from grass-pastured animals is more nutritious than that from animals fed primarily grain, especially in terms of beneficial omega-3 fatty acids[8] and a nutrient called conjugated linoleic acid (CLA), an important omega-6 fatty acid that is found in milk from grass-fed animals in concentrations up to five times the amount found in milk from grain-fed animals.[9]

As a result of rapid urbanization, particularly during the nineteenth century, many dairies expanded their herds to meet rising demand for milk, while simultaneously pasture land was getting crowded out. This forced urban dairies to search for more space-intensive methods. Meanwhile a domestic liquor-distilling industry began to develop in the United States, which produced lots of waste in the form of spent grains known as "swill" or "slop." The urban dairies found in the distilleries' by-product a cheap alternative to pastures for feeding their cows. The two industries joined together, first in New York City, and slop dairies became widespread around the United States by the 1830s.

Slop diets kept cows lactating, but it made them unhealthy. "The milk was so defective in the properties essential to good milk that it could not be made into butter or cheese," writes naturopathic doctor and dairy farmer Ron Schmid, author of *The Untold Story of Milk*.[10] Instead of keeping cows outside grazing in pastures as cows always had been, the new dairy industry confined their cows and fed them slop. Their feces were concentrated rather than dispersed, and they wallowed in it. Nonetheless the milk produced by the slop dairies was popular, because it was cheap. By 1852 three-quarters of milk sales in New York City were of slop milk. Problems were developing as well, specifically rising mortality rates among infants, leading to debates over "the milk problem."

Two distinct milk reform movements emerged in the 1890s. One, advocated primarily by medical doctors, called for "certified milk." The "milk cure" was a long-established healing regime prescribed by many medical doctors of the time, and good-quality milk was regarded by the profession as an important factor in maintaining health. Milk certifying commissions were formed by medical associations in many areas. The commissions established hygiene and care standards for farms, performed inspections, and gave their seals of approval to milk from farms meeting the standards.

The other reform movement advocated pasteurization as the most effective means of making the milk supply safe. The two contrasting approaches to safe milk—certification and pasteurization—are not mutually exclusive. It is possible to have a regulatory scheme in which some or most milk is pasteurized (and clearly labeled as such), while other milk that meets some specified standard can be sold raw (and clearly labeled as such). Such is the situation in California and several other states today, and historically, both regulatory schemes overlapped in most places.

Pasteurization is simple, and it dramatically improved infant survival rates. A powerful advocate for pasteurization was New York philanthropist Nathan Straus, a partner in Macy's department store. Straus funded the establishment of "milk depots" around New York, where slop milk was pasteurized and sold cheaply starting in 1893. Between the milk depots and the new system of chlorinating the New York City water system, the epidemic of infant mortality rapidly receded. The diseased milk from the slop dairies was rendered safer by pasteurization, but still it lacked the nutrients, enzymes, and bacteria found in raw milk from healthy pastured cows. Pasteurization was and is "a quick, technological fix."[11]

Quick technological fixes have their appeal. New York's success with pasteurization spurred its rapid spread. In 1908 President Theodore Roosevelt, an old friend of Straus, ordered a study of milk pasteurization, and the Surgeon General declared: "Pasteurization prevents much sickness and saves many lives."[12] A 1911 National Commission on Milk Standards recommended mandatory pasteurization—except for certified milk. By 1917 pasteurization was legally required or officially encouraged in forty-six of the fifty-two largest U.S. cities, and over time, systems of milk certification gradually died out in most places.

The rise of mandatory pasteurization solidified the myth that raw milk is inherently dangerous—regardless of the conditions of the animals it comes from. This has become dogma. The people charged with protecting the public health are so thoroughly indoctrinated with the idea that raw milk is inherently dangerous that raw milk is always the presumed culprit if someone who has drunk it falls ill. "Allowing the sale of raw dairy products goes against everything I ever learned and everything that public health stands for," said Suzanne Jenkins, head epidemiologist at the Virginia Department of Health, in 2004.[13] Public health authorities have a difficult time recognizing that the quality of the milk is determined by how the animals are kept.

As the pasteurization-promoting Straus said, "If it were possible to secure pure, fresh milk direct from absolutely healthy cows, there would be no necessity for pasteurization. If it were possible by legislation to obtain a milk supply from clean stables after a careful process of milking, to have transportation to the city in perfectly clean and closed vessels, then pasteurization would be unnecessary."[14] A hundred years later, we have refrigeration, and it *is* possible to obtain pure, fresh milk that meets all of Straus's criteria. When healthy cows are removed from confinement and allowed to graze in pastures, their milk is healthy and safe.

Unfortunately, most places do not permit or regulate the retail sale of raw milk. In most of the United States and much of the rest of the world, it is simply illegal to buy or sell raw milk. As more and more people learn about the benefits of raw milk and want to start drinking it, a grassroots underground has emerged, linking consumers directly to dairy farmers with small, pastured herds.

The Grassroots Raw Milk Movement

I've been astounded by how widespread the raw milk underground has become. It really is a grassroots movement because obtaining raw milk, in most places, involves community-organized effort bringing people together for a purpose, and generally that purpose involves breaking the law. It's happening all over. The *New Yorker* reported in 2004, "In a Hell's Kitchen basement the other day, Manhattan's first shipment of raw milk—unpasteurized, unlicensed, unhomogenized, and illegally transported across state lines—was delivered to the grateful, if wary, members of a private raw milk coven."[15] An Atlanta raw milk organizer I know is part of a "totally illegal" goat milk co-op: "I split the drive once every five weeks with five other women to a farm that's one hour away. We buy raw milk, cheese, and yogurt she makes."

In many places a gray area exists between raw milk that is specifically illegal and that which is specifically legal. It is in this quasi-legal realm that much raw milk distribution takes place. For example, in Australia real milk is being distributed and sold as beauty products: "body milk" and "body cream." There is no law prohibiting this and no way to control what people do with their body milk when they get it home. Where I live, in Tennessee, as in several other states, farms may sell raw milk directly off the farm "for pet consumption only." A Wisconsin cheesemaker is marketing her raw cheeses as "fish bait."

The most widespread means of circumventing laws prohibiting the sale of raw milk is to redefine the relationship between the parties so that no sales transaction takes place. Generally the way this works is that a group of consumers will enter into a "cow-share" or "goat-share" contract with a farmer, whereby they technically own the animal and pay the farmer to maintain it on their behalf. In this way the sales transaction is eliminated, and so laws restricting the sale of raw milk are not actually broken. The economic exchange is for a service, which the farmer provides by feeding, caring for, and milking the animals. Raw-milk drinkers from an area often enter into a share together and take turns picking up the milk. This is a great food-consciousness and community-building exercise: shareholders get to know each other, and they all get to experience the farm and the farmer and the animals at regular intervals. And they get good, real, raw milk.

Grassroots raw milk distribution networks like this are happening all over the United States. The Web site of the Weston A. Price Foundation's Campaign for Real Milk lists hundreds of contacts around the United States. Though the details of state laws vary widely and are shifting somewhat (see pages 172–174), people everywhere want access to better milk.

Interest in raw milk has been growing thanks in large part to a woman named Sally Fallon. Sally has devoted herself to spreading the nutritional teachings of Weston A. Price, an Ohio dentist who in the 1930s traveled the world exploring the relationship between diet and health and wrote the book *Nutrition and Physical Degeneration* (1939). Price's studies of isolated populations still practicing traditional diets led him to the conclusion that traditional diets—featuring milk and other animal fats with enzymes intact as well as live ferments, and excluding processed foods and refined sugar—held the keys to human health.

Weston Price's research was respected but relatively obscure until Sally Fallon began popularizing it in her 1999 book, *Nourishing Traditions: The Cookbook That Challenges Politically Correct Nutrition and the Diet Dictocrats*. She formed the Weston A. Price Foundation (WAPF) with the ambitious mission of "restoring nutrient-dense foods to the human diet through education, research, and activism." The foundation now has more than three hundred local chapters in the United States and more than fifty chapters abroad, mostly in Canada and Australia, but also in Brazil, China, and elsewhere. Sally's work has galvanized a grassroots movement of people organizing access to real milk and other farm products at the local level.

The first time I met Sally Fallon was at a conference of the Northeast Organic Farming Association in 2003. Sally delivered a keynote address that posed the question, "What kind of economic and political system would we have as a consequence of making food choices that are truly healthy and fundamentally supportive of optimal development and superb well-being, instead of merely convenient?"[16] In exploring this question, she made it vividly clear that she is much more than a nutrition guru.

Sally Fallon has a radical analysis, and her dietary ideas are interwoven with an economic and political vision. Her vision of health encompasses not only individual nutrition but community well-being, with milk as the centerpiece of an economic revival. The farmers producing raw milk and dairy products are finding prosperity providing raw milk from pastured cows directly to consumers. The direct-to-consumer raw dairies stand in stark economic contrast to the standard arrangements that are driving small dairy farmers out of business at an alarming rate: purchasing all the inputs (such as grain, rBGH, and antibiotics), then selling the milk to bulk processors, who pasteurize, homogenize, package, and market the milk and receive most of the profits. Providing healthy milk directly to consumers is dramatically more lucrative for the farmers. It takes prosperity back from the mass processors and returns it to the farm and the community.

"The one major impediment to this happy picture," says Sally, "is the anti-raw milk agenda—scare-mongering propaganda and compulsory pasteurization laws." But rather than accepting these laws as prohibiting a raw milk revival, she sees the possibility that they can actually benefit farmers and appealed to the assembled organic farmers to join the raw milk underground:

> In fact, now that we are rolling back the propaganda and creating more and more customers for raw milk and related products, these pasteurization laws can actually work to the benefit of farmers. If people can't get raw milk in stores, they will make the effort to come to the farm, or pay you for the service of delivering your products to their doorstep. The farm-share

system also allows you to provide other value-added products which health laws prevent you from selling directly—farm-butchered meat, sausage, baked goods, and so forth could be "provided," not "sold," to farm-share owners.

Like community-supported agriculture, this is a structural revolution.

The people who are part of this growing market for raw milk defy any easy political categorization. The raw milk scene is very "family values"— because the people who get most passionate about milk are mothers. "Passionate moms will win!" is Mark McAfee's raw milk movement mantra. Sally Fallon is a passionate mom who became a nutrition crusader as a result of what she learned while trying to feed her kids well. S., the organizer of the Nashville-area raw milk underground, is another passionate mom. She's a Christian who homeschools her two kids, and for a while she embellished her e-mails with a quote from George W. Bush: "The proper response to difficulty is not to retreat, it is to prevail." I'm not accustomed to being allied with people who find inspiration in Bush, but I am never one to demand total ideological agreement.

S. sent an e-mail to Tennessee raw milk enthusiasts recommending that we support a Republican candidate for governor who had been sympathetic to the legislative effort to legalize on-farm raw milk sales. "According to my sources, if all the raw milk supporters out there got busy and started supporting her we could see some real progress made for the raw milk bill," wrote S. "I know some of you are Democrats, but I guess how you vote will depend on how much you want to see raw milk legalized in this state. You may have to hold your nose and vote for the Republican gubernatorial candidate this time, if raw milk is important to you." Raw milk is important to me, but not more important than environmental protection, or health care, or the rights of queers and immigrants to exist, or of women to control their own bodies, or of workers to organize into unions. Even if I were a single-issue voter, raw milk wouldn't be that issue.

It's interesting how an issue such as raw milk, which is a question of freedom from regulations ostensibly designed for consumer protection, challenges peoples' political ideologies and alignments. Is the state really just trying to protect milk drinkers? How much influence do the milk processors—the major organized stakeholders—have in blocking

legal reforms that would regulate direct farmer-to-consumer raw milk
sales? How much freedom should people have to reject the prevailing
public health dogma and assume the risk of drinking raw milk? Is the
answer different if they are feeding it to their children?

Though we have not explored the differences in our political values,
S. and I find common ground to stand upon. Our shared interest in the
availability of raw milk—as well as a shared sense of the absurdity of the
very concept of the state prohibiting the trade of a food in its unadulterated form—speaks to the broad appeal of issues related to food
quality. "How can we buy raw oysters, sushi, and other raw things at
restaurants, and not have the freedom to buy fresh milk off the farm?"
asks S. "Official health restrictions are discriminating and arbitrary."

Shifting Legal Terrain

In California and a few other states, raw milk retail sales are legal.
Federal laws prohibit the interstate trade of raw milk. Individual state
laws, and in some cases further restrictions placed by counties and
municipalities, make up a complex and unwieldy regulatory patchwork.
In twenty states raw milk sales for human consumption are prohibited
altogether. In some states raw milk, or sometimes only raw goat's milk but
not cow's milk, may be sold "for animal consumption." In some places
raw milk, or sometimes only raw goat's milk, may be sold directly from
the farm, in limited quantities; in Illinois and Oklahoma, customers must
provide their own containers. In Kentucky and Rhode Island, sales of raw
goat's milk are legal with a doctor's prescription. The state-by-state sum-
mary of raw milk laws around the United States that follows is current as
of publication. For the latest information on the legal status of milk in different locales consult www.realmilk.com/happening.html.

Alabama	Illegal; for animal consumption only with license
Alaska	Shares okay; also for animal consumption
Arizona	Sales okay with license and warning label
Arkansas	On-farm sales up to 100 gallons per month okay
California	Sales okay with license, except in Humboldt County

Colorado	Shares okay; milk for animal consumption must be dyed
Connecticut	Sales okay with license
Delaware	Illegal
District of Columbia	Illegal
Florida	Illegal except for animal consumption
Georgia	Illegal; for animal consumption only with license
Hawaii	Illegal
Idaho	Sales okay with license
Illinois	On-farm sales okay; customers must bring their own bottles
Indiana	Shares okay
Iowa	Illegal
Kansas	On-farm sales okay; must be labeled "ungraded raw milk"
Kentucky	Illegal; only exception is goat's milk by physician's prescription
Louisiana	Illegal
Maine	Retail sales okay with license; on-farm sales okay without license
Maryland	Illegal
Massachusetts	Sales okay with license
Michigan	Illegal; shares tolerated
Minnesota	On-farm sales protected by constitution, but contested
Mississippi	On-farm sales of goat's milk okay if less than ten lactating goats
Missouri	On-farm sales and direct delivery okay with license
Montana	Illegal
Nebraska	On-farm sales okay
Nevada	Sales okay with license; however, no such licensed dairies exist
New Hampshire	On-farm sales okay
New Jersey	Illegal
New Mexico	Sales okay with license
New York	On-farm sales okay with license
North Carolina	Illegal
North Dakota	Illegal except for animal consumption

Ohio	Illegal
Oklahoma	On-farm sales okay; customers must bring their own bottles
Oregon	Retail and on-farm sales okay for goat's and sheep's milk
Pennsylvania	Sales okay
Rhode Island	Illegal; only exception is goat's milk by physician's prescription
South Carolina	Sales okay with license
South Dakota	On-farm sales and direct delivery okay with license
Tennessee	Illegal except for animal consumption
Texas	On-farm sales okay with license
Utah	On-farm sales okay with license
Vermont	On-farm sales okay
Virginia	Illegal; some shares tolerated
Washington	Sales okay with license
West Virginia	Illegal
Wisconsin	On-farm sales and shares okay
Wyoming	Illegal

In some states where raw milk sales are prohibited, cow-share or goat-share programs are sanctioned and may openly operate and promote themselves. Elsewhere they are tolerated or function in secret or semi-secret, under the radar. In several notable cases authorities have taken action against farmers providing milk through on-farm sales or share programs, though in many of those cases the farms have ultimately prevailed in appellate rulings.

In the stories of law enforcement prosecuting dairies over raw dairy sales, there is a repeated theme of zealous officials overstepping their authority. Texas law explicitly permits on-farm raw milk sales, but that didn't prevent state health officials from raiding White Egret Farms in Austin and, a year later, based on no specific violations, issuing an "emergency order" prohibiting White Egret's sale of raw milk cheeses. White Egret Farms owner Lee Dexter is not only a dairy farmer and cheesemaker but also a microbiologist formerly employed by the USDA. She contested the order, and after two days of testimony a judge lifted it, stating that the health department "had held the farm liable for violations against regulations that were not yet in effect, did not prohibit the activity cited, were not applicable, or did not say what the [department] interpreted them to say."[17] White Egret Farms continues to sell its unprocessed milk and raw cheeses. "We prevailed because we used good science and our constitutional rights," Lee reflects.[18]

In Wisconsin, "America's Dairyland," the state agriculture department engaged in a campaign of deception and espionage in its unsuccessful effort to shut down raw milk cow-share programs. Officials agreed to sanction a cow-share at Clearview Acres, a Hayward, Wisconsin, dairy farm, and in negotiating the contract, they proposed inadequate safety and testing requirements, which farmer Tim Wightman replaced with his own more demanding protocols. Internal documents later revealed that the department had acted in anticipation of people getting sick from raw milk, so they could shut the whole program down.

The agency sent a spy to buy a share, who secretly picked up milk weekly and had it tested for over a year for the presence of *Listeria* and *Salmonella*. Officials complained when the tests kept turning out negative, according to documents released during legal proceedings. "So basically, the Wisconsin agency responsible for food safety has been caught deliberately promoting raw milk sales with improper safety protocols in an attempt to cause an outbreak of illness," concludes Wightman.[19] His healthy pasturing practices, and his insistence on safety protocols, foiled the plan with safe milk. That didn't stop the agriculture agency from trying to shut down Clearview Acres as "an imminent public health hazard," even though no pathogens had ever been detected and no one had ever gotten sick. But the courts backed Clearview Acres and ordered that the cow-share be allowed to continue. Wisconsin's cow-shares currently have about 1,100 members.

Advocates have had successes in convincing officials in some places that raw milk can be produced safely. In 2003 Colorado authorities proposed regulations making cow-shares explicitly illegal—after permitting them for nearly a decade—but they dropped the plan after meeting with cow-share participants and experts. Similarly in Connecticut, where raw milk sales are legal when licensed by the state, legislation was introduced to prohibit them. Targeting the legislative committee considering the bill, "dairy farmer Deb Taylor rounded up her customers and met with committee members, explaining in friendly terms the importance of raw milk sales for her livelihood and for their health," reports the Campaign for Real Milk Web site. "Many committee members were sympathetic and the bill died in committee."

In other places advocates have faced state officials who refuse to consider facts that contradict the dogma that raw milk is inherently dangerous, as well as powerful economic interests that have a stake in factory milk production and mandatory pasteurization. Virginia recently adopted new, more restrictive raw milk rules, and in my home state of Tennessee, a bill to legalize and regulate raw milk sales was defeated in the state senate agriculture committee.

Sadly, dairy farms are disappearing from the Tennessee landscape at an alarming rate. According to the USDA's National Agricultural Statistics Service, my state has lost 98 percent of its dairy farms since 1965, and they continue to disappear at a rate of at least one hundred operations per year.[20] At a state senate agriculture committee hearing I attended in 2005, Lawrence County farmer Franklin Sanders testified at the hearing: "In a county once covered with independent free-holders—self-sufficient farmers and small business owners—most people have become propertyless employees." In Sanders's view, echoing Sally Fallon's, raw milk is an element of reversing this process. The economies of scale of factory milk production have driven down prices, requiring farmers to grow or get out. This is the model that mandatory pasteurization promotes: bulk tank collection and processing, rather than small farms. Selling milk directly to consumers without an intermediary enables the small dairy farm to be economically viable. "The Raw Milk Bill does not ask to grant anyone special, new privileges," testified Sanders, "but would only restore a farmer's ancient common law right to sell his own produce."

Related to debates over milk pasteurization, yet distinct, are debates over cheese pasteurization. Most cheese aficionados, myself included, agree that raw milk cheeses are more flavorful than their pasteurized counterparts. New York cheese guru Steve Jenkins, author of the book *Cheese Primer*, describes pasteurized Brie and Camembert cheeses as "pretenders—inauthentic impostors bearing their names."[21]

In the United States the FDA has imposed a national standard: cheese must be made from pasteurized milk unless it is aged for at least sixty days, in which case it may be made from raw milk. This exemption is an acknowledgment that the acidic environment that forms naturally over time—which is what enables aged cheeses to be preserved—does not allow the growth of pathogenic bacteria. Effectively, this exemption means that hard cheeses such as cheddar may be sold raw, but not soft cheeses such as Brie or Camembert, which have shorter aging periods.

Despite the fact that virtually all cheese-related illnesses occur in pasteurized cheeses, the FDA's Center for Food Safety and Applied Nutrition is exploring the elimination of even the aged-sixty-days exemption and requiring across-the-board cheese pasteurization. The United States has also pushed, unsuccessfully, to establish mandatory cheese pasteurization as the international standard for trade at the Codex Alimentarius Commission, an international entity that sets standards for food trade.

In the European Union, where mandatory pasteurization was proposed and debated in the early 1990s, policies have mostly taken a different turn. Many European lands have strong and proud living regional cheesemaking traditions and widespread appreciation of the various qualities embodied in different cheeses. Researchers at the French Institut National de la Recherche Agronomique compared the same cheeses made from raw and pasteurized milk and concluded that "pasteurization modifies the biochemistry and microbiology of ripening, and the flavor and texture of cheese."[22] Rather than mandating pasteurization as the only safety net against cheese contamination, the European Union created a broad regulatory framework based on microbiological risk assessment. Some laws of E.U. member states actually *forbid* pasteurization, for example the French Appellation d'Origine Controlée ("Name of Controlled Origin") laws, which dictate that certain cheeses must be made exclusively from raw milk. "Milk must come from herds in good health that have regular sanitary controls," says Jean Garsuault, president of L'Institut International du Fromages.[23] "The milk must be collected, transported, stocked, and transformed within a short period of time, applying strict hygienic rules."

Recipe: Sour Cream and Cottage Cheese from Raw Milk

Though I relish any opportunity to patronize nonsanctioned markets, I have not had to resort to civil disobedience for access to raw milk. I've had the privilege of living with a small herd of goats for thirteen years now. For me the connection to these goats—at present Sylvia, Lovegoat, Lynnie, Lentil, Luna, Lydia, and the reigning queen of the herd, Persephone—has been a great and unanticipated benefit of community living. On my own I would never have the wherewithal to sustain the twice-daily ritual of milking. I like to do other things too much, and I love travel and spontaneous adventure. However, since I share the milking with other people in our collective, it's rare that I milk more than one or two days a week, and when I go away there are others to keep things going. Food production and community building go hand in hand. Sharing the awesome responsibility of milking goats has enabled me to participate in their care without being in any way burdened.

I love these goats. I talk to them, and I wrestle with them, too. Their individual personalities and their capricious collectivity have given my life an additional dimension that it did not have without them. They are our symbiotic partners here on this land. They "browse" the mountainside munching on leaves, lichens, flowers, and seedpods, incorporating that rich phytochemical diversity—which we humans are unable to access directly—into their delicious milk. We try to take good care of them, and they provide us with milk that couldn't be fresher or more local.

The milk flow is seasonal. In the late winter it can taper off to almost nothing as pregnant goats are "dried up" and milk production is reduced by more limited grazing opportunities and the hard work of staying warm. Spring brings new kids and a renewed milk flow, which increases into the summer—at which point we get up to five gallons a day—just as the summer's relentless heat and bugs send people off on travels and reduce our human population to its annual minimum. Inevitably we run out of refrigerator space to store the milk, and as milk accumulates we turn it into kefir, cheese, yogurt, and sour cream.

One advantage of raw milk over pasteurized milk is that rather than "spoiling" into something putrid or rotten, it sours in a fairly predictable way that generates most of the dairy products we know and love. Milk that has not undergone pasteurization is host to *Lactobacillus* and other types of lactic-acid-generating bacteria. As it ages, the milk becomes more acidic. This acidity both protects the milk from potentially disease-causing bacteria and curdles the milk, coagulating fats and separating them from the watery but still protein-rich whey. The familiar dairy products all occur along this spectrum of milk acidifying itself.

Milk can also be cultured. Culturing milk involves adding to it specific live microorganisms. Yogurt is the product of culturing, made by introducing to milk, via a spoonful of a previous batch, various lactobacilli and a specific coagulating bacteria, *Streptococcus thermophilus*, that is active only at temperatures around 110°F (43°C). Kefir is another cultured milk, a tart and often effervescent drink that is sometimes described as "the champagne of milks." The culture for kefir comes not from a previous batch of kefir but from symbiotic colonies of bacteria and yeast; these small, rubbery white "grains" look like something between curds of cottage cheese and cauliflower florettes.

In different culinary traditions around the world, milk (from many different animals) is cultured with a variety of starters that evolved in those different regions. These cultures are not incidental culinary novelties; they are manifestations of complex coevolutionary processes of coexistence and integration. We, the plants and animals we eat, the cultural practices of obtaining and utilizing them, and the bacterial and fungal cultures that we use to flavor and preserve foods, are all interdependent elements of this ongoing evolutionary process. These cultured milks can then be transformed into cheeses, endlessly manipulated with temperature, salt, humidity, molds, and flavors. Every cultured milk and every cheese started as a spontaneous wild fermentation, which people selected and perpetuated. Like the phytochemical micronutrients that reflect the land and its plant growth in the milk, the unique microbial culture of the land is embodied in the ferment. Though flavors will vary with temperatures and local microbial populations, often the product of a spontaneous wild fermentation is delicious.

Sour cream and cottage cheese are the products I most often ferment from milk. This recipe is simply raw milk that is no longer fresh—day two or three or four without refrigeration—without doing a thing. I call the resulting product sour cream, though classic sour cream would start with cream rather than milk and would introduce a specific

Lactobacillus culture. My fellow communard and cheesemaker Laurel has found that leaving the souring milk a day or two longer results in the formation of firmer curds, which we call cottage cheese. These fermented forms of milk, also known as clabber, are truly the path of least resistance.

As rich condiments, raw milk sour cream and cottage cheese can excite the plainest of foods, such as a baked potato. I grew up eating sour cream (with salt and pepper) on French toast, and I love it in chili, soups and stews, and cold summer soups like shav (see recipe, page 156) and gazpacho.

So here's how I make sour cream: I pour raw goat's milk into a pot or widemouthed glass jar. The advantage of glass is that you can see what's happening beneath the surface. A wide mouth is important because you need to be able to get into it later with a spoon to gently scoop out the coagulated milk. Leave the milk out on the kitchen counter at room temperature and covered so that flies can't get in.

After one to four days (depending on the temperature) the milk will visibly separate, such that the milk fats float above the whey. Scoop out the milk fats gently—rough handling can cause them to dissipate—and enjoy them as sour cream. If you wait instead and leave the milk to ferment a day or two longer, the fats solidify further into curds of cottage cheese. Often by this point the milk will develop a film of mold on the surface. Mold is a common surface phenomenon on ferments—including not only dairy but sauerkraut, miso, and others—unless they are protected from exposure to air. Foods that have had surface molds scraped from them are perfectly safe. Simply scrape off and discard any mold. Gently scoop curds into a colander and/or cheesecloth, drain liquid off, salt to taste, and enjoy the cottage cheese.

From 1 quart of goat's milk you'll get about 2 cups of sour cream or cottage cheese. Cow's milk is different than goat's milk in that unless it is homogenized—which it won't be if it's raw—its cream rises to the top in its fresh state. The cream will rise right away, before it sours, which takes a day or two. The soured cream of cow's milk, too, is absolutely delicious.

Sour is not a static state. As days and even weeks pass (at ambient temperatures), the sour cream turned cottage cheese gets more sour, and quite extreme flavors can be achieved if that is what you desire. When your ferment reaches a pleasing level of sourness, move it to the refrigerator. If the flavors that develop spontaneously are not to your liking, try clabbering your milk in a warmer spot. Or culture the milk with a starter culture, which brings greater predictability.

Please note that if you try clabbering *pasteurized* milk, you are unlikely to have successful or appetizing results. The lactobacilli present in raw milk come into dominance easily and inhibit competitors. Pasteurized milk, on the other hand, is a microbial vacuum, a blank slate open to whatever bacteria should come along. To ferment pasteurized milk with good results, it is important to use starter cultures such as yogurt, kefir, or their many more obscure cousins from different parts of the earth.

Raw Food Revival

Beyond milk, a raw food movement has been spreading in recent years consisting of people eating primarily or exclusively raw foods. As is the case with milk, every raw product of agriculture contains enzymes and bacteria that help to digest it. Raw food goes to the nutritional source, rejecting the very act of cooking, and in some cases defying deeply ingrained taboos in order to consume food with a maximum amount of nutrients and enzymes intact.

There are many different approaches to raw food, from vegan to primarily carnivorous. The original modern-day raw foodist was Ann Wigmore, who popularized sprouts, wheatgrass juice, and a fermented sprouted-grain beverage called rejuvelac in the 1960s as part of her "living foods" diet. In big cities today a high-priced raw haute cuisine has emerged; some inventive culinary artists have taken prepared raw foods to great heights.

Other raw foodists feel that such elaborate concoctions are contrary to the simplicity of food in its raw state. Friends of mine in Australia embrace a raw ideology they call Instincto—or Instinctive Eating. James and Philippe eat primarily fruit—and incredible quantities of it. They also eat raw vegetables, nuts, fish (even prawns), meat, and salt (not *on* the food but *as* a food). They'll eat greens and avocadoes and tomatoes, but while James might toss them together into a salad (with ocean water for dressing), Philippe will eat them only as individual foods. Instinctos use their sense of smell to decide what to eat. They eat as much as they want of each food before moving on to the next. But mostly, at least in summer in Australia, they eat fruit.

I never ate anywhere near as much fruit in my life as I consumed the week I spent staying with James and Philippe at their Instincto retreat center in New South Wales. Each feeding would generate several plates piled high with skins and seeds. When I was visiting, mangoes were in season, and I stuffed my face with at least half a dozen mangoes a day. I discovered lychees for the first time there. Lychees are about the size of golf balls, and out of their hard, red, spiky skins pop succulent balls of sweet white flesh. At Instincto I could satisfy my desire with dozens of these delicious fruits each day. It felt great eating all that fruit. I love cooked food and flavors and textures way too much to give them up, but my brief time eating the Instincto way was no sacrifice. Having enough fruit to fill you up is a luxurious existence. It left me feeling sated and nourished.

The most extreme raw variation I've encountered is called the Primal Diet, the brainchild of a fellow named Aajonus Vonderplanitz.[24] The Primal Diet revolves around raw dairy, eggs, and meat, as well as raw meat that has been fermented, which Vonderplanitz calls "high meat." To facilitate the appropriate stomach pH level for effective digestion of raw meat, this diet counsels avoidance of vegetable fibers and relies upon vegetable juice as a fiber-free source of vegetable nutrients. Cailen Campbell, who was following this diet and filled me in on its details, looked great. He told me he eats salads consisting of chunks of raw meat tossed with slices of raw butter. It's a quirky, eccentric diet, but Cailen looked incredibly healthy.

Raw flesh can be very compelling. How else could sushi and sashimi and steak tartare enjoy such enduring popularity? As kids, my siblings and I always tried to sneak some of the meat our parents were cooking before it was cooked, and they always tried to stop us. My friend Orchid, whose diet has become mostly raw, procured a bit of local pasture-raised beefalo on one of his visits and served it up raw. After probably twenty years of not eating raw red meat, scared by the potential risks, I decided to throw caution to the wind and try some. I planned on having only a tiny taste, to be daring and challenge myself. That raw meat tasted so right to me that I filled up a bowl and ate a big serving, and then went back for seconds.

Though raw meat is delicious and, like other raw foods, densely packed with digestive enzymes, I am skeptical about the sustainability of any primarily meat diet. Meat calories take more land and resources to produce than plant-source foods. Sustainable food systems can *include* meat, but in most environments, the conditions for producing large quantities of meat for dense populations require excessive resources and they pollute. In a similar vein, many other raw foodists subsist on vast quantities of imported fruit out of season, depending heavily upon the global food trade and prioritizing personal health over local food production and broad sustainability.

Yet these extreme dietary ideas—and the culinary renegades who practice them—still have important contributions to offer to movements for sustainability. Raw food is nutritionally important. Salads of iceburg lettuce and cardboard tomatoes do not satisfy our need for raw nutrients. Though I remain devoted to the pleasures and comforts of cooking, of hot food, and of starchy foods, I strongly believe that most of us would do well to incorporate more raw foods, and a greater variety of raw foods, into the mix.

Recipe: Vegetable-Nut Pâté

Personally, I have felt quite inspired by some of the food coming out of the raw cuisine movement. Eating daily in a communal kitchen shared with a steady stream of visitors, I am exposed to many emerging culinary influences. I especially love pâtés, which translate simply to "pastes" and can be created from a great variety of herbs, vegetables, seeds, nuts, and even fruits, in a whole spectrum of textures. Pâtés are best served with something to spread them on, or dip into them with, such as vegetable crudités, chips, bread, or flax crackers (see the recipe on page 184). They can also be used as a creamy layer in sandwiches, omelettes, nori rolls, spring rolls, and other such constructions.

I am indebted to my fellow communard Lapis Luxury, an irrepressible kitchen experimentalist, for introducing me to the simplicity, diversity, and flexibility of pâtés. Any seeds or nuts can become a pâté; they are best and most digestible if they are presoaked. The seeds or nuts are then ground with vegetables, herbs, fruits, spices, and other flavorings (not necessarily raw) such as miso (in which the beans are cooked prior to their lengthy fermentation) or well-cooked chickpeas (to give the pâté a hummus-like quality). In fact, if you change the proportions in the recipe for chickweed pesto from chapter 1 (see page 34), using more seeds and less weeds, you can turn it into a pâté.

A food processor is the easiest way to grind the ingredients into a paste, though chopping with a knife, followed by grinding with a mortar and pestle, works fine too. Blend vegetables to a pulp first, adding water or other liquid (such as pickle brine, tamari, olive oil, vinegar, or wine) as needed. Then add soaked seeds or nuts (for more information on soaking, see page 71) and other ingredients, striving to achieve a texture thick enough to hold its form. Taste as you go and adjust proportions, salt, and spices as needed. Form the pâté into a mound (or other cute shape) on a beautiful plate and decorate it with herbs and flowers. During my "pâté du jour" period, when I was making experimental pâtés every day, the most popular offering turned out to be okra–dulse–lamb's-quarters–cashew pâté (dulse is a seaweed; lamb's-quarters is a common weed). Some of my other favorite pâté combinations are tomato–herb–miso–walnut, arugula–sunflower seed–kimchi juice, and beet–carrot–pickle brine–cashew. If some of these ingredients seem weird, don't use them; incorporate foods you like. Simmer, another fellow communard, made a delicious sweet pâté with raisins and maple syrup for her birthday. Lapis has made great pâtés using flowers and sprouts. Don't be afraid to go wild with unusual flavor combinations. If you add live-culture starters such as pickle brine, kimchi juice, or miso, you can ferment pâtés for a few days to develop tangy cheesiness.

Recipe: Flax Crackers

Flax crackers are the best crackers ever. My two professional raw chef friends, Tanya and Orchid, taught me how to make these. Raw foodists can be very particular about the maximum temperatures their foods are exposed to, so many of them use thermostat-controlled dehydrators to make these crackers. Dehydrators are great tools, but you don't need to run out and buy one. Improvise by adapting existing technology. Since I lack both a dehydrator and sufficient electrical power to run one, this recipe dehydrates the crackers in a home gas oven with a pilot light. Other options would be dehydrating under a fan, using air circulation rather than heat to dry the crackers; under the sun on a clear day; or, in a pilotless oven, by using a light bulb as a source of heat.

Soak whole flaxseeds in an equal volume of liquid. Three cups of each will yield one large (18 x 24-inch) tray of crackers. For soaking liquid you can use water and/or a flavorful liquid such as kimchi juice, pickle brine, tamari, vegetable or fruit juice, wine, or vinegar. You can also add other solid flavorings, such as shallots or onions, garlic, dill or other herbs, Thai curry paste, or anything you can imagine. Spice and salt to taste.

The flax seeds will absorb all the liquid within a few hours and form a slimy, mucilaginous mass. Oil a large cookie sheet as lightly as you can. Spread the soaked flax mixture in as thin a layer as possible without creating holes, using a rubber spatula or your hands. Wet the spatula or your hands as you spread the flax mixture to prevent it from sticking. Place the tray in the oven or other dehydrating chamber. You can use a thermometer to gauge the temperature of the oven and leave the door ajar if necessary to keep it under 110°F (43°C), the temperature at which enzymes begin to be destroyed. In a shared kitchen it is imperative to leave a sign over the oven controls so no one heats the oven and accidentally bakes the raw crackers!

Once the top surface of the flax dries into a skin, which takes about eight to twelve hours, invert the sheet of crackers directly onto a wire-mesh cooling rack, which allows air circulation from beneath, so it can continue dehydrating with greater surface area exposed. After eighteen to thirty-six hours, depending upon temperature and air circulation, the crackers will be dry and crispy. Break them into dipping- and spreading-size pieces and enjoy them with pâtés or plain. These crackers are so flavorful they can stand on their own.

Recipe: Massaged Kale

Kale is an enigma to many people. When it is raw, most seem to find it overly tough, bulky, fibrous, and strongly flavored and will eat just a taste. When cooked, it is more tender, but at the cost of lost nutrients.

Massaging kale and other heavy leafy greens offers a way to break down the tough fibers without diminishing the nutrient content. Orchid first introduced me to the simple secrets of massaging kale. As we were doing it, I realized that the massaging action accomplishes exactly the same thing as the pounding of cabbage into a crock for sauerkraut: breaking down plant fibers and releasing juices. It is really a manual mastication to initiate cellular breakdown or, in other words, predigestion.

Start with any variety of kale (or collards) and shred the leaves as finely as possible, across the stem. Dress the greens with flavorful liq-uids: olive oil, vinegar, tamari, citrus juice, pickle brine, wine, honey, hot sauce, or chili paste. Add other ingredients as desired: grated or julienned carrots, radishes, or Jerusalem artichokes; chopped tomatoes, peppers, or pickles; raisins; walnuts or other nuts; and other herbs and seasonings (Orchid likes black pepper, chili powder, and nutritional yeast). "This salad is very malleable," says Orchid. "Experiment with different oils and seasonings and bring lovely, delicious kale into your daily diet."

Mix the vegetables and dressing together with clean hands, and then start squeezing! Grab a fistful of vegetables in each hand and squeeze hard. Squish the vegetables in your hands to crush them and express their juices. This is something kids can help with. Keep mixing the veg-etables into the marinade and squishing and squeezing for a few min-utes, until the greens appear wilted and saturated with marinade. Taste and adjust seasoning, if necessary. Massaged kale is tender and deli-cious when fresh, but it can also be stored for days in the refrigerator; as the kale marinates, the flavors will meld.

Action and Information Resources

Books

Alexander, Joe. *Blatant Raw Foodist Propaganda!* Grass Valley, CA: Blue Dolphin Press, 1990.

Cousens, Gabriel. *Conscious Eating.* Berkeley, CA: North Atlantic Books, 2000.

Douglass, William Campbell, M.D. *The Milk of Human Kindness is Not Pasteurized.* Marietta, GA: Last Laugh Publishers, 1985.

Fallon, Sally, with Mary G. Enig. *Nourishing Traditions: The Cookbook That Challenges Politically Correct Nutrition and the Diet Dictocrats.* Washington, DC: New Trends, 1999.

Jenkins, Steve. *Cheese Primer.* New York: Workman, 1996.

Price, Weston A. *Nutrition and Physical Degeneration.* Lemon Grove, CA: Price-Pottenger Nutrition Foundation, 1939.

Salatin, Joel. *Holy Cows and Hog Heaven: The Food Buyer's Guide to Farm Friendly Food.* Swoope, VA: Polyface, 2004.

Schmid, Ron. *The Untold Story of Milk: Green Pastures, Contented Cows, and Raw Dairy Foods.* Washington, DC: New Trends, 2003.

Underkoffler, Renée Loux. *Living Cuisine: The Art and Spirit of Raw Foods.* New York: Avery, 2003.

Vonderplanitz, Aajonus. *The Recipe for Living without Disease.* Los Angeles: Carnelian Bay Castle Press, 2002.

Organizations and Other Resources

American Cheese Society
304 West Liberty Street, Suite. 201
Louisville, KY 40202
(502) 583-3783
www.cheesesociety.org

A Campaign for Real Milk
www.realmilk.com

G.E.M. Cultures
30301 Sherwood Road
Fort Bragg, CA 95437 USA
(707) 964-2922
www.gemcultures.com

Institut International Du Fromage
19 rue Pierre Loti
92340 Bourg-la-Reine
France
33 (0)1 46 60 06 06

Institut National de la Recherche Agronomique
147 rue de l'Université
75338 Paris Cedex 7
France
33 (0)1 42 75 90 00
www.inra.fr

Living and Raw Foods
www.living-foods.com

Organic Pastures Dairy Company
7221 South Jameson Avenue
Fresno, CA 93706
(559) 846-9732
www.organicpastures.com

PaleoDiet.com: The Paleolithic Diet Page
www.paleodiet.com

Virginia Independent Consumers and
    Farmers Association
PO Box 915
Charlottesville, VA 22902
www.vicfa.net

Weston A. Price Foundation
4200 Wisconsin Avenue NW
Washington, DC 20016
(202) 363-4394
www.westonaprice.org
www.realmilk.com

CHAPTER 6

Food and Healing (or, Beware the Neutraceutical)

here exists a strong link between the food we eat and the state of our health. That much is obvious. Sever people from traditional food practices and feed them overprocessed fats and sugars and their health—including mental health—will eventually suffer. The biggest killer epidemics of our time—heart disease, cancer, and type 2 diabetes—are all related to diet. There are many different ideas about the precise nature of the food-health connection; however, it is widely agreed that dietary factors can both contribute to disease and healing. Grandmothers, from time immemorial, have nurtured our growth and treated our ailments with chicken soups, miso broths, herbal brews, and various other concoctions intended to comfort and heal. These grandmothers and other wise women (and sometimes men) are passing on wisdom received through intergenerational tradition and reinterpreted through experience and adaptation to a rapidly changing world. This is "folk medicine," and we are all folks. Just as people have always been integrated into the natural world as we seek sustenance, so have we been integrated into the natural world in our quest for well-being and healing.

This connection to nature as a source of food and medicine is always in a broader context and always unique in its details. Traditional diets and healing practices are quite varied; they are at the core of what makes cultures distinct and unique. Scientific rationalism seeks generalized, universal, verifiable answers, such as the correct or best diet. "How can I achieve optimal health?" is the million-dollar question. Best-seller lists are full of prescriptive diets, many related to slimming, all attempting to guide humans toward some ideal of optimal health.

I personally reject the idea of any prescriptive system for "optimal health," and I think that many of the nutrition and lifestyle gurus out there exploit and feed our culture of narcissism, the desire for idealized beauty, perpetual youth, and eternal life. Health is an ebb and a flow. It's wonderful to feel healthy and strong, and easy to take that state for granted. We all get sick sometimes, and we all are going to die.

Diet is absolutely a powerful tool for healing and staying healthy. However, there is no single best means of doing this. Many people have survived what doctors declared "incurable" cancers using macrobiotics, a simple grain-based diet in which foods are pressure-cooked, steamed, baked, or fermented but rarely, if ever, eaten raw. Equally dramatic cures have been achieved by people switching to all-raw diets. Some people find healing in a vegan diet; others follow their cravings back to meat at some moment of their lives when they feel the need to build strength. I agree with Annemarie Colbin, the author of *Food and Healing*, whose nondogmatic approach to nutrition influenced me long ago, and who said, "There is no one diet that is right for everyone all the time."[1] After all, human beings are extremely adaptable, able to survive and thrive in many different climates, and this adaptability has yielded very different diets and very diverse healing practices all around the world.

Sometimes I think life might be easier with simple, straightforward, absolute answers, or a panacea, as heralded in Aajonus Vonderplanitz's *The Recipe for Living Without Disease* or Dr. Hulda Clark's classic *The Cure for All Diseases*. Who knows? Perhaps Vonderplanitz is correct that an all-raw, meat-centered diet is the solution to what ails us. Or perhaps Dr. Clark is correct that the chemical benzene—present in virtually anything processed by machine—is the root cause of most of our health problems and that we should go to great lengths to avoid exposure to it. However, I cannot believe that any single factor can be the cause of all disease. Such reductionism arouses the depth of my skepticism and makes me run the other way. The spectrums we all live through, periods of well-being and disease, are clearly multifactorial, with many and varied causes.

Denial of the Obvious:
The Twisted Chemical-Medical-Industrial Complex

Despite our popular culture's obsession with food and its effects on the body, our official health-care system barely acknowledges that a link even exists between eating and health. Most U.S. medical schools do not require any courses in nutrition; the topic receives a total of eighteen hours of attention in the average four-year medical program.[2] Indeed, most medical education, and our health-care system as a whole, is organized around a corporate agenda of pharmaceutical and diagnostic products. These technologies can be powerful and effective. But the whole health-care system is built around heroic treatment of symptoms, while ignoring nutrition, which underlies every individual's health and well-being, or lack thereof.

Nutritionists I've encountered in the medical system mostly dispense soy-based, nutrient-enhanced energy drinks, as if these neutraceutical products were the singular solution to poor eating habits. And what could be more antithetical to healing than the overprocessed junk they serve as food in most hospitals? Our medical system denies that food has any qualities beyond a uniform set of quantifiable "macronutrients." Fortified, reconstituted food products are regarded as the equivalent of fresh, nutritious whole foods. Synthetic nutrient encapsulation in the form of supplements is another presumed equivalency. The idea that synthetic powders in a capsule could really give us everything that food does is a delusion. Yet people spend billions of dollars—nearly $5 billion in 2003 in the United States alone—on vitamins and supplements.[3]

The same erroneous assumption of equivalence underlies chemical fertilization of the soil. If a chemical additive contains the essential plant nutrients of nitrogen, phosphorus, and potassium in appropriate proportions, then it is assumed to be the equivalent of feeding the soil manure and leaves and kitchen scraps. It just isn't so. The soil is alive, and our bodies are alive, and these complex life processes require a huge variety of micronutrients in order to thrive. They cannot properly sustain themselves on the limited nutrients provided by synthesized chemicals. In both cases, the chemicals give rise to the need for more chemicals. Techno-problems are addressed with techno-solutions, which inevitably create unanticipated techno-problems, and so on, ad infinitum. The pharmaceutical corporations that promote drugs as the greatest hope for better health are not so very different from the chemical corporations that promote high yields from chemical agriculture.

In its 2005 *Report on Human Exposure to Environmental Chemicals*, the Centers for Disease Control tested for the presence of 148 toxic compounds (of an estimated 80,000 in commercial use today) in the blood and urine of 2,400 people. Thirty-eight of the compounds were being tested for the first time ever in a large sample. Among them, neurotoxic pyrethroids (used in pesticides) were found to be widespread, as were hormone-altering phthalates (used in plastics—including food packaging—and "beauty" products).[4]

Pyrethroids and phthalates, like many of the chemicals identified, were found in greater concentration in children than in adults. When young people's developing bodies and minds are encumbered by chemically induced hormonal shifts and neurotoxins, this suggests a big problem. Even developing fetuses receive a steady dose of chemical exposure. The Environmental Working Group analyzed umbilical cords collected by the Red Cross and found the presence of an average of two hundred known toxic chemicals in them, pumped from mother to fetus.[5] Fetal development is when life is at its most vulnerable. Fetuses and infants do not possess the blood-brain barrier, which in older children and adults prevents some toxins from leaving the blood and entering brain tissue, and therefore, when they are exposed to certain chemicals, "they are exquisitely vulnerable to vanishingly small amounts," says biologist Sandra Steingraber.[6]

The classic approach to toxicology, which seeks to determine at what level a particular substance causes harm, was established in the sixteenth century, when a monk named Paracelsus coined the phrase "the dose makes the poison." But at different stages, such as gestation and infancy, as well as adolescence and old age, sensitivity to toxins can be much greater. According to Steingraber, "Timing makes the poison as much as the dose . . . there are times in our human development when some biological event is unfolding, and if a toxic exposure occurs during that time, you have a disproportionate risk for harm." This heightened risk is recognized by the U.S. Environmental Protection Agency's *Guidelines for Carcinogen Risk Assessment*: "The risk attributable to early-life exposure. . . can be about ten-fold higher than the risk from an exposure of similar duration occurring later in life."[7]

All of the evidence suggests that the continued widespread use of synthetic chemicals has great costs and is damaging to human health. Unfortunately the present course seems likely to continue because there are great profits to be made in the business of pharmaceuticals and pesticides, and of course "free trade" cannot be restricted. Chemical agriculture feeds the market for chemical medicine; the search for magic bullets intensifies, as profits in both industries soar and we and our earth get sicker and sicker.

Consider this: In 1989, for the first time, the U.S. economy directed greater resources toward health care than toward food. In 1960 the average household spent 17.5 percent of its income on food and 5 percent on health care. In 2003 the average household spent less than 10 percent on food and more than 15 percent on health care.[8] As we spend less and less on food, we spend more and more on health care, and many of these health-care expenses are caused by the poor quality of the food we are eating. One study I came across systematically calculated the "diet-related medical costs" of six diseases—coronary heart disease, certain cancers, stroke, diabetes, hypertension, and obesity—and found that they exceeded $70 billion in 1995.[9] A more recent calculation, by the U.S. Centers for Disease Control in 2005, found that annual health-care costs associated with obesity alone amount to $78.5 billion.[10] If we spent more on food—that is, if we valued quality in food more highly, becoming more connected to the sources of our food, the land, and local producers—we wouldn't need to spend nearly so much on health care.

Despite the huge chunk of our economy that fuels it, our high-tech health-care system is not always safe or effective. A 2000 study published in the *Journal of the American Medical Association* calculated that the third leading cause of death in the United States, behind heart disease and cancer, is the medical system itself, by way of unnecessary procedures, hospital-acquired infections, medical error, and adverse

Recipe for a Health-Care Crisis (and Enormous Profits) By Sally Fallon

Ingredients:
  Greed
  Envy
  Ignorance
  Manipulation
  Cunning
  Extortion
  Lies
  Fraud

Instructions:

Conspire to convince the populace that the natural whole foods that have nourished mankind for millennia (such as eggs, butter, whole raw milk, and red meat) are dangerous and unhealthy.

Train the medical profession to advocate antibiotics, vaccinations, fluoride, and fabricated foods as scientifically proven methods for preventing illness.

Ignore or suppress healing methods that work; claim that real diseases have no cure or do not exist.

Define normal human conditions such as menopause and average cholesterol and blood pressure levels as illnesses, which must be treated with expensive drugs that create serious side-effects.

Stew, broil, half-bake, or boil as the occasion requires.

Serves 260,000,000

Excerpted from "The Oiling of America," PowerPoint presentation, Weston A. Price Foundation conference, November 12, 2005. Used by permission.

drug reactions. The journal of the medical establishment acknowledged that the U.S. medical system causes 225,000 iatrogenic (caused by medical care) deaths per year.[11] Another 2003 analysis calculated as many as 750,000 iatrogenic deaths in the United States each year,[12] suggesting the possibility that the health-care system itself is the greatest single threat to our health. Both counts agree that 106,000 of these annual iatrogenic deaths involve reactions to prescribed drugs. Like pesticides, PCBs, and all the other synthetic chemicals in our lives, these magic-bullet solutions can be dangerous. And they impact not only the individuals who take the drugs but all of us via their growing presence in the water supply from unmetabolized drugs in human and livestock excrement as well as household, hospital, and industry disposal.[13] Pharmaceuticals become pollution.

Your health is not at the top of any corporation's agenda—not a pharmaceutical corporation or an agricultural chemical corporation or a food-processing corporation or a seed corporation. The primary agenda of corporations is return on their shareholders' investment. If they can get you to drink three liters a day of their soft drink, which will surely have health ramifications over time, they will. If they can get your doctor to prescribe—and your insurer to pay for, and you to take—their revolutionary new wonder-drug that will mitigate the problems caused by all the soft drinks, they will. Corporations always try to present themselves as being socially concerned. Indeed, they may possibly even be run by decent people with good intentions, and many fund important philanthropies. However, such gestures of goodwill are by definition secondary to their primary mission.

My Own Fall into Pharmaceuticals

After all my ranting about the superiority of whole-food nutrition to pharmaceutical symptom control, it may surprise you to learn that in my own healing odyssey I've taken prescription medicines every day for seven years, in an anti-HIV "cocktail" of protease inhibitor and antiretroviral drugs. I am a bundle of contradictions, and in a period of health crisis, when nothing seemed to be stopping my downward spiral and death seemed potentially close, I opted for medications I had seen help other friends with AIDS. The drugs seemed like my best chance, and in some situations, they are.

AIDS crept up on me slowly. I had several role models who had lived with HIV for years without getting sick, and I intended to be one of them. I was determined to demonstrate that an active outdoor country life, with fresh, homegrown, organic food, good springwater, and positive thinking, would save me from developing AIDS. After a decade of living quite well with the HIV-positive death prophecy and refusing drugs that some doctors pushed very aggressively, I found myself sinking into a state in which I felt hopeless, disconnected from people, lethargic, and unmotivated. I had less and less energy, and my outlook was grim.

As I languished in this state of uncharacteristic despair, sometime in the spring of 1999 I lost my appetite. It was the strangest thing. I have always enjoyed a tremendous appetite, always been thinking about my next meal, always derived extraordinary pleasure from food. It seemed consistent with my general state of misery that I developed a persistent nausea that made food in general unappealing. Suddenly the smell of food could make me gag. I'd take tiny portions and not be able to finish them, and sometimes I couldn't eat at all. When I went to the doctor I discovered that I had lost fifteen pounds.

I thought a change of environment might do me good and set off to visit friends in Maine. The drive from Tennessee to Maine depleted my energy profoundly. Once I arrived at Ed's house, I was barely able to get myself off the couch. I felt wiped out all the time. I couldn't walk far— and only very slowly. I had no reserve of energy to call upon when I needed to exert myself, say to lift something heavy. I felt like an old man—like my grandfather before he died at age ninety-four. I'd gingerly push myself off the couch, requiring my arms for this maneuver, gener- ally only for meals, and afterward I'd quickly return to the couch to rest my neck, sore from the hard work of sitting in an upright position.

I experienced frequent light-headedness. My balance felt precarious. On one occasion I blacked out and fainted; on many others I felt the faintness coming on and lay down before I fell. I also became aware that I was losing mental acuity. Having been a math whiz from a very young age, it stunned and terrified me to discover that I had to think long and hard to do the subtraction to keep my checkbook balanced. I started having other weird symptoms as well. One day I experienced chest tight- ness and worried that I might have some heart infection. Urination was difficult. I felt like I was falling apart, descending into the abyss of AIDS.

Still I resisted the obvious medical options. I didn't want my life to become "medically managed" for the duration. I hated with pas- sionate conviction the idea that for the rest of my life I'd be taking high-tech synthetic chemical drugs, with unknown long-term side effects, that had been developed by corporations driven by profit. These drugs are antithetical to everything I believe and the values I've devoted myself to. I regarded them as dangerous, potentially more damaging than the virus itself. As long as I felt healthy, I never even considered the drugs.

From their earliest introduction in the late 1980s, I had doubts about the anti-HIV drugs. They were enthusiastically embraced because people with AIDS were dying in droves. The sick were scared, and desperate for something, anything. But when otherwise healthy HIV-positive people started taking the early high doses of AZT, it often made them ill. The drug caused crippling nausea, anemia, muscle pain, and weakness. Many previously healthy people suffered debilitating symptoms from this drug.

In addition, I wasn't completely sold on the lone-assassin HIV theory. I believed, as I continue to believe, that the story of AIDS is more complex and multifactorial than a single rogue retrovirus. Some factors must account for the many anomalies, like the people who test positive for HIV but never develop AIDS, and others who develop AIDS symptoms but never test positive for HIV. What are those factors? Are they genetic? Behavioral? Environmental? In the AIDS activist group ACT UP[14] that I was part of in the late 1980s, we saw that expressing rage, feeling solidarity, and believing in the possibility of change were all therapeutic cofactors that helped people stay healthy. What other factors might explain individuals' widely varying disease progression?

Unfortunately, the discussion of HIV causality has grown extremely polarized. The mainstream medical establishment, as well as the AIDS service providers for the most part, view questioning the conclusion that HIV is *the* cause of AIDS as preposterous and in complete contradiction with reality. They suggest that because effective strategies for long-term treatment have been devised according to this model, it must be correct. My knee-jerk skeptic's question is, What if HIV is not the whole story? What if the varied symptoms we categorize as AIDS are triggered by other factors as yet undetermined? Knowledge is imperfect and always evolving.

The public face of HIV skepticism devolved into its own dogma, as certain that HIV does *not* cause AIDS as the medical establishment is that it *does*. HIV dissidents became known as "denialists." I'm left feeling wary of both dogma and counterdogma, angered by the arrogant certitudes of both camps, still questioning and trying to remain open on the middle road.

But as I watched myself spiral downward and my situation felt increasingly desperate, I had to do something. I decided on a last-ditch herbal therapy for intestinal parasites, on the theory that this was a condition other than generic AIDS which could be causing my wasting. The herbal regime was extreme. It gave me diarrhea and made me feel even weaker.

After years of refusing the pills, I felt I had no choice but to try them. My rejection of them was based on ideology. Though my ideas hadn't changed, my reality had. I had classic AIDS wasting and it seemed that my brain function was deteriorating. I didn't know what else to do or where else to turn. My rejection of the pills was no longer a healthy person's rejection of a suspect diagnostic category and treatment but a sick person's refusal of what appeared to be my best chance for recovery and survival. Though I am very devoted to ideas, and it is a noble thing to die for one's ideas, I was not ready to die for these ideas. If the perverse technology of my time could keep me alive, I'd gladly swallow my words along with handfuls of pills. I embraced flexibility, let go of my rigid ideas, and started taking Viracept and Combivir.

I anticipated that my body would reject the pills, as my mind had for so long. As I prepared to swallow that fateful first dose, I made sure a receptacle was nearby to receive the convulsive vomiting I imagined would immediately follow. Of course it was anticlimactic. The pills went right down, and taking them became an easy twice-a-day routine. Not that I didn't experience side effects; in fact, my first weeks on the "cocktail" were full of intestinal distress. I was bloated, horribly constipated (though I had been told to expect diarrhea), and felt like I was carrying a lead weight in my gut. I'd been warned that the drugs could be difficult to adjust to, and that initial side effects often go away after a couple of weeks. But I had no way of knowing whether these painful sensations were from the drugs or from some scary opportunistic infection, and, if they were from the drugs, whether they would really go away or how much I could tolerate. As I pondered these questions I kept taking the pills—on "the road to adherence" as a promotional video phrased it—and waiting for them to work their magic. It was difficult for me to imagine my vigor restored.

Then, slowly, I felt better. The nausea subsided and my appetite returned; I discovered great pleasure, once again, in the realm of food. One day I felt like going out for a walk. I picked up an ax and found the strength to chop some wood. I experienced erections for the first time in many months. I was shocked at how "normal" I was beginning to feel, and as time has passed much of my strength, stamina, and resilience have returned to me. Years later, I sometimes think about stopping the drugs, or at least taking a break from them, but thus far I have not done so. I am scared to. I'd prefer not to find myself back in that harrowing downward spiral. My ambivalence about being a pharmaceutical miracle notwithstanding, I am happy to be alive.

Just as I myself am a critic of the drugs I take, so I have encountered many critics of my decision to take the drugs. One of my friends, an herbalist and healer, refused to treat me because he felt I was killing myself with the drugs. His judgment was not helpful; I needed his encouragement and healing skills. He softened and came around to treating me. A friend in crisis needs to be supported, even if you think they are making wrong decisions.

Having publicly identified myself in my book *Wild Fermentation* as a person living with AIDS and taking antiretroviral medications, I receive a steady trickle of mail from well-intentioned people who feel it is their duty to let me know what a terrible mistake I have made. You are "suffering from some self-deception," wrote a reader named Peter. "If you have HIV/AIDS you have nothing, and have let yourself be fooled by lies and disinformation. . . . Whatever caused your condition or suffering, it was never any HIV."

What really irks me is the tone of absolute certainty. Peter evidently sees everything clearly and suffers no self-deception. He knows. One of my biggest pet peeves (I have many) is when meteorologists predict a 100 percent chance of rain. I would feel so much better if they expressed a 99.9 percent chance and left open the door to the possibility that their knowledge is not all-encompassing. I myself still question the drugs I am on and wonder how long my liver can sustain them. I question the lone-assassin HIV theory and wonder what as yet unidentified cofactors might be involved. However, these are abstract questions compared to the all too real experiences that got me on the drugs in the first place. I can believe that my recovery was a "placebo effect" or that the right herbal treatment or lifestyle change or dietary regime might have worked instead; but, for better or worse, it was the medical treatment that was most accessible, and it seemed to me like my best bet.

This experience has given me occasion to reflect on the dramatic treatment decisions that people are forced to make at times of health crisis. Take a deep breath. Don't panic. Stressing out will not improve the outcome. Go through the experience with courage and do what you have to do. One form of treatment does not have to preclude others. Health-care decisions are difficult and can be overwhelming. There is generally not a single best answer. Be kind to yourself and be kind to other people. Be open to guidance from intuition or unexpected sources. One important source of guidance for me comes from plants, and the plants that I love and that love me have made it abundantly clear that their nourishment and medicine are still sustaining me right alongside the six pills of synthesized chemicals that I swallow every day. Chickweed and burdock and milk thistle and cleavers and yellow dock and persimmon care for me no less because of my chemical ingestion and dependence on the medical-industrial complex.

And dependent I am, dependent on patented technology that comes at a high price. The drugs I take cost an astronomical $1,500 each month. Even though most of the basic molecular research for these drugs has been publicly funded, drug manufacturers use the research costs to justify high prices, while showing greater rates of profit than any other industry. I can afford this $50-a-day habit only by virtue of the willingness of the state to keep transferring this sum to the pharmaceutical corporations, which seems unlikely to continue for long. As I write this, in 2005, Tennessee's state health-care program, TennCare, is being dismantled. Some 325,000 people, including many of my friends living with HIV and AIDS, lost their coverage altogether; the lucky remaining recipients (myself included) have had their prescription drug coverage significantly reduced.

My friend SPREE, who was precariously close to death ten years ago when the protease-inhibitor drugs were first released, now depends upon eighteen different prescription medications. He has been terminated from TennCare, denied coverage for the drugs that have kept him alive all this time. He's managing to buy some, and he obtains others through bureaucratic ingenuity and considerable effort, but sometimes he has been unable to procure all the medications he needs. Who knows how SPREE will fare? I also wonder whether, by the time you are reading this in a year or more, the "safety net" will still provide me with these expensive drugs. Will the shrinkage of government services—other than homeland security and the war on terrorism—make health coverage for people with chronic illnesses a thing of the past? Even if you have oodles of money, if you have HIV you can't buy an individual insurance policy, at least not here in Tennessee. The only way SPREE and I and other friends with HIV got accepted into TennCare in the first place was by applying for private policies and being rejected. Now the system is tossing us aside. Will my medical miracle come to a budget-driven demise? Whatever decisions you make, it's sure nice to have choices.

Grassroots Health Activism

We are all dependent and vulnerable when health-care systems and practices revolve around corporate pharmaceuticals, diagnostics, and hospitals. The globalized pharmaceutical-driven medical system is no more sustainable than the globalized chemical-driven food industry. The food industry creates health crises that are business opportunities for the chemical industry. The earth and our bodies suffer, while corporate earnings skyrocket. Health care—like food—must be reimagined as community-based. We have to create accessible local health-care alternatives, as well as health-care education and the sharing of health-care information and skills, wherever we are.

Community-based traditions of plant healing were systematically destroyed in the witch hunts of the Inquisition. According to Barbara Ehrenreich and Deirdre English, "In the Witch-hunts, the Church explicitly legitimized the doctor's professionalism, denouncing non-professional healing as equivalent to heresy: 'If a woman dare to cure without having studied, she is a Witch and must die.'"[15] This action by authorities seeking to expand their power severed many traditional practices and drove surviving practices and practitioners underground. It also made people dependent on professionals. Health care departed from the realm of community self-sufficiency and entered the realm of experts. In the words of activist and author Starhawk, "Activities and services that people had always performed for themselves or for their neighbors and families were taken over by a body of paid experts, who were licensed or otherwise recognized as being the guardians of an officially approved and restricted body of knowledge."[16]

This is not a simple historical act that took place hundreds of years ago. It is a process that continued through the ages of colonialism and imperialism, as occupiers banned various indigenous healing practices. It also continues in our time, with laws that restrict plant knowledge and usages (see chapter 7) and ongoing cases of biopiracy, which force people to pay for biological resources that they have traditionally used for free (see pages 46–47). As we've seen in the preceding chapters, this same process of replacing community-based self-sufficiency with dependence on centralized systems has also been happening with food and seeds, and our future hinges on whether we are able to reverse this trend.

I am encouraged by meeting many people who are creating community-based health care by learning and practicing various healing traditions. My friend L. recently completed her training in acupuncture. Every Monday she runs a clinic from her rural home ten miles down the road from us, with payment on a sliding scale. I love going to see her and getting "needled." I love to feel the energetic impulses released by the needles, and after each treatment I feel reborn. L. has a gentle and reassuring bedside manner, and it is such a pleasure to watch an old friend grow into a new role as a community healer.

Any community is healthier when it has access to healers. Likewise, any healing path can be a form of activism and community empowerment if the skills and knowledge are shared in ways that are accessible to people with limited resources. Lisa's rural acupuncture clinic is an example of this, as are the peer-trained medics who help keep people safe and healthy at demonstrations, direct actions, and other organized events. A group called Katuah Medics offers a twelve-day course combining a wilderness first-responder program with protest medicine (such as treating pepper spray and tear gas) and herbal first aid. According to the group's description of the training, "Whether you are involved in direct action environmental protest, mass action street demonstrations, or extended, community resistance campaigns—and even, recently, solidarity relief with disaster victims—emergency medical training has proven a very valuable skill in our collective toolbox."[17]

Knowledge of the healing powers of common plants especially lends itself to easy diffusion and holds out the potential for anyone to become an empowered lay generalist. Just as gardening and eating wild plants empower you and integrate you into your environment, so does learning to access these plants as healing allies. Very often the very plant you need is right outside your door.

Susun Weed, an herbalist whose books have influenced me greatly, writes of three healing paths: scientific, heroic, and wise woman. The medical system—with double-blind, placebo-tested pharmaceuticals, endless specialization, and high-tech diagnostics—is a manifestation of the scientific tradition. Many healing systems commonly referred to as "alternative" make up what she terms the heroic tradition, or "the way of the savior," in which the patient is told by the healer, "Trust me," and healing is accomplished through purification and other means of error correction. The wise woman tradition contrasts with these two expertise-based healing traditions, in that the person to trust is *yourself*.

Not every health problem can be adequately treated by home remedies. It's important to know your limits and to learn to recognize when more expert intervention is necessary. But most routine health concerns can be treated at home. "Most of the health caring done worldwide, and most of the health care in your own life, is part of this third, invisible tradition," writes Susun. "The wise woman tradition of health care focuses on prevention and on remedies which are accessible, inexpensive, effective, and safe. It is time now to recognize and support the wise old woman in ourselves, our communities, and the global village."[18] The wise woman way is not restricted to women; even men can find the wise woman inside ourselves. We each need to empower ourselves, and together we need to empower our communities, with more healing skills.

As I was writing this chapter, a small sore started festering on my foot. My friend Merril took a look at it and thought it was either a bite from a venomous brown recluse spider or a staph infection. Merril is a gardener who makes the fullest use of what she grows of anyone I know, constantly drying herbs for both culinary and medicinal purposes. She dressed my sore with echinacea root powder, showed me how she did it, and sent me home with extra powder. The infection quickly cleared up; in a week all signs of it had disappeared. And now I have a technique to effectively treat a festering sore.

My friend Granite saved my life several years ago with a gallon of water. I had just been released from the hospital, where I'd been for testing related to an abscess growing on the wall of my intestine. In the hospital I was subjected to a battery of invasive internal explorations, and then I was sent home on triple-antibiotic drug therapy. I was scared and compliant and so happy to be home, but that first night at home was endless and sleepless. My kidneys hurt so badly that I couldn't get comfortable, and I really felt ready to give up and die. Granite saw how miserable I was and brought me a gallon of water. He sat with me while I drank the whole thing, and it flushed my kidneys. The pain subsided and life went on. As it turned out, the abscess persisted for as long as I took the antibiotics (several months!), then mysteriously disappeared a couple of weeks after I stopped. Hallelujah! The point of this story is that water—hydrotherapy—enabled me to endure those toxic drugs, and this simple treatment solves many conditions. The lesson learned is that people around us, like Granite and Merril, often have knowledge and skills to help us. We need to share and spread these healing skills.

I have no greater healing skill to share than simple techniques for the fermentation of vegetables. Sauerkraut, kimchi, and pickles will not cure every ailment, but they will contribute to overall well-being. Whether you are the healthiest person in the world, are facing a life-threatening health crisis, are living with a chronic disease, or are just aging like everyone else, live-culture (unpasteurized) fermented foods improve digestion, absorption of nutrients (especially minerals), and immune function. Fermenting vegetables preserves them with their nutrients intact, "predigests" those nutrients into more accessible forms, and generates *additional* nutrients, both vitamins and obscure micronutrients only just beginning to be identified and understood.

Live ferments also contain lactobacilli and other related bacteria, which repopulate and diversify the intestinal microflora. Our bacterial symbionts provide us with immunological protection by creating a densely populated, biodiverse, and thus competitive bacterial ecology in which pathogens have a difficult time establishing themselves. This is well established in medical and scientific literature, and it has been confirmed by my own experience and anecdotes from people I meet.

People regularly report that eating live-culture ferments generates improvements in all sorts of digestive disorders. I've also heard reports of cancers resolved by live-culture ferments. In Australia, a Russian-born woman told me about healing her husband's skin cancer by applying topical sauerkraut poultices. This treatment came to her in a dream, shortly before her husband was scheduled for surgery. In her dream she saw her grandmother applying a sauerkraut poultice. The wise woman tradition spoke to her through her dream, reviving the wisdom of her grandmother in spite of the disruption of migration and the passage of many decades. Her husband's cancerous growth disappeared after a few days of kraut poultices, and he never needed to undergo surgery.

Bacteria are not our enemies; however, our culture has declared a foolish all-out war on them, overdeploying antibiotic drugs, chlorinated water, and antibacterial cleaning products. The war on bacteria is like the war on terror or the war on drugs: an unwinnable exercise in futility. Winning the war on bacteria would be our demise. Though certain bacteria can cause disease under the right (or for us, wrong) conditions, bacteria are our partners in life. They are our ancestors and they can be powerful allies in healing.

Isn't it curious that we use the word *culture* to describe both the bacteria in yogurt and sauerkraut as well as language, art, science, and the totality of human endeavor? Cultured foods are not culinary novelties. They are found in infinite variation in culinary traditions around the world and are often invested with profound symbolic meaning. The earliest writings all refer to ferments, and folklore around the world has long associated good health and longevity with such diverse live-culture ferments as sauerkraut, kimchi, miso, yogurt, kefir, and vinegar.

Medical science has documented the healing power of live cultures in hundreds of controlled studies, and today probiotics are among the fastest-growing segments of the nutritional supplement market. But any nutrient you can obtain in a pill or a powder you can get better from a whole food. Fermenting with spontaneously occurring local organisms integrates us into the web of life of our environment and adapts us to the local microbial ecology.

Fermented foods and drinks have always been a community-based production, up until the past few generations. As I have traveled with my *Wild Fermentation* road show, I have met hundreds of people who shared recollections of a grandparent with an annual fermentation routine. Like so many survival and self-healing skills, fermentation needs to be revived as something people do on a community scale.

Most ferments available commercially today are pasteurized for ease of transport and long shelf life. The pasteurization, however, destroys the beneficial bacteria. I am pleased to report that there is a small revival of community-based vegetable fermentation happening, and "artisanal" sauerkraut has been added to Slow Food USA's Ark of Taste. What you get from local ferments is local culture, quite literally: the unique community of microbial subspecies that inhabit a particular place. The local *Lactobacillus*, and the motley company it's found with, replenish your gut microflora, which probably need regular replenishment, given the prevalence of broad-spectrum antibacterial chemicals. The particular lactobacilli that inhabit your environment are uniquely adapted to that particular place. There is no simpler way to invite these bacterial allies into our lives and share them with the people around us than by becoming food producers and fermenting some vegetables ourselves at home.

Recipe: Vegetable Fermentation Further Simplified

A head of cabbage forgotten on an obscure shelf of your pantry will not spontaneously transform itself into sauerkraut. Vegetables left exposed to air start to grow molds, and if left long enough, those molds can reduce a head of cabbage to a puddle of slime, bearing no resemblance whatsoever to crunchy, delicious, and aromatic sauerkraut.

The simple key to successful vegetable fermentation is to make sure your vegetables are submerged in liquid. That's it, the big secret. Usually the liquid is salty water, also known as brine, but fermentation can be done without salt, or with other liquids, such as wine or whey. Typically, when fresh vegetables are chopped or grated in preparation for fermentation—which creates greater surface area—salting pulls out the vegetable juices via osmosis, and pounding or tamping the vegetables breaks down cell walls to further release juices, so no additional water is required. However, if the vegetables have lost moisture during long storage, occasionally some water is needed; if brine hasn't risen to submerge the weighted vegetables by the following day, add a little water. In the case of vegetables left whole (cabbage heads, cucumbers, green tomatoes, string beans, okra, zucchini, eggplant, peppers—try anything), the vegetables should be submerged in brine.

The huge variety of vegetable ferments you can create all exist along the spectrum from shredded and salted to whole and submerged in a brine. Sometimes you use elements of each style, as in kimchi recipes that call for soaking vegetables in a brine to soften them and leach out bitter flavors, then pouring off excess brine and mixing in spices. In some cases the liquid is what we're after, flavored by the vegetables and fermentation.

Pretty much any vegetable can be fermented. Use what is abundantly available and be bold in your experimentation. Seaweeds are a wonderful addition to ferments, as are fruits, though mostly fruit ferments go through their process very quickly. I've even made delicious sauerkraut with mashed potatoes layered in with the salted cabbage, as well as kimchi with sticky rice layers. The sharp fermented starches are delicious. The spicing of vegetable ferments is quite varied, too. Kimchi typically includes red chili peppers, garlic, ginger, and scallions. Sauerkraut might include caraway seeds (my favorite), juniper berries, apples, or cranberries. New York–style sour pickles are spiced with dill, garlic, and sometimes hot peppers. To keep cucumbers crunchy, add to the brine some grape leaves or leaves of horseradish, oak, currant, or cherry.

How much salt do you use? Traditionally vegetables have been fermented with lots of salt. In addition to pulling water from the vegetables, salt hardens pectins in the vegetables, rendering them crunchier, and discourages the growth of bacteria other than lactobacilli. By inhibiting competing bacteria, salt enables the vegetables to ferment and to be stored for longer periods of time. Since preservation has historically been one of the important motivations for fermentation, ferments have tended to be quite salty. But for health-conscious people interested primarily in flavor and nutrition, less salt can be better. Salt lightly, to taste. It is easier to add salt than to take it away, but if you oversalt, you can dilute by adding water and/or more vegetables. There is no magic proportion of salt the process requires—it's just personal preference. As a starting point, try 3 tablespoons of salt per 5 pound of vegetables. More salt will slow the fermentation process; less (or none) will speed it up. Ferments with less salt may be more prone to surface molds. You can leave out the salt or use various mineral-rich substitutes such as celery juice (my favorite salt-free variation) or seaweed. Just be sure the vegetables are submerged in the liquid.

Some people promote the idea that salt-free sauerkrauts contain more beneficial organisms than salted krauts. I don't believe that. The most specific beneficial bacteria we're after, *Lactobacillus*, is salt-tolerant and abundantly present even in salty krauts; arguably, salt-free ferments are more biodiverse, but this diversity often results in mushy textures. Though it is possible to ferment vegetables without salt, a little salt results in far superior flavor and texture—and just as much beneficial bacteria. So again, salt to taste.

What kind of vessel should you use to hold your ferment? Avoid metal, as salt and the acids created by fermentation will corrode it. Heavy ceramic cylindrical crocks are the ideal fermentation vessels, though they can be hard to find and expensive. Glass containers work well, especially those with a cylindrical shape or with a wide mouth, and so do nesting bowls. Crock pots with ceramic interiors make effective fermentation vessels and can often be found in thrift stores. In a pinch, you can use plastic, but even food-grade plastics leach toxic chemicals.

The reason a cylindrical shape is desirable is for ease of weighting down the fermenting vegetables to keep them submerged rather than floating to the top. I generally use a plate that just fits inside the vessel, weighted down by a full jug of water, and I drape a cloth over the top of the vessel to protect against flies. I call this the "open-crock" method. Containers in other shapes can work with improvisation, or you can manually press the vegetables to submerge them in the liquid.

If the vegetables float to the top and remain exposed to air, they are likely to develop mold. Sometimes, especially in hot weather, your ferment may develop a film of white mold on its surface. This is very common and will not hurt you or the kraut. Scrape off the mold as best you can, don't worry about particles that mix into the vegetables, and enjoy the delicious ferment beneath. Specially designed Harsch crocks eliminate this problem by creating an oxygen-free airspace around the ferment. These German crocks are elegant but expensive. Another way to avoid mold is by weighting the ferment in the vessel with water contained in a double layer of plastic bags. The water will spread to cover the entire surface, protecting it from aerobic surface molds. The downside of this method, of course, is that your food comes into prolonged contact with plastic, which leaches chemicals into the food. I prefer to use the open-crock method and remove mold as necessary.

Whatever type of vessel you use, pack the vegetables into it with some force (unless they are whole), in order to break down cell walls and release juices. I use a blunt wooden tamping tool. You can improvise with a piece of wood or your fist, or you can manually massage and squeeze the vegetables, as described in the recipe for massaged kale (see page 185). Once the vegetables are weighted down, the salt will continue to pull moisture from the vegetables for many hours yet. If, by the following day, the vegetables are not submerged, add a little water.

How long do you ferment the vegetables? I wish I had an easy answer to this question. "Ferment until ripe," many recipes advise, but ultimately you will have to decide when it is ripe. Sour flavor—from lactic acid—develops over time. Longer fermentation translates to tangier flavor. This happens more quickly in warm temperatures than in cool ones. If you start your ferment at harvest time, in the autumn, as temperatures are dropping, it can ferment for six months or longer. This is how people survived before refrigeration and globalized food. Many people, however, prefer the flavor of a mild ferment to that of a strongly acidic one. When you are first experimenting, taste your ferments early and often. Serve some after three days, then three days later, and again three days after that. Familiarize yourself with the spectrum of flavors that fermentation can create and see what you like.

Manufacturing and Marketing Confusion

For the first time ever demographers are seeing a decline in U.S. average life expectancy.[19] The food most of us eat is of such poor nutritional quality that it is killing us. And food-processing and marketing corporations spend billions of dollars promoting lies and confusion about nutrition.

In fact, nutritional truth is very simple: Whole foods are more than the sum of their parts. Eating the whole apple offers more complete nutrition than drinking the juice pressed from the apple. Each food's many nutritional qualities are contextual; that is, they exist in a complex web of relations with all the other properties of the food, including qualitative factors determined by how it was produced.

Profitability truth is simple, too: processing adds value to food. Farmers have long processed agricultural products into "value-added" foods such as pickles, cheeses, wines, cured meats, and jams. As we have seen in chapter 4, more and more farm-based and home-based food processing is being outlawed. Food processing has moved from the community scale to the global scale. The more processed the food, the greater the potential for profit. Each stage of processing is an opportunity for marginal earnings—and for nutrient loss. The handful of global food processors and marketers want you to consume more of their products.

Confusion reigns in the marketing wars among products aimed for our bodies. One contemporary strategy that both exploits and feeds this confusion is the phenomenon of functional foods, or neutraceuticals. In these engineered food products, whole foods are deconstructed and fragmented, and certain of their parts are then conjoined with medicinalized nutrients, which are often deconstructed from other foods. For example, chocolate and other candies are now being marketed with added nutrients. Candy giant M&M/Mars has launched a new division: Mars Nutrition for Health & Well-Being. Its CocoaVia line of chocolates, fortified with sterols from canola oil, is being marketed as a functional food for cardiovascular health; two servings a day are recommended for maximum benefit.

Such health claims have been permitted on food labels only since 2002. Prior to that, health claims on labels had to be based on scientific evidence and evaluated by the FDA. The new policy, supported by the food-processing industries, permits health claims regardless of scientific evidence, so long as they are accompanied by a disclaimer in small print qualifying the claims with language such as "limited and inconclusive."

So ketchup is now being marketed as an antioxidant, based on the presence of lycopene in tomatoes, and retail coolers are full of high-fructose-corn-syrup-based soft drinks augmented by echinacea, guarana, ginseng, ginkgo, and various other herbs and nutrients. Fortification with herbal extracts and nutrients marks these drinks as "healthy" and "nutritious," yet even extracts of the most potent medicinals cannot possibly salvage high-fructose corn syrup from its nutritional (and economic) void.

High-fructose corn syrup is today the most widely consumed of processed foods. It is present in sodas and almost anything mass-produced and sweet, especially beverages. Corn is wholesome, so presumably corn syrup is too, right? And fructose sounds fruity, so it must be a more benign sugar than cane sugar, right? Wrong on both counts. High-fructose corn syrup is popular as an ingredient because it is marginally cheaper than cane sugar (at least with corn subsidies and sugar import tariffs in place, which the World Trade Organization is not likely to permit much longer). Fructose is also sweeter than glucose, so it enables more sweet flavor to be concentrated.

The process of converting corn into high-fructose corn syrup is complex and involves many steps. It's not something you can make at home. The transformation requires fermentation by the fungus *Aspergillus*, the same organism used to make miso, saké, and amazaké. Liquid chromatography is used in the process, and at two different steps, genetically modified enzymes are introduced. A lot of work goes into transforming that corn into fructose. The process was first engineered in the late 1960s and then steadily refined. High-fructose corn syrup consumption in the United States rose more than 1,000 percent from the 1970s to 2000[20]; today in the United States, average consumption of high-fructose corn syrup is more than fifty-five pounds per person per year, nearly ten pounds more than the average consumption of refined cane and beet sugar.[21]

Unfortunately, fructose does not metabolize as easily as glucose. "Every cell in the body can metabolize glucose," says Dr. Meira Field of the U.S. Department of Agriculture, who studied rats on a high-fructose diet. "However, all fructose must be metabolized in the liver. The livers of the rats on the high-fructose diet looked like the livers of alcoholics, plugged with fat and cirrhotic."[22] According to a study published in the *American Journal of Clinical Nutrition*, fructose fails to stimulate a number of key chemical signals that regulate appetite and food intake. "There is a distinct likelihood that the increased consumption of [high-fructose corn syrup] in beverages may be linked to the increase in obesity," the authors conclude.[23]

Experience tells me that sweet drinks can be powerfully addictive. I rarely drink them these days, but I am no purist, and I know that after I drink a soda or other beverage sweetened with high-fructose corn syrup, all I want is another one. As we know from the tobacco industry, addiction is the ultimate marketing scheme.

Rivaling high-fructose corn syrup as the miracle of modern food processing most responsible for our collective health crises is hydrogenated vegetable oil. Hydrogenation is a chemical manipulation of fat molecules that makes otherwise liquid oils hold a solid form. This process was pioneered early in the twentieth century to create improved vegetable-based imitations of butter (margarine) and lard (shortening). These imitations were initially marketed as such, replacing traditional animal sources by reason of shortages, lower prices, or (later) perceived health benefit (for more on the vilification of animal fats, see chapter 8). The U.S. Food, Drug, and Cosmetic Act of 1938 regulated these foods by defining them as imitations: "There are certain traditional foods that everyone knows, such as bread, milk and cheese, and that when consumers buy these foods, they should get the foods that they are expecting . . . [and] if a food resembles a standardized food but does not comply with the standard, that food must be labeled as an 'imitation.'"[24]

Once they were introduced, these highly processed imitations came, in just a few decades, to be more widely consumed than the animal fats they were imitating. Today virtually all processed foods contain hydrogenated vegetable oils, and their consumption more than tripled from the 1960s to the 1990s. Oil processors and their sponsored science were able to convince the public that hydrogenated vegetable oils are healthier than animal fats, even though heart disease and cancer are rare in traditional cultures using animal fats, and the rise in prevalence of these diseases has paralleled the introduction and spread of hydrogenated oils.

The story of the imitations' fast rise to dominance of the American food supply sounds just like the story of genetically modified foods (see chapter 2). Both were accomplished by regulatory coups in which corporate agendas guided policies that presumed nutritional equivalence between the newfangled creations and traditional foods—those coups carried out by the revolving door between food-processing industry lobbyists and regulators.

Peter Barton Hutt, a Washington, DC, lawyer who long represented the edible oil industry, was appointed general counsel to the U.S. Food and Drug Administration (FDA) in 1971. He argued that the word *imitation* in the 1938 food law was outmoded, that it ignored advances in food-processing technology that produced foods "not necessarily inferior to the traditional foods for which they may be substituted." Until this point, the law always considered certain traditional foods as *real*, in contrast to imitations. The 1970s revisions to the law eliminated this distinction. Fabricated and fortified fragments of foods became the legal equivalents of traditional whole foods. Once the food-processors' lawyer completed his term of government service, the word *imitation* had virtually disappeared from FDA regulations, and realness in food has since become increasingly elusive.

The process of hydrogenation creates fat molecules that are fundamentally different from the saturated and unsaturated natural fats found in traditional foods. Mary Enig is a lipid biochemist who has studied trans fats for decades and challenged the idea that hydrogenated vegetable oils are healthier than animal fats. In an essay she coauthored with Sally Fallon, they explain:

> Most of these man-made *trans* fats are toxins to the body, but unfortunately your digestive system does not recognize them as such. Instead of being eliminated, *trans* fats are incorporated into cell membranes . . . your cells actually become partially hydrogenated! Once in place, *trans* fatty acids with their misplaced hydrogen atoms wreak havoc in cell metabolism because chemical reactions can only take place when electrons in the cell membranes are in certain arrangements or patterns, which the hydrogenation process has disturbed. . . . Altered partially hydrogenated fats made from vegetable oils actually block utilization of essential fatty acids, causing many deleterious effects including sexual dysfunction, increased blood cholesterol and paralysis of the immune system. Consumption of hydrogenated fats is associated with a host of other serious diseases, not only cancer but also atherosclerosis, diabetes, obesity, immune system dysfunction, low-birth-weight babies, birth defects, decreased visual acuity, sterility, difficulty in lactation and problems with bones and tendons.[25]

Dr. Enig's critique of trans fats has become increasingly accepted. "Today, most scientists and nutrition experts agree that trans fat is America's most dangerous fat," wrote the *New York Times* in August 2005, as New York City asked restaurants to voluntarily switch from hydrogenated to nonhydrogenated oils.[26]

The rising consumption of anti-nutrients such as hydrogenated oils and high-fructose corn syrup is contributing to a rapid decline in American health. The path of least resistance is eating overprocessed synthetic junk. What else do many people know? "There is profit in poisoning the population, and lethal food peddling, unlike lethal drug peddling, is legal," observes *The Nation*. "A go-getting, job-creating ad agency entrepreneur can make a hell of a lot of money teaching children how to grow fat and kill themselves."[27] A third of Americans are currently obese (as defined by a body-mass index of 30 or more), double the rate of thirty years ago.[28] One Harvard University study concluded that each additional soda a kid drinks on a daily basis increases his or her risk of obesity by 60 percent.[29] Obesity causes 325,000 American deaths annually, more than motor vehicles, illegal drugs, alcohol, and firearms combined[30] (though not quite half as many as iatrogenic causes).

Considering obesity as an epidemic is not about condemning fat or overweight people. Certainly the cult of thinness is an oppressive force all unto itself. Healthy bodies come in many different shapes and proportions, and as a culture we need to recognize that. Nonetheless, at the macro level of demographics, the explosion in obesity rates suggests serious social problems. Obesity at this unprecedented scale is a result of sedentary lifestyles and dietary changes, largely manufactured by the food-processing and marketing industries. Another factor in the growing levels of obesity may be the organophosphate chemicals used in agriculture, which slow metabolism.[31]

The plague of obesity, and its twin diabetes, is not evenly distributed among the population. Native Americans exhibit dramatically high rates of diabetes. They have not always lived with this disease; their indigenous diets and lifestyles sustained them well and protected them from it. However, as their traditional foods have been replaced with the hydrogenated, high-fructosed, anti-nutrient foods that are the staples of the standard American diet, a vulnerability toward obesity and diabetes has emerged in Native communities. More than 17 percent of

Native American adults are diabetic, double the rate of the adult U.S. population as a whole. African-Americans, Latinos, and Asians also show higher-than-average rates of diabetes and obesity.[32]

Beyond being cut off from traditional diets, people with fewer economic choices generally have easier access to aggressively marketed junk foods than to fresh, wholesome foods. This is true in rural areas as well as in inner cities. Affluent areas may have Trader Joe's and Whole Foods, but poor people get convenience stores. Food processors spend $33 billion annually promoting their products in the United States,[33] with much of this advertising targeted at kids. Marketing anti-nutrient foods is a brilliant strategy, because you eat them and you're still hungry, still craving more. The insidious nature of junk-food marketing is well illustrated by soft-drink "pouring rights" in schools. Pouring rights are exclusive contracts between soft-drink marketers and schools, or school districts, or entire cities, where the schools get cash (and some free soft drinks) in exchange for the soft-drink manufacturer having exclusive marketing rights. Carbonated soft drinks are the ultimate anti-nutrients, vehicles for high-fructose corn syrup and even more troubling artificial sweeteners. Yet their consumption just keeps increasing. Soda production in the United States was fifty-four gallons per person in 2004, or about 576 twelve-ounce servings,[34] more than a soda and a half per person per day. "Our strategy is ubiquity," boasts a Coca-Cola spokesperson. "We want to put soft drinks within arm's reach of desire."[35]

A manufacturer having pouring rights in a school means that the manufacturer has not only vending machines stocked with its brands— but its logos pasted throughout the school, sales quotas, and incentives for higher-than-target sales, turning school administrators into brand-loyal pushers of high-fructose corn syrup and students into captive audiences. "It must be the dream of marketing executives," speculated an *Advertising Age* op-ed. "The law requires your future customers to come to a place 180 days a year where they must watch and listen to your advertising messages exclusively, your competitors are not allowed access to the market. The most important public institution in the lives of children and families gives its implied endorsement to your products."[36] In one telling incident, a Georgia school held a "Coke Day" rally, and an iconoclastic student who wore a Pepsi tee-shirt that day was suspended.[37] In response to the twin epidemics of obesity and diabetes, parents and public health activists in some localities are putting an end to pouring rights and banning junk food in schools altogether. Seattle enacted such a ban in 2004; New Jersey and Maine have passed similar bans that will be implemented in 2007, and bills have been introduced in Congress to establish such a ban in schools nationwide.

Desperate to divert public scrutiny away from the harmful effects of their products on children's health, soft-drink manufacturers have begun sponsoring health education programs in schools. Coca-Cola is spending $4 million to bring its "Live It!" curriculum to middle schools, Pepsi is sponsoring a program called "Balance First" in elementary schools, and Ronald McDonald is visiting schools in the role of "ambassador for an active, balanced lifestyle." "What better way to deflect attention from your unhealthy products than to promote exercise?" asks Michele Simon, director of the Center for Informed Food Choices.[38]

The junk food giants have been the targets of many notable political actions. McDonald's in particular has inspired opposition because it uniquely epitomizes globalization, with all of the homogenization and diminishment of culture that comes with that. The Slow Food movement was born of Carlo Petrini's rage against McDonald's, and French farmer José Bové drew international notoriety for a 1999 action in which members of his local Farmers' Confederation and Union of Ewe's Milk Producers dismantled a McDonald's in Millau, France. Every year since 1985, October 16 (United Nations World Food Day) has been a day of anti-McDonald's actions; this practice was initiated by Greenpeace in 1985 and by 1999 had spread to 345 cities in twenty-three countries.[39]

Helen Steel and Dave Morris—the "McLibel Two"—participated in some of the London anti-McDonald's actions, standing in front of a McDonald's handing out a Greenpeace flyer titled "What's Wrong with McDonald's? Everything They Don't Want You to Know." The flyer criticized McDonald's from many perspectives, including the poor nutritional content of its food, its deceptive marketing practices, its destructive environmental impact, and its poor labor practices. In 1990 Steel and Morris were sued by McDonald's for libelous statements in this flyer. British libel law places the burden of proof on the accused, who must demonstrate that the contested statements are true, rather

Corn as Commodity By Betty Fussell

Today the corn synthesizers can transmute substances at will. "The primary message," the National Corn Growers' Association declared in 1987, was that "anything made from a barrel of petroleum can be made from a bushel of corn." . . . Joining the chorus are the nation's nine giant wet-millers, the kings of corn processing known as the Corn Refiners Association, the archdeacons of pumping and squeezing, who proclaim, "Corn refiners constantly search for new technologies and more uses which will squeeze even more value out of every bushel of American corn."

Today, the way to squeeze money out of corn is to squeeze the molecule and manipulate its structure in the tee (for total) commodification of corn, in which farmers are replaced by marketers, millers by refiners, and machinists by biochemists. From the perspective of industrial farmers, corn is of value only as it can be transformed chemically into whatever commodity is most in demand. The methodology of nineteenth-century chemistry underlies the refining of corn as it does the refining of oil: analyze the system, fragment the parts, quantify the parts and synthesize at will. In such a system organic plants are but raw material for the processor, who fabricates products for which the manufacturer creates demand. Equally, consumers are raw material for processing and consumption by the manufacturer. The consumer becomes the consumed.

Excerpted from *The Story of Corn: The Myths and History, the Culture and Agriculture, the Art and Science of America's Quintessential Crop* (New York: North Point Press, 1992). Used by permission.

than on the allegedly libeled party to prove that the statements are false (as in the United States). McDonald's spent an estimated £310 million in legal fees pursuing the case; Steel and Morris represented themselves in court, and their defense of the truth of the criticisms of McDonald's contained in the flyer text resulted in the longest trial in English history, lasting 314 days.

The court's ruling was mixed. It found many of the flyer's statements to be unambiguously true: McDonald's *has* "pretended to a positive nutritional benefit which their food (high in fat and salt, etc.) did not match"; *does* "exploit children" with its advertising strategy; *is* "culpably responsible for animal cruelty"; and *does* "pay low wages." Nonetheless, the court was not convinced that every single statement on the flyer was correct and ordered Steel and Morris to pay McDonald's £40,000 in damages. The pair refused to pay McDonald's and appealed the decision. The appeals court found that further flyer statements were true; for instance (as the 2004 documentary *Super Size Me* later starkly illustrated), "if one eats enough McDonald's food, one's diet may well become high in fat, etc., with the very real risk of heart disease."

But the court still upheld the damages, so Steel and Morris appealed to the European Court of Human Rights. Sometimes higher authorities, with broader jurisdictions, are better able to grasp the big picture than local officials more beholden to specific financial or ideological interests. In 2005, fifteen years after the trial first began, the European Court ruled that the trials had been unfair, that the protestors' freedom of expression had been violated, and that no damages were due to McDonald's. The court championed the "strong public interest in enabling campaign groups and individuals outside the mainstream to contribute to the public debate by disseminating information and ideas on matters of general public interest such as health and the environment."

From neutraceuticals to McDonald's, the food marketing industry twists facts and manipulates consumer desires—with grotesque results. The results are no less grotesque when marketing and advertising drive our health-care choices. The growing trend toward advertising pharmaceutical products directly to consumers—ask your doctor about (fill in the blank)—begs people to tap into the deep well of pain and malaise and perhaps pursue a particular product as a solution. In 2003 pharmaceutical manufacturers spent more than $3 billion on direct-to-consumer (DTC) advertising,[40] a practice that was considered unethical until the 1980s.

Total expenditures for prescription drugs, expressed as a percentage of gross domestic product, almost tripled between 1980 and 2000, the period in which DTC drug advertising became widespread.[41] (They had remained constant from 1960 to 1980.) The Pharmaceutical Research and Manufacturers of America claims that DTC drug advertising "enhances consumer knowledge" and "improves public health." But two Harvard medical professors, both former editors of the *New England Journal of Medicine*, counter that "DTC ads mainly benefit the bottom line of the drug industry, not the public. They mislead consumers more than they inform them, and they pressure physicians to prescribe new, expensive, and often marginally helpful drugs, although a more conservative option might be better for the patient."[42]

Predictably enough, the most-advertised drugs become the most prescribed. According to an analysis in the journal *Health Affairs*, prescriptions for the fifty most heavily advertised drugs rose an average of 25 percent between 1999 and 2000, while prescriptions for less heavily advertised drugs rose an average of only 4 percent.[43] The most-advertised drug at the dawn of the new millennium was Vioxx, which treats symptoms of arthritis. The ads paid off, with twenty million people taking Vioxx in the United States between 1999 and 2004.[44]

Unfortunately for Vioxx's manufacturer, Merck, the self-described "global research-driven pharmaceutical company dedicated to putting patients first,"[45] that cash cow had to be recalled after a study determined that the drug dramatically increases the risk of heart attack for the people who take it. The *Wall Street Journal* reported that Merck knew as early as 2000 about the problem but worked hard to conceal it by distorting statistics.[46] By the time Vioxx was recalled in 2004, the FDA estimates that more than 27,000 people had died from it.

Health care by corporate advertisement is McMedicine. McFood feeds McMedicine, and we need to liberate ourselves from both profit-driven monsters. Our well-being is not on their agendas; selling things to us is. We must reclaim our health and our power, both as individuals and as communities. We all must be healers—for ourselves and for the people we know. Information is plentiful if you know how to seek it out. In fact, in the search for health-care information you will always find contradictory opinions, from doctors, drug or nutraceutical ads, herbalists, acupuncturists, nutritionists, or diet gurus. Many people feel like they're drowning in information. Ultimately it is up to you to decide which paths to follow. Vibrant health is not the result of a single factor. Healing doesn't come about by rules or dogma; it's about learning what works for you. My own health care regime is a patchwork that includes pharmaceuticals and acupuncture, but along with them weed-eating plant medicine and homegrown food. For me loving the plants is a healing in itself. They nourish and heal me every day, and they give me the comfort of knowing that in the end my fate (like that of all life forms) is to nourish them. The earth has abundant food and medicine to sustain us.

Action and Information Resources

Books

Colbin, Annemarie. *Food and Healing: How What You Eat Determines Your Health, Your Well-being, and the Quality of Your Life*. New York: Ballantine Books, 1986.

Cook, Christopher D. *Diet for a Dead Planet: How the Food Industry Is Killing Us*. New York: New Press, 2004.

Cooper, Ann, and Lisa M. Holmes. *Bitter Harvest: A Chef's Perspective on the Hidden Dangers in the Foods We Eat and What You Can Do about It*. New York and London: Routledge, 2000.

Duke, James. *The Green Pharmacy*. Emmaus, PA: Rodale Press, 1997.

Eisenstein, Charles. *The Yoga of Eating: Transcending Diets and Dogma to Nourish the Natural Self*. Washington, DC: New Trends, 2003.

Enig, Mary. *Know Your Fats*. Silver Spring, MD: Bethesda Press, 2000.

Fallon, Sally, with Mary G. Enig. *Nourishing Traditions: The Cookbook That Challenges Politically Correct Nutrition and the Diet Dictocrats*. Washington, DC: New Trends, 1999.

Fitzgerald, Randall. *The Hundred Year Lie: How Food and Medicine are Destroying Your Health*. New York: Dutton, 2006.

Fussell, Betty. *The Story of Corn: The Myths and History, the Culture and Agriculture, the Art and Science of America's Quintessential Crop*. New York: North Point Press, 1992.

Nabhan, Gary Paul. *Why Some Like It Hot: Food, Genes, and Cultural Diversity*. Washington, DC: Island Press, 2004.

Nestle, Marion. *Food Politics: How the Food Industry Influences Nutrition and Health*. Berkeley: University of California Press, 2003.

————. *Safe Food: Bacteria, Biotechnology, and Bioterrorism*. Berkeley: University of California Press, 2003.

Pichford, Paul. *Healing with Whole Foods*. Berkeley, CA: North Atlantic Books, 1993.

Price, Weston A. *Nutrition and Physical Degeneration*. Lemon Grove, CA: Price-Pottenger Nutrition Foundation, 1939.

Sams, Craig. *The Little Food Book: You Are What You Eat*. New York: Disinformation, 2004.

Schlosser, Eric. *Fast Food Nation: The Dark Side of the All-American Meal*. Boston: Houghton Mifflin, 2001.

Simon, Michele. *Appetite for Profit: Fighting Corporate Control and Spin in the Nutrition Wars*. New York: Nation Books, 2006.

Stitt, Paul A. *Beating the Food Giants*. Manitowoc, WI: Natural Press, 1982.

U.S. Centers for Disease Control and Prevention. *Third National Report on Human Exposure to Environmental Chemicals*. Atlanta, GA: U.S. Centers for Disease Control and Prevention, 2005. Available online at www.cdc.gov/exposurereport.

Weed, Susun S. *Wise Woman Herbal: Healing Wise*. Woodstock, NY: Ash Tree, 1989.

Films

McLibel. Directed by Franny Armstrong. London: Spanner Films, 2005; www.spannerfilms.net.

Super Size Me. Directed by Morgan
    Spurlock. New York: Morgan Spurlock
    and The Con, 2004; www.super
    sizeme.com.

Organizations and Other Resources

ACT UP/New York
332 Bleecker Street, Suite G5
New York, NY 10014
(212) 966-4873
www.actupny.org

Center for Informed Food Choices
PO Box 16053
Oakland, CA 94610
www.informedeating.org

Environmental Working Group
1436 U Street NW, Suite 100
Washington, DC 20009
(202) 667-6982
www.ewg.org

Everybody In Nobody Out
PMB #142
1815 MLK Parkway, #2
Durham, NC 27707
(919) 402-0133
www.everybodyinnobodyout.org

Health Care for All
30 Winter Street, 10th Floor
Boston, MA 02108
(617) 350-7279
www.hcfama.org

McLibel Support Campaign
5 Caledonian Road
London, N1 9DX
United Kingdom
44 (207) 713 1269
www.mcspotlight.org

Tennessee Health Care Campaign
1103 Chapel Avenue
Nashville, TN 37206
(615) 227-7500
www.tenncare.org

Universal Health Care Action Network
2800 Euclid Avenue, Suite 520
Cleveland, OH 44115-2418
(216) 241-8422
www.uhcan.org

Urban Nutrition Initiative
Franklin Building Annex
3451 Walnut Street, Suite P-117
Philadelphia, PA 19104
(215) 898-1600
www.urbannutrition.org

CHAPTER 7

Plant Prohibitions: Laws against Nature

eyond outlawing traditional small-scale modes of food production and requiring that the products of agriculture be
processed in specific ways (as with milk and cider), the legal
apparatus has seen fit to outlaw certain plants altogether. This
is a logical trajectory for a rule of law that divides the earth into property and seeks constantly to assert its power over the natural world.
Perhaps other potentially dangerous manifestations of nature should be
prohibited as well, such as excess sunlight, or aging, or thinking lewd
thoughts. The challenge before us, suggests Winona LaDuke, is "to
transform human laws to match natural laws, not vice-versa."[1]

The existence of borders is a vivid example of states asserting their
power over the flows of multitudinous forms of life. All the rhetoric
about free trade across borders applies only to global traders and their
goods—not to average people. The cruelest fact of borders is that they
keep loved ones apart and force millions of people all over the world
to live in fear of discovery and deportation. Borders are designed to
limit the flow of animals, seeds, plants, and microbes, our partners in
life as well as in agriculture, many of which are themselves also foods.
A 2005 public television documentary, *The Meaning of Food*, contained a poignant scene in which a group of customs inspectors in an

international airport in the United States show and discuss foods that
they have confiscated from people entering the country.

> These are things that they might not be able to purchase in our
> country. . . . Some of them will tell you that the food over there
> is better than the food in the United States. . . . People in
> essence don't know what they're bringing; they just know that
> they're bringing food from my grandmother's garden. . . . That
> could be Grandpa's famous recipe for salami. . . . My auntie
> made it. . . . We always get the great-great-grandmother who
> has probably been dead for fifteen years. . . . Or these are the
> potatoes that grow in Grandpa's field. . . . This is from the
> sacred tree, you must let me pass with this, it was passed down
> through many generations (the customs inspectors laugh). . . .
> Sometimes there's more food in their bags than clothing. They
> just feel the need to bring something from back home here.
> They want to have a connection to where they came from, and
> each time they bring food from there and they eat it at home
> they have that connection.

Ever-vigilant border inspections must stop immigrants who crave a
connection to their roots from biologically corrupting our national
purity. Candies aren't prohibited; only foods that are in some sense
alive.

Ironically, the importation of exotic plants has been the driving force
of globalization from the very beginning. The quest for spices—the
exotic aromatic seeds of the Orient—drove the European sea exploration. Sugar and its associated stimulants (coffee, chocolate, and tea)
could be grown only in tropical lands, motivating colonial conquests
and the African slave trade.[2] "The history of colonialism is a history of
the struggle to capture and monopolize botanical resources,"[3] write
Cary Fowler and Pat Mooney. "The surplus value of all the new and
increased production accrued to those who orchestrated the plant
transfers. Wherever the plants ended up, the money was safely routed
to London, Paris, and other capitals of the North."[4] This historical
process brings to mind once again the term *biopiracy* (see page 46–47).
The earth's plant diversity and the knowledge of plant use accumulated

by cultures everywhere are freely exploited and moved about by global traders. Meanwhile the borders are sealed from the grassroots free trade of seeds and plants, and laws render the practice of certain types of plant knowledge illegal. Apparently we must be protected with ever-growing vigilance from the threat of "invasive species" and forbidden plant phytochemicals.

Controlling Dispersion

Now more than ever before, control over biological resources is concentrated, with a handful of patented seed varieties dominating global markets, and in that concentration lies great vulnerability. Economic losses caused by "invasive alien species" is equivalent to an estimated 5 percent of the global gross national product, totaling about $1.4 trillion a year.[5] "Biosecurity" is the urgent concern of a growing cadre of executives, consultants, regulators, and lobbyists.

Government jurisdictions in many places use laws to attempt to protect local crops, as well as wilderness areas, from potential invaders. "Nonindigenous invasive species may pose the single most formidable threat of natural disaster of the twenty-first century," predicts a report from the NASA Office of Earth Science and the U.S. Geological Survey.[6] Many conservationists and environmentalists have joined in the war on invasive species.

No doubt about it, introduced species can come to dominate ecosystems. The most dramatic evidence of this simple fact is the expanse of monoculture fields across "America's breadbasket." Some introduced species become naturalized or go feral. In the woods here in Tennessee, we regard the ailanthus tree as an invader, spreading by its root system, fast-growing, crowding out native hardwood trees, and of no practical value (known to us). A few miles down the road you can see groves of dense kudzu vine, another introduced species considered invasive in this region.

Certainly people have introduced plants into many places where they later became problems. But often the reasons introduced plants take over have less to do with the plants themselves than with ecosystem disturbances that create the opportunity for a newly introduced plant to

proliferate. Many people who know far more than I do feel very passionately that invasive species must be more effectively controlled. I am
willing to support the idea that in specific instances such controls are
warranted. However, increasing centralized control over the dispersal of
plants means less grassroots empowerment for immigrants, travelers,
and independent horticulturalists and botanists. Controls must be specific and narrow—not broad and all-encompassing.

Freedom demands that borders be as porous as possible. Open borders allow for cross-pollination and exchange; ironclad borders are
expressions of totalitarian control. And generalized prohibitions on
"invasive aliens" are oversimplistic and inflammatory. "Alien species do
not come from Mars," the popular science magazine *Discover* reminds
us; "they are not 'other.' They are very much of us, by us; we are the
main agent of their spread."[7] There must be a more neutral vocabulary
we can use to address the problematic species that neither sensational-
izes nor generalizes "alien" as bad and "native" as good.

Seeds migrate via birds and the wind, so "native" is not a static state.
Is a species that migrated one hundred thousand years ago a native?
What about ten thousand years ago? Plant and animal species ranges are
always in flux. And people have greatly speeded their spread.
Everywhere people have ever gone on this earth—by foot, by horse, by
ship, by train, by car, and by plane—we have carried and dispersed,
intentionally as well as accidentally, plants and other types of organisms.
If we're going to talk about invasive species, then we have to recognize
that we—*Homo sapiens*—are the major invasive species all around the
earth, and many other species have accompanied us in our accelerating
mobility. Evolutionary biologist Stephen Jay Gould asked the question,
"Is it more 'democratic' only to respect organisms in their natural
places? How, then, could any non-African human respect himself?"[8]

The legal enforcement of nativism in plants and microorganisms is
ultimately not so very different from the enforcement of nativism in
people. The generalization of "aliens" as the problem, rather than the
identification of specific problems, is an expression of xenophobia, or
fear of that which is strange or foreign. "Demon species are then used
to tar the entire class of alien plants with guilt by association," observes
Michael Pollan.[9]

Sometimes people have reacted strongly against the xenophobia of invasive-species eradication programs. "Plants and trees without the proper papers to show their pre-Mayflower lineage are called 'invasive exotics' and are wrenched from the soil to die," commented San Francisco official Leland Yee in response to an invasive-species eradication proposal. "How many of us are 'invasive exotics' who have taken root in the San Francisco soil and thrived and flourished?"[10] Biologist and seed propagator David Theodoropoulos, the crusading author of *Invasion Biology: Critique of a Pseudoscience*, observes of eradication programs, "Ideas are imparted of the correctness of human domination of the earth, justification for total human control over natural processes, the appropriateness of the extermination of species within a landscape, and using acts of mass killing as a means of problem solving."[11]

It turns out that a movement promoting native plants and disparaging aliens emerged earlier in the twentieth century. It was in Hitler's Germany. In the Nazi era native plantings known as "blood-and-soil-rooted"[12] gardens "became the landscape architect's swastika."[13] The Central Office of Vegetative Mapping initiated plant eradication programs against nonnative species. In 1942 it declared a "war of extermination"[14] against *Impatiens parviflora*, a perceived invasive threat. The botanists exhorted, "As with the fight against Bolshevism, our entire Occidental culture is at stake, so with the fight against this Mongolian invader, an essential element of this culture, namely, the beauty of our home forest, is at stake."[15]

I love many native as well as introduced plants, and I work hard to push back certain plants, both natives and introduced species, especially in the garden. I have met many dedicated conservationists who work to promote the revival of native plants or curtail the growth of invasive plants. I certainly do not mean to imply that any of them are motivated by a fascist agenda. Mostly I am concerned about the eroding rights of ordinary people to transport seeds, plants, and fruits across borders.

Further distancing ourselves from the natural world with more and more legal restrictions only intensifies the root problem of people trying to control nature. "We must learn to *let go*, and allow other beings to express their volition, to thrive and prosper outside of our control," writes Theodoropoulos.[16] The global traders who have always moved people, animals, plants, and pests around the globe now find themselves needing to protect their biologically fragile "free trade" commodity system by restricting the free trade of plants. The casual grassroots dispersion of plants is defined as dangerous. A person crossing a border with the family's heirloom seed, a seedling, or a fruit from the Old Country, is considered a criminal.

The concept of invasive species has become the organizing principle of policies that rule U.S. borders and much of the world. Regulatory bureaucracies everywhere have responded to perceived invasion threats. Canada's 2005 Weed Seeds Order defines various categories of "noxious weeds"—among the long list are chickweed, cleavers, heal-all, plantain, and yellow dock—that are prohibited beyond threshold limits in seed imports.[17] In 2006, Massachusetts added 140 new species to its list of invasive plants prohibited from importation or sale in the state, among them wineberries[18] (which I think are wonderful precisely because they naturalize and propagate so effortlessly). Laws in Australia require landowners to report sightings of noxious weeds to "local control authorities" within twenty-four hours. "Occupiers of land must take whatever actions are required to control noxious weeds on the land they occupy," according to the New South Wales Department of Primary Industries. If a private landowner does not comply:

> The authority may compel the occupier to take actions by issuing a notice specifying the control measures to be taken. The authority may also initiate a prosecution and/or issue an on-the-spot fine. Failure to comply may allow the authority to enter the property and control the noxious weed/s as specified in the notice.[19]

And South Africa in 2004 implemented a new policy to "close the door" on alien plant introductions, requiring that anyone wishing to bring any new plant into the country have extensive risk assessment performed at his or her expense.[20]

Sensational threats of alien invasions justify and expand bureaucracies. We must protect the nation from invasive aliens! In 1999 President Clinton issued an executive order creating a National Invasive Species Council (NISC), an interagency group to coordinate federal policies and encourage state and local governments to act against invasion threats.

One issue under discussion by the NISC and analogous bodies in governments and supracorporate entities (such as the World Trade Organization) is the question of a "clean list" versus a "dirty list."

The existing U.S. system is an example of a "dirty list," whereby certain listed plants (and other organisms) are prohibited for various reasons. A "clean list" is a more restrictive regulatory approach that, instead of listing prohibited species, lists permitted species. Everything else is prohibited. No other species may be imported or grown without first undergoing extensive (and expensive) risk assessment. And there is really no established way of predicting the risk of invasiveness. As a first step toward exploring such a regulatory strategy, the NISC is developing a "prototype assessment process upon which subsequent regulation could be based."[21]

Theodoropoulos, who first drew my attention to this issue, warns that this is a "government seizure of power."[22] If this concept of presumptive danger became the law, peoples' relationships with plants would be dramatically more constrained by the state.

> Grass-roots seed-saving organizations, conservationists propagating rare plants or butterflies, ecological restorationists, native plant enthusiasts and landscape designers, permaculturists, taxonomists and biological researchers of all kinds will find their hands tied, as all living materials will require expensive "risk assessment" and approval by bureaucrats. Gardeners will be prohibited the majority of the world's plants, and ethnic vegetables, herbs, and spices will be banned, denying people their cultural heritage. . . . Family farms and other smallholders who are found with any one of millions of prohibited species on their land will find themselves fined, sprayed, and billed for the costs of extermination.[23]

And while traditional plant varieties without corporate sponsors would lack the documentation needed to make the clean list, genetically modified seeds—which aren't subjected to any meaningful risk assessment—would continue to cross the borders unimpeded. Though U.S. plant prohibitions remain structured as a dirty list rather than a clean list, invasive-weed eradication programs continue to grow.

In 2004 the Noxious Weed Control and Eradication Act became law, mandating U.S. Department of Agriculture (USDA) grants "for the control or eradication of noxious weeds." Herbicide manufacturers have long promoted all kinds of plant eradication programs—because the easiest method of eradication in most cases is to apply herbicides. Fear-mongering about weeds and invasive threats sells herbicides, and government policies of plant eradication sell even more herbicides. Chemical corporations fund Exotic Pest Plant Councils and other supposedly grassroots groups.[24] It's hard to be sure who you are listening to sometimes. "Environmentalism and protection of natural habitats . . . are susceptible to being co-opted by groups whose intentions may not reflect the benevolent concerns of the majority of their followers," observes author Charles Lewis. "It is important that we take nothing at face value but try to learn who is speaking, what they stand to gain or lose, and what they really are saying."[25] Some environmental activists have labeled the herbicide-funded Exotic Pest Plant Councils "astroturf activists" to distinguish the corporate-sponsored eradication campaigns from true grassroots activism.[26] Groups like these are eligible for the new USDA noxious-weed eradication funding stream, resulting in more public funds transferred to the chemical corporations, more pollution, and more assertion of human control over the natural world; meanwhile, some of our most important plant allies make the noxious weed lists.

We must resist the centralized control of biological resources and cherish the biota in all its glorious diversity. Challenge the oversimplistic idea that alien plants are bad and native plants are good. Cultivate an awareness of plant communities in your ecosystem. Become part of the grassroots revival of plant knowledge and the grassroots exchange of seeds and plants.

The World's Most Notorious Prohibited Plant: Marijuana

No plant has ever faced greater resources devoted to its eradication than cannabis, also known as marijuana. According to the United Nations Office of Drugs and Crime, "In terms of both volume and geographic spread, cannabis herb is the most interdicted drug in the world."[27]

Worldwide reported cannabis seizures in 2003 amounted to nearly fifteen million kilograms.[28] The plant's distinctive serrated leaf is as well known as any corporate logo, and with a slash through it, it appears as a wordless symbol of "zero tolerance" on police cars and public buildings.

Periodically as I write in late summer, the chirping of the birds I hear from my desk is drowned out by the chop-chop-chop of National Guard helicopters overhead, searching for marijuana plants. The helicopters have been flying over for the past couple of weeks, as harvest time approaches. All my friends are too scared of losing their land to grow marijuana, but evidently some Tennesseans must not be, because it is estimated to be the state's largest revenue-producing crop.[29] It's now two weeks after Hurricane Katrina devastated New Orleans, and National Public Radio is reporting that the rescue operation there was hindered by how overstretched the National Guard is. Meanwhile, this is what some of the National Guard is doing, combing the rural Tennessee landscape in fine detail, searching (invasively) for the demon (noxious) weed and the people who would dare defy the law. The aggressive enforcement of the current prohibition on marijuana is really just an effort to demonstrate the power of the state, instill fear and respect, and turn millions of ordinary people into criminals. Returning to the theme of human laws versus natural laws: how flawed and antithetical to nature is a law that incarcerates thousands and spends billions to stop a plant, especially one with a long history of usefulness?

Cannabis has a long history of cultivation and use. It is generally considered to be the earliest of cultivated fiber plants, important for fishing line and nets, ropes, sails, clothing, and paper. The development of shipping industries depended so heavily on the cannabis fiber hemp that globalization would not have been possible without this plant. Even after cannabis became prohibited in 1937, when the United States entered World War II there was a renewed demand for hemp for military purposes. The USDA undertook a "Grow Hemp for Victory" campaign, and farmers and their sons who grew it were exempted from military service.[30]

Cannabis also has ancient uses as medicine. It appears in the earliest known materia medicas from the Chinese, Ayurvedic (Indian), and Greek traditions. Cannabis seed has always been eaten as food, and we now know that it is rich in protein and essential fatty acids. In addition, cannabis has been used in many cultures to alter consciousness, and this use is thought of variously as medicinal, spiritual, recreational, or criminal.

Before it was prohibited, cannabis was very widely grown and used in the United States primarily for fiber. Hemp cultivation was mandatory in the English colonies from 1611, by order of King James I. The prosperous agrarian founding fathers of the United States grew it; George Washington himself once lamented in his journal that he had failed to separate the male plants from the females early enough to prevent fertilization.[31]

In the nineteenth century European and American physicians and pharmacists took note of the ways that cannabis was used as medicine in India. It began to be listed in various pharmacopoeias and formularies and became popular as medicine. The *United States Pharmacopoeia* of 1850 lists cannabis as a treatment for neuralgia, tetanus, typhus, cholera, rabies, dysentery, alcoholism and opiate addiction, anthrax, leprosy, tonsillitis, incontinence, snake bites, gout, convulsions, insanity, and uterine hemorrhaging. Cannabis was used primarily in tincture form, which was widely incorporated into "patent medicines" with proprietary formulas. "Doctors were keen to prescribe [cannabis] because the only other effective painkiller they could offer was highly addictive opium and, it was soon realized, cannabis-based extracts were not physically addictive," writes historian Martin Booth. "Cannabis appeared to have no adverse side effects whatsoever other than feelings of euphoria, drowsiness and hallucinations."[32]

Cannabis also has a history of being enjoyed recreationally in the United States. It was marketed in the form of maple-syrup "Ganjah Wallah Hasheesh Candies," as a snuff, and as "Indian cigarettes." At World's Fairs and International Expositions from the 1860s through the early 1900s, visitors seeking horizon-expanding experiences could visit the popular Turkish Hashish Smoking Exposition. "In the decades after the U.S. Civil War, cannabis use in America became accepted," writes Booth. "It was seen neither as anti-social nor as a serious weakness of character, such as was considered alcohol abuse."[33]

So how did this safe, widely used, socially acceptable plant come to be outlawed? Through my explorations of history, I have come up with a threefold explanation: the protection of profits, bolstered by racism and xenophobia, and perpetuated by law enforcement's need to have threats to justify its invasive activities and expansive nature. The primary beneficiary of the 1937 outlawing of cannabis was the timber-invested paper industry and the chemical manufacturer DuPont, which produced chemicals for the wood-pulp papermaking process. Pharmaceutical manufacturers also had an interest in cannabis prohibition, for they were starting to produce aspirin and other synthetic drugs used to treat many of the same conditions for which cannabis was in widespread medicinal use; and alcohol manufacturers saw recreational cannabis use as a threat to their market, which was still under attack by the forces that had created the U.S. alcohol prohibition from 1920 to 1933.

The wood-pulp paper companies faced the most immediate threat from cannabis. Hemp was another, much more quickly renewable source of pulp for making paper. The major limitation of using hemp for papermaking had historically been the laborious and time-consuming process of stripping apart the fibers. Though many clever agrarian tinkerers had created hemp-processing machines, the hemp decorticator, patented in 1919, was the first that proved to be effective at the industrial scale. It enabled paper to be produced not only from the hemp fibers themselves but also from the hemp "hurds," the by-product from which the fibers are separated. The wood-pulp paper industry was threatened by the potential of a modern hemp paper industry. Cannabis prohibition would eliminate the competition and protect their timber investments. The largest wood-pulp paper manufacturers also happened to be major newspaper publishers, and they were well positioned to advance their anti-hemp agenda.

California newspaper magnate William Randolph Hearst was ready with his chain of newspapers to promote the grave "marijuana" threat. Using the Mexican slang name for cannabis rendered the danger foreign and new, despite widespread familiarity with cannabis in the United States. "New Dope Lure, Marijuana, Has Many Victims," announced a typical Hearst headline from the 1930s.[34] "Hearst, through pervasive and repetitive use, brought the word 'marijuana' into the American, English-speaking consciousness," writes Jack Herer, author of *The Emperor Wears No Clothes*.[35]

The anti-marijuana news reports exploited existing racial prejudices and fears, focusing primarily on Mexican and African-American users, with sensational stories that the drug would corrupt America's youth and make people disrespectful, sexually aggressive, and violent. "The American public was ripe for anti-marijuana press exploitation," writes Martin Booth. "Prohibition had been extremely unpopular, and anything that diverted attention away from it was welcome. Apart from not being able to get a glass of whiskey, the public was also worried by the crime wave Prohibition had set in motion; indeed, it gave a far greater boost to organized crime than anything before."[36] Fears of crime, coupled with xenophobic racial fears, gave a certain urgency to the marijuana menace. "All Mexicans are crazy," stated a Texas legislator in a marijuana prohibition debate, "and this stuff is what makes them crazy."[37]

The first director of the federal Bureau of Narcotics, Harry J. Anslinger, became fixated on marijuana and skillfully orchestrated a "Reefer Madness" campaign of anti-marijuana misinformation and propaganda. The following excerpt, from an article with the sensational title "Marijuana—Assassin of Youth," which was published under Anslinger's name in *The American Magazine* in 1937, is fairly typical of his tone:

> Not long ago the body of a young girl lay crushed on the sidewalk after a plunge from a Chicago apartment window. Everyone called it a suicide, but actually it was a murder. The killer was a narcotic known to America as marijuana, and to history as hashish. Used in the form of cigarettes, it is comparatively new to the United States and as dangerous as a coiled rattlesnake. How many murders, suicides, robberies, and maniacal deeds it causes each year, especially among the young, can only be conjectured. In numerous communities it thrives almost unmolested, largely because of official ignorance of its effects.[38]

According to Booth, Anslinger was "out to get the drug and all connected with it, almost at any cost and often with blunt disregard for the truth of any facts that were contrary to his argument."[39] Interestingly, Anslinger was appointed by (and related by marriage to) Treasury

Secretary Andrew Mellon, who was banker to DuPont, manufacturer of the wood-pulp papermaking chemicals.

In 1937, with little fanfare, Congress effectively prohibited cannabis by enacting the Marijuana Tax Act. The law was not an outright ban but rather a prohibitively high excise tax with onerous reporting requirements. The American Medical Association (AMA) opposed the bill and stated in its testimony that it had only days earlier realized that "marijuana" was the same plant as "cannabis," which they regarded as an important medicinal plant.[40] Yet on the floor of the House of Representatives, when the sole discussion of the bill was a question asking how the AMA felt about it, the congressman shepherding the bill lied and reported that the AMA was behind it.[41] The bill passed without further debate, and law enforcement bureaucracies have built a huge industry around marijuana prohibition ever since.

Marijuana arrests in the United States are currently at their highest levels ever: 755,186 in 2003,[42] with the vast majority (88.6 percent) for possession.[43] I know many people who have been arrested on marijuana charges, and many more, myself included, who have been searched and harassed just for suspicion of possession. Let me tell you about the experience of my friend B., who was arrested in 2004 and convicted of selling an ounce of marijuana. B., who was seventy-five years old at the time, enjoyed smoking marijuana (before his two-year court-supervised probation began), but he was never a dealer. An acquaintance of his approached him with the story that his brother was battling cancer and needed marijuana to quell the nausea and discomfort of chemotherapy. Being a sympathetic soul, B. got him a bag. Unfortunately for B., his "friend" was outfitted with a recording device and B. was the target of a police sting operation. It turned out that the "friend" was facing criminal charges of his own and had been offered a deal in court if he would help target a dealer. Despite the preposterous circumstances, B. was convicted of a felony, was fined thousands of dollars, lost the right to vote, and is on probation for two years.

It could be worse. At least B. is not in jail. In 2000, 63 percent of marijuana sale convictions in the United States led to prison time, as did 51 percent of marijuana possession convictions.[44] In Tennessee a prison sentence for selling or even possessing a single ounce of marijuana can be as long as six years.[45] In Montana or Oklahoma a person selling it can be imprisoned *for life*.[46] Some 27,900 people were incarcerated in 2003 for marijuana offenses.[47]

The cost of this enforcement is high. Economist Jeffrey A. Miron calculated that in 2000 state and local governments spent $5.1 billion on marijuana enforcement, and the federal government spent $2.6 billion.[48] If marijuana were legalized, regulated, and taxed, he calculates that not only would governments save $7.7 billion, but the sales would generate additional tax revenues between $2.4 billion (if marijuana were taxed like all other goods) and $9.5 billion (if marijuana were taxed at rates comparable to those for alcohol and cigarettes).[49] Miron's findings were so stark that they prompted Nobel laureate economist Milton Friedman and five hundred other economists to send a letter to President Bush in 2005 urging an "open and honest debate" on marijuana prohibition: "We believe such a debate will favor a regime in which marijuana is legal but taxed and regulated like other goods."[50]

To mitigate the costs of the war on marijuana, asset forfeiture laws give law enforcement agencies the power to seize the property of individuals convicted, or even just accused, of marijuana and other drug crimes. Cash-strapped police forces can supplement their budgets by taking possession of marijuana offenders' homes and land. "Law enforcement agencies focus resources on enforcement of drug laws because of the financial gains for the agencies arising from forfeitures," observe the authors of *The Economic Anatomy of a Drug War*.[51]

What is the impact of all this aggressive anti-marijuana law enforcement? "Little evidence indicates this spending accomplishes the government's stated goal of reducing marijuana use," concludes Miron.[52] Though the marijuana prohibition makes millions of people criminals, marijuana use is as common as ever. According to the 2002 National Survey on Drug Use and Health, ninety-five million Americans, more than one in three, have used marijuana at some point in their lives. Around twenty-six million, or nearly 10 percent, are estimated to have used marijuana within the past year, and fifteen million are estimated to have used it within the past month.[53] Some estimates calculate marijuana as the biggest cash crop in the United States, of greater total value than either corn or soybeans, the two biggest legal plant commodities.[54] In 2003 more than 87 percent of high-school seniors reported that marijuana is "fairly easy" or "very easy" to obtain.[55]

So many people have personal experience with marijuana that it is widely understood to be benign, the greatest risk being that of discovery, not only by the law but by job-related drug testing. "Penalties against possession of a drug should not be more damaging to an individual than the use of the drug itself," said President Jimmy Carter, endorsing marijuana decriminalization in 1977.[56]

Through the 1970s most marijuana in the United States was imported. Ironically, the war on drugs stimulated domestic production by making it difficult, and thus expensive, to smuggle marijuana across the border. Homegrown marijuana was also encouraged when U.S. and Mexican authorities sprayed Mexican marijuana fields with the toxic herbicide paraquat, sparking concern over the safety of smoking Mexican marijuana. The Reagan administration targeted domestic marijuana growers with infrared air surveillance, forcing growers to decentralize into small operations and spurring innovations in indoor cultivation. Today much U.S. marijuana is grown in hermetically sealed grow rooms with hydroponics and carefully regulated light, temperature, and carbon dioxide levels. One result of the high-tech direction that marijuana growing has taken is that its potency has increased dramatically. Michael Pollan attended a convention of marijuana growers in Amsterdam, where he reflected: "It dawned on me that *this* was what the best gardeners of my generation had been doing all these years: they had been underground, perfecting cannabis."[57]

The current U.S. marijuana prohibition—exported worldwide via the 1961 United Nations Single Convention on Narcotic Drugs—is not the first time use of this plant has been outlawed. Among the heresies Pope Gregory IX sought to eradicate as the Inquisition got under way in 1231 was witchcraft, comprising largely the knowledge of and skills for using plants, including cannabis.[58] Plant healers have often faced persecution from central religious authorities. Chapter 6 explored this theme in relation to grassroots health care and the process by which knowledge of healing became professionalized by means of the outlawing of traditional healing practices. Witches were burned, but the plants themselves the Pope did not attempt to eradicate. "The plants were too precious to banish from human society," explains Michael Pollan; "cannabis, opium, belladonna, and the rest were simply transferred from the realm of sorcery to medicine."[59]

Marijuana is effective medicine. In the period when I felt the most depleted after long-persisting nausea, marijuana eased the nausea and kept me eating, and without it, I wonder whether I would be alive today. During this time I was up in Maine, in the midst of that state's medical marijuana referendum, and I talked to the doctor I saw up there about cannabis. He said that the medical literature confirmed the benefits I was reporting to him, and he noted my use of marijuana in my records; however, he felt that marijuana's legal status was still too tenuous for him to recommend it as a treatment. Maine's medical marijuana referendum passed, and ten other states have legalized the medical use of marijuana (Alaska, Arizona, California, Colorado, Hawaii, Nevada, Oregon, Rhode Island, Vermont, and Washington). In California, where medical marijuana has been effectively institutionalized, a number of people I know have received marijuana "prescriptions" from doctors and fill them at state-licensed "buying clubs."

I am glad that the people who need it are being granted legal access to this effective medicine. However, as a grassroots health-care activist, I believe that people should have access to safe and effective plant medicine without requiring a doctor's intervention. This is not a dangerous refined chemical warranting strict control by highly educated experts; it is a plant with far less toxicity than most over-the-counter treatments available for self-prescription. Just as the Inquisition suppressed grassroots plant knowledge and concentrated it under the control of the medical profession, so the current efforts to medicinalize marijuana disempower the lay generalist healer in favor of a doctor's prescription.

The pharmaceutical industry has already synthesized THC (tetrahydrocannabinol, the primary known psychoactive phytochemical in cannabis) and markets it as the prescription drug Marinol. It seems twisted to me that our government demonizes the cannabis plant and jails people for its cultivation, while it grants a patent for a drug mimicking the plant and approves the drug's sale by prescription. The discovery in the 1990s that the brain produces its own endogenous cannabinoids has spurred much new research aiming to synthesize other cannabinoid compounds. "New product opportunities will arise from more precise targeting of cannabinoids to specific illnesses and from the discovery and application of new cannabinoid products," speculates the Web site of GW Pharmaceuticals' Cannabinoid Research Institute.[60]

Some cannabinoid research aims to develop drugs containing the "medicinal" qualities of marijuana without the mind-altering ones. In my experience, the mind-altering qualities of marijuana are integral to its medical benefits. The way it relieves pain and nausea is by distracting the mind away from the pain and nausea. Distracting the mind of a sick person, enabling him or her to space out and not focus on the illness, can be a great and uplifting gift.

There was a time when I used to feel dismissive of marijuana activists. Dana Beale, one of the original Yippies[61] whom I saw in New York City activist circles into the 1990s, used to come to ACT UP meetings seeking support for various marijuana freedom campaigns. Though I have always supported marijuana freedom, I can remember judging Beale's agenda, for many issues seemed more urgent than "stoner" rights. They still do. But now, after devoting myself to gardening and the exploration of diverse plant usages, I have come to regard this issue as being much more fundamental than the right to get high. Suppression of plants and suppression of plant knowledge are anti-life assertions of a central authority seeking to control and disempower people, as with the Inquisition. People who resist this control and keep plant knowledge alive and seed varieties going are heroes. Sometimes laws that are antithetical to the truth must be broken.

Recipe: Extracting Cannabis into Oil or Butter

Though cannabis is most often smoked, at least in the United States, it also has a long history of being enjoyed as food. Many regions of the world have developed elaborate culinary traditions for the preparation of cannabis food and drink. Eating cannabis rather than smoking it spares your lungs, though because it metabolizes and takes effect much more slowly, dosage is more difficult to regulate.

Generally the way people cook with cannabis is to extract the THC into butter or oil. THC is oil-soluble, so it can be easily extracted into fats, but not into water. THC is most concentrated in cannabis flower buds, but it is found in lower concentrations throughout the rest of the plant. Cooking with cannabis butter or oil is an ideal way to make use of the leaves and stalks of the plant, after the flower buds have been separated and trimmed for smoking.

A disclaimer: Cooking with cannabis—like any possession or use of the plant—is illegal, except for medically sanctioned purposes in eleven states. The following recipes are intended for legal medical usage and are not encouragement to break the law.

My friend S.—who lives in California, where she uses legal medical cannabis to control her fibromyalgia—makes cannabis snacks for several of the organized cannabis-buying clubs in the Bay Area. S. collects discarded leaves and stalks and cooks them into butter and olive oil, which she incorporates into various delicacies. She uses $1\frac{1}{2}$ pounds of leaf for 5 pounds of butter or oil. If you grow your own cannabis or know someone who does, leaves and stalks are inevitable by-products that are abundantly available. If you have only buds available to you, use $\frac{1}{4}$ to $\frac{1}{2}$ ounce per pound of butter or oil.

The simplest method is direct extraction. First, grind the dry plant material to expose maximum surface area. Then sauté the well-ground plant material in butter or oil, very gently, for an hour or more. After sautéing you can strain out the plant solids and use just the infused butter or oil, or you can allow the butter or oil to remain coarse and leave the cannabis fibers in it. Fiber gives your digestive system a good scrub.

S. uses a more involved method, which I will describe for the adventurous connoisseur. S. has cooked far more cannabis than anyone else I know, and she is emphatic that the best way to extract the THC is by water extraction. This involves slowly and gently cooking the cannabis in butter or oil that is mixed with water. The addition of water enables you to cook the brew longer without any danger of burning, and S. says that it enables a fuller extraction of THC. Be aware that this is a strongly aromatic process which S. does legally—in accordance with state but not federal law—in her urban California neighborhood.

For water extraction, place the plant material in a cooking pot, cover it with water, add the butter or oil, and gently heat on a stovetop. Once the brew begins to bubble at the sides—before it comes to a full boil—

lower the heat, insert a heat distributor (a metal plate, often of several layers, that absorbs and spreads the heat) between the burner and the pot, cover the pot, and gently cook. S. recommends cooking for eighteen hours for a full extraction. If this is not practical, cook as long as you can.

As in salad dressing, the oil (or melted butter) will float to the top. When you are done cooking, you need to separate the cannabis oil from the water and spent plant fiber. The *easiest* way to separate out the plant fibers is to pour the cannabis-oil-water brew through a strainer and squeeze out as much of the liquid as you can. Unfortunately, some of the precious butter remains trapped in the spent plant material. S. says the *most effective* way of separating out the plant fibers without losing any oil is to fashion something akin to a French coffee press, a porous disc that presses the plant fibers to the bottom of the pot, under the water and out of the oil. Hardware cloth (a steel mesh available in hardware stores) or an aluminum pie plate with holes poked in could be cut to shape for this purpose. Use a spoon or other implement to press the disc down, trapping the plant fibers beneath it, and hold them at the bottom of the pot. Then move the whole pot, with the disc weighted down, to the refrigerator and cool it to congeal the oil or butter. Once the fat is congealed, carefully scoop it out, leaving behind the water and plant material to discard.

Use your butter or oil however you like. Spread it on toast, bake with it, or cook anything you like with it. Use just a little to start, until you gauge the potency and appropriate dosage. In contrast with smoking cannabis, which affects the brain within minutes, your body needs some time to metabolize the THC when you eat cannabis, so it doesn't take effect as quickly. In the interim, it is sometimes tempting to eat more; be aware that it is easy to eat too much cannabis. An overdose won't kill you, but it can make you feel disoriented, disabled, and uncomfortable. Start with a small amount, then wait two or three hours to see how it affects you before eating more. Always keep cannabis in a safe place, and clearly marked, to prevent people from unknowingly eating it.

Recipe: Savory Vegetable Strudel

Ingredients (for four strudel rolls)
1 box frozen phyllo pastry sheets
3 large onions
1 pound greens
1 head garlic
1 cup raisins or other dried fruit
1 sweet potato
3 slices dry bread
1^1/2 cups butter or oil, with or without cannabis
^{1}/4 to ^{1}/2 pound feta or other cheese (optional)
Salt to taste

Gertrude Stein's companion Alice B. Toklas was famous for her cannabis brownies, and most of the cannabis food I have been offered in my life has been in the form of brownies, cookies, chocolate truffles, and other sweets (including ice cream). But the last thing a sick person needs is all that sugar. Sugar suppresses white blood cell activity and immune function. I personally think savory foods are a better vehicle for medical marijuana. I love serving savory strudels of phyllo dough stuffed with sautéed vegetables, cheese, and dried fruit. This dish is delicious and may certainly be enjoyed without the cannabis, substituting unadulterated butter or oil.

The only special ingredient you need for this recipe beyond cannabis butter or oil (see the previous recipe) is a box of frozen phyllo pastry sheets. Follow the directions on the phyllo package regarding slow thawing in the refrigerator and how to remove individual sheets, to avoid having them stick together or become brittle. Phyllo sheets come in different sizes and thicknesses. A pound of phyllo sheets can wrap four or more strudel rolls, enough to feed eight as a meal or more as a snack or side dish.

The strudel stuffing can be improvised from common ingredients. Coarsely slice three large onions and chop about 1 pound of greens: spinach and/or lamb's quarters, cabbage, kale, or collards work well. Peel and chop a head's worth of garlic cloves. Plump raisins and/or other dry fruit by pouring hot water over 1 cup of the fruit and letting it sit, covered, for fifteen minutes. Peel a sweet potato, chop it, and steam until soft. Cut a few slices of dry bread into about 1 cup of small croutons.

Sauté the onions in ¼ cup of butter or olive oil until they are lightly caramelized. Add greens and sauté only until wilted. Then add the garlic, soaked fruit (drained first), sweet potatoes, croutons, and salt to taste. This, along with cheese, which you'll add later, is the stuffing for the strudel. Add other seasonal vegetables or special treats if you like: roasted peppers or eggplant, carrots or turnips, broccoli, okra, artichoke hearts, sausage, or just about anything else.

To assemble the strudel, unwrap the thawed phyllo sheets and carefully peel off the top sheet. Lay it on a towel and brush generously with butter or olive oil. The phyllo layer absorbs that oil, and it keeps the sheets crispy and distinct, so that they don't stick to each other and melt into a single mass. Lay another sheet on top of the first and brush it with butter or oil. Continue until five sheets are stacked and brushed. This should take about ¼ cup of butter or oil. Then spread a strip of stuffing about 2 inches wide down a long side of the stacked sheets, leaving about 1 inch at either end to fold in and contain the strudel. Crumble cheese over the stuffing, if you wish. I use our homemade goat cheese, but feta or any crumbly cheese—or any cheese, really—is fine. You can also use homemade sour cream or cottage cheese (see page 178 for the recipe). Begin to roll the strudel, using the towel to lift up the phyllo and filling, and fold it over. Tuck in the ends of the roll, then roll until the entire phyllo stack is wrapped around the stuffing. Brush the outside with butter or oil. Move the roll to a greased cookie sheet. Repeat for more rolls. Bake at 350°F (175°C) for thirty to forty-five minutes, until golden brown. Slice and serve hot or cold.

Alternatively you can present these as individually wrapped phyllo triangles. Cut a sheet of phyllo dough into strips about 3 inches wide. Brush a strip with butter or oil. Place a teaspoonful of stuffing and a bit of cheese at one end of the strip. Fold a corner of the strip over the filling diagonally to the other side. Then fold up the other corner, folding along the edge of the previous fold, and continue folding up the triangle until you reach the end of the strip. Brush the outside of each triangle with butter or oil, then place on a cookie sheet and bake for fifteen to twenty minutes.

Enjoy this savory strudel as an hors d'oeuvre or as a main dish. Remember, start with just a small serving of cannabis food. And be sure you have other food around, so that if the cannabis stimulates your appetite, you'll have snacks other than more of it.

Policing Plant Knowledge and Usages

Cannabis is illegal, but in actuality its status is more complex and nuanced than that. In ten states it is legal within certain limits with a doctor's recommendation, though the Supreme Court has affirmed that the federal government may still enforce its prohibition even in states in which medical marijuana is allowed. Hemp fibers are legal to import into the United States. They come primarily from Canada, which legalized and started licensing hemp growing in 1998. Canadian farmers plant more acres in hemp every year; in 2005 they produced the crop on an estimated 24,000 acres.[62] The European Union even subsidizes hemp growers to encourage production. North Dakota, Hawaii, Kentucky, Maine, Montana, and West Virginia have all passed laws to license hemp growers, in anticipation of a relaxation of federal anti-hemp laws. These states are even considering a lawsuit challenging the federal hemp ban. "It's legal for us to import the stalks and the seed and turn them into clothes and food, but it's not legal for us to grow it," observes North Dakota Agricultural Commissioner Roger Johnson. "What's the sense in that?"

The official U.S. war-on-drugs position on hemp is "Just Say No!" In 2001 the Drug Enforcement Agency (DEA) announced a ban on the importation and sale of hemp food products, including those containing hemp seeds, which up until that time had been legal to import and sell provided they were sterilized (usually by irradiation) so they could not be used to grow cannabis plants. In fact, the seeds of cannabis contain only traces of THC but much protein and oil, with both medicinal and nutritional value. Our government shouts "Free Trade!" when other nations restrict imports of genetically modified foods because of safety concerns and challenges their right to restrict trade at all. But this same government tried to restrict imports of hemp.

The Hemp Industries Association, retailers, and a Canadian hemp exporter sued the DEA to stop the hemp seed ban. The Ninth Circuit Court of Appeals allowed hemp product sales to resume in 2002 and reversed the DEA action in 2004, with a unanimous ruling that the DEA had exceeded its authority. The court even ordered the DEA to pay a portion of the plaintiffs' legal fees (much of it reimbursing Dr. Bronner's Magic Soaps), and the government declined to appeal the ruling to the Supreme Court.[63]

All the plants condemned as illicit drugs actually have strangely convoluted legal status. Cocaine is made from the leaves of coca (*Erythroxylum coca*), a plant indigenous to highland regions of South America. The drug cocaine was first refined from coca leaves in 1860 by a German chemist. The chemist's transmutation of the plant rapidly sealed its fate. Traditionally the leaf of the plant had been simply chewed raw or roasted and ground into a fine powder. Coca leaves are a food containing not only a small amount of the numbing alkaloid cocaine but also vitamins, minerals, protein, carbohydrates, and fibers. The whole plant is much more than just the isolated active ingredient. This plant is essential nourishment for the people who depend upon it, not a recreational drug. In addition to all these nutrients, coca leaves contain compounds that regulate glucose metabolism and are thought to help those who eat it digest carbohydrates.[64]

Before the end of the nineteenth century, just a few decades after its invention, cocaine began to be regarded as an addictive and dangerous substance. It is. The Pure Food and Drug Act of 1906 established cocaine as a controlled substance in the United States. Coca-Cola had to remove cocaine as an ingredient in its popular beverage. But it kept using the coca leaves as a source of flavoring in its secret formula. According to ethnobotanist Wade Davis:

> To this day coca leaves are brought into the United States by the Stepan Chemical Company of Maywood, New Jersey, the only legal importer in the country. Once the cocaine has been removed and sold to the pharmaceutical industry, the residue containing the essential oils and flavonoids is shipped to Coca-Cola. The company is not especially proud of this fact, but it ought to be, for it is the essence of the leaves that makes Coca-Cola the "real thing."[65]

So exceptions to the coca ban are granted for Coke and pharmaceutical manufacturers. Unfortunately the diverse highlands peoples whose traditional cultures revolve around this plant have not been granted similar exemptions. The anti-cocaine panic led to anti-coca laws. Ever since, various government and international initiatives—in our time, the American war on drugs—have sought, unsuccessfully, to eradicate the plant. Exclusive rights to the use of fragmented elements of the plant are granted to corporations; but then, in yet another case of biopiracy, peoples' rights to use the same plant in traditional ways are taken away. "The real issue is cultural identity and the survival of those who traditionally have revered the plant," concludes Davis. "Take away access to coca, and you destroy the spirit of the people."[66]

The legal situation with regard to opium poppies (*Papaver somniferum*) is even more convoluted. As with marijuana and coca, the active compounds in poppies have been isolated, synthesized, and widely incorporated into the pharmaceutical pharmacopeia. "Yet although the medical value of my poppies is widely recognized," writes Michael Pollan, reflecting in *Harper's Magazine* about his poppy-growing experience, "my failure to heed what amounts to a set of regulations (that only a pharmaceutical company may handle these flowers; that only a doctor may dispense their extracts) and prejudices (that refined alkaloids are superior to crude ones) governing their production and use makes me not just a scofflaw but a felon."[67]

Poppies are not banned outright in the United States. Many seed catalogs sell *Papaver somniferum* seeds, and many people grow them perfectly legally in their gardens. Poppy seeds have many culinary (nonnarcotic) uses and are widely used in baked goods. Dried poppy seedpods, which can be easily ground into a powder and steeped in water to produce a potent opium tea, are popular in floral arrangements and are commercially available. What renders growing opium poppies or possessing their seedpods illegal is if it is done "knowingly or intentionally."[68] In true Orwellian fashion, ignorance is security and knowledge is dangerous.

Jim Hogshire, the author of a do-it-yourself guide called *Opium for the Masses*, knew too much and brazenly shared his knowledge. One day a police SWAT team raided his Seattle apartment (his book constituting probable cause for the search warrant), found several bunches of dried poppies he had legally purchased from a florist, and arrested Hogshire and his wife on felony drug charges. Hogshire reports that a police officer waved a copy of *Opium for the Masses* in his face and asked, "With what you write, weren't you expecting this?"[69] It was Hogshire's exercise of free speech that rendered his activities illegal. "Whether or not the opium poppies in your garden [or indeed, purchased from a florist] are illicit depends not on what you do, or even intend to do, with them but very simply on what you know about them," concludes Pollan.[70]

This distinction, in which knowledge places people in legal jeopardy, is appearing in more drug laws. In 2005 Louisiana enacted a law making it a crime "for any person knowingly or intentionally to possess a material, compound, mixture, or preparation intended for human consumption which contains a hallucinogenic plant." The law names thirty-nine different hallucinogenic plants and fungi, many of them common weeds.[71] If datura grows in your yard, no problem. If you accidentally serve it in a salad and people get sick, still no problem, at least in terms of criminal liability. But in Louisiana, if you were in possession of a book of ancient witchy knowledge, with recipes for extracting datura into a flying ointment, that same weed in your yard becomes criminal due to your knowledge, and you could find yourself doing ten years with hard labor.

The aromatic roots of the sassafras tree, one of the original sources of flavoring in root beers, is also subject to legal restrictions. Human consumption of sassafras roots and essential oil was banned by the U.S. Food and Drug Administration in the 1960s after the active compound, safrole, when isolated, was determined to be carcinogenic in laboratory animals. But is brewing tea or root beer from a plant root really the equivalent of ingesting high concentrations of an isolated active compound? "There is no question that pure alkaloids and essential oils . . . can cause cancers and precancerous changes, severely injure, and even kill," writes Susun Weed. "However, the scientific tradition claim that the crude plant itself is harmful, not just the oil or alkaloid, is questionable."[72] Processes of refinement transform plants into chemicals, drugs, and essential oils. It's ridiculous to try to regulate crude plants in the same manner as the various concentrated products into which they may be made.

Some of the concentrated substances that can be refined from plants are dangerous or addictive. This reality I do not dispute. But plants themselves are not drugs. The current war on drugs perpetuates the underlying dynamics of the Inquisition and various other witch hunts throughout history. It is a war against community-based plant knowledge on behalf of the industries (pharmaceutical), professions (medical), and authorities whose powers are increased by our disempowerment. We must safeguard and assert our rights to associate, as amateurs, with a diversity of useful plants. As David Theodoropoulos exhorts, "Exchange, propagate, plant, and release."[73]

Recipes: Sassafras Tea and Roots Beer

Sassafras was regarded as one of the wonders of the New World by the colonizers. Many peoples of eastern North America used the leaves, flowers, and roots of the tree as food and medicine. Sassafras's distinctive taste and smell were exotic in Europe, and in the early years of colonial settlement sassafras was one of the major exports from the New World that arriving ships brought back with them on the homeward passage.

Spanish physician Nicolas Monardes waxed poetic in 1574 about the medicinal uses of this tree: "The Spaniards did begin to cure themselves with the water of this tree and it did in them great effects, that it is almost incredible . . . they were healed of so many griefs and evil diseases that to hear of them what they suffred and how they were healed it doeth bring admiration and they which were whole drank it in place of wine, for it doeth preserve them in health."[74] Peter Holmes's more contemporary herbal, *The Energetics of Western Herbs*, credits sassafras with stimulating circulation; relieving joint and muscle pain; promoting sweat, urination, and menstruation; draining fluid congestion; dissolving stones; reducing fevers; stimulating digestion; and healing the skin.[75]

Sassafras has a long tradition of use as a spring tonic tea, for which the bark of the root is boiled, often along with other roots. A little bit of sassafras goes a long way. Dried sassafras root bark is commercially available where other herbs are sold, or you can find a sassafras tree and

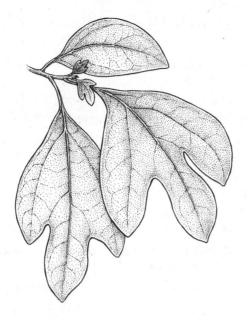

Sassafras. ©Bobbi Angell. Used by permission.

harvest some yourself. The lowest-impact way to harvest sassafras is to find a dense grove of sassafras seedlings, each displaying miniature versions of the tree's distinctive handlike leaves. Thin the seedlings by digging up a few. The roots of seedlings can be used in their entirety, once they have been cleaned and chopped. I've also harvested roots from mature sassafras trees that blew over, roots and all, in storms. If you harvest roots from mature living trees, be gentle. Dig for roots at least six feet away from the trunk in order to limit the damage to the tree. You know a sassafras root when you hit it because it releases a powerful, distinctive, sweet aroma. Break through the root with your shovel once you hit it. Leave the end that is attached to the tree, and pry, pull, and coax out of the earth as much as you can of the rest of the root. Scrub the roots clean, then shave off the root bark with a vegetable peeler or knife, leaving the pithy core of the root. You can dry the root bark and store it in a jar, or you can use it fresh.

For tea, simmer the sassafras root bark very gently for about half an hour. It takes cooking to get roots to release their flavors, but a full boil will cause the volatile oil to evaporate. See how you like sassafras flavor on its own. Experiment with adding other roots. Try burdock, yellow dock, dandelion, licorice, ginger, and others. Sassafras tea served warm with milk and sugar makes a once-popular beverage called saloop.

You can also turn your sassafras tea into root beer, or better yet, roots beer. My friend Frank Cook, who spent time in the Jamaican bush learning how people there use plants, reports that people he met mixed the roots and other parts of more than twenty different plants to make a "roots beer."

My favorite method for getting the roots beer bubbling is called a ginger bug, which takes up to a week to get going. Grate about 2 teaspoons worth of fresh ginger, or in a pinch you can use ground dried ginger. Combine the ginger and about 2 teaspoons of sugar (or other sweetener) with 1 cup of tepid water. Stir. Leave the bug in a warm spot, loosely covered but not airtight. Stir as often as you think of it, several times a day. Add ginger and sugar every day until your bug is good and bubbly. Then it is ready to use. Keep feeding it daily until you use it, or slow it down by placing it in the refrigerator.

When you are ready to ferment, make a sweet roots tea. For a gallon of root beer use maybe 4 to 6 ounces of mixed roots. Gently simmer the roots, as described above for making sassafras tea. Sassafras tea is a great base, but I think the flavor of root beer is enhanced by multiplicity and complexity. Licorice is a great accent, but it's very strong, so use it sparingly. Ginger is a great accent, too. Burdock is mellow, earthy, and sweet. Sarsaparilla (*Smilax*) is a wonderful flavor. Experiment with other roots and plants. Once the tea is brewed, cool it to body temperature and strain out the plant material.

Mix sweetener into the strained tea. Many recipes will tell you to mix in sweetener while the tea is hot so it will dissolve more easily, but I like to use at least some "live" sweeteners, such as raw honey. So I preserve the raw nutrients by adding it after the tea has cooled to body temperature, and with a little stirring it will dissolve easily. Just as mixing the roots adds complexity and mystery to the root beer, so does mixing different sweeteners. My favorite mix is raw honey (from our bees), accented by sorghum molasses (a food tradition that endures around these parts), maple syrup, and just a touch of strong-flavored blackstrap molasses. You could use sugar if you like, but these less refined sweeteners contribute more flavor to the root beer. Don't use stevia, which some people use as a sweetener, because it is not a carbohydrate and will not feed the fermentation organisms. Use about 2 cups of sweetener for a gallon of root beer, more or less. Start with less and let taste be your guide. Make your wort a touch sweeter than you wish your finished root beer to be, as some of the sugar will be consumed in fermentation.

Now add the vigorously bubbling ginger bug to the sweetened wort and stir. Transfer the wort to a glass or ceramic vessel (*not* metal), loosely covered to protect the wort from flies and dust but not airtight. Leave the wort in a warm spot and stir periodically for a day or so, until it becomes actively bubbly. Then it is ready to bottle.

Homemade sodas are carbonated by sealing them in airtight bottles while they are actively fermenting. This traps the carbon dioxide generated by the fermentation process in the bottle, under pressure. But if the soda or beer ferments too long inside the bottle it can become over-pressurized. Bottles have been known to explode, and when a bottle is opened the pressure can easily spray the contents everywhere. Modest carbonation is more useful than extreme carbonation.

I like to bottle homemade sodas in used plastic 2- and 3-liter soda bottles. They are abundantly available for free everywhere and require no special gadget to seal them, and best of all you can easily feel how pressurized they are becoming, which you cannot do with glass. On the downside, they release chemicals into whatever is stored inside them. Absolutely you can bottle root beer and other sodas in glass bottles, so long as they are sealable and designed to withstand the pressure of carbonation.

Ferment soda in the bottles for about a week—less if it's really warm, more if they are in a cold spot. If you are using plastic, you will feel the bottle becoming firmer and less yielding to your touch. That's the building pressure. When the soda has fermented long enough, move it to the fridge. The cold slows down fermentation to an imperceptible rate, so you can store the bottles there for a while. Also, when you open cold bottles they spew less and you lose less soda. Remember that carbonation can be explosive. Wrap bottles in a towel before opening them (for safety, just in case the bottle actually explodes, which does happen), and open them over a sink. One of the fringe benefits of writing and teaching about fermentation is that lots of people want to share their ferments with me, and along with wonderful homemade sodas in many unusual flavors, I have witnessed some explosive brews!

A note on alcohol: Many people who are interested in natural sodas talk in terms of "lacto-fermented" beverages to distinguish them from alcohol-fermented beverages. The reality of this ginger-bug method is that it appears to yield a mixed culture, a starter that is a community of microorganisms, including both *Lactobacillus* (bacteria) and *Saccharomyces* (yeast), along with probably others as well. In the fermentation some modest amount of alcohol is produced by the yeast, along with lactic acid from lactobacilli. If you desire to minimize alcohol content, minimize the fermentation time. Or try another starter, such as whey or kefir grains, though these too probably generate some alcohol. Sugars attract yeast, and except perhaps under extremely controlled conditions, it is unlikely that sugars can be fermented without some alcohol production.

Action and Information Resources

Books

Bey, Hakim, and Abel Zug, eds. *Orgies of the Hemp Eaters: Cuisine, Slang, Literature, and Ritual of Cannabis Culture*. Brooklyn, NY: Autonomedia, 2004.

Booth, Martin. *Cannabis: A History*. New York: St. Martin's Press, 2003.

Davis,Wade. *One River: Explorations and Discoveries in the Amazon Rainforest*. New York: Simon & Schuster, 1996.

Fowler, Cary, and Pat Mooney. *Shattering: Food, Politics, and the Loss of Genetic Diversity*. Tucson: University of Arizona Press, 1990.

Grinspoon, Lester, M.D. and Bakalar, James B. *Marihuana: The Forbidden Medicine*. New Haven, CT: Yale University Press, 1997.

Herer, Jack. *The Emperor Wears No Clothes*. Van Nuys, CA: HEMP, 1990.

Hogshire, Jim. *Opium for the Masses*. Port Townsend, WA: Loompanics, 1994.

McKenna, Terence. *Food of the Gods: The Search for the Original Tree of Knowledge—A Radical History of Plants, Drugs, and Human Evolution*. New York: Bantam Books, 1993.

Pendell, Dale. *Pharmako/Dynamis: Stimulating Plants, Potions and Herbcraft*. San Francisco: Mercury House, 2002.

————. *Pharmako/Poeia: Plant Powers, Poisons, and Herbcraft*. San Francisco: Mercury House, 1994.

Pollan, Michael. *The Botany of Desire*. New York: Random House, 2001.

Rasmussen, David W., and Bruce L. Benson. *The Economic Anatomy of a Drug War*. Lanham, MD: Rowman & Littlefield, 1994.

Schivelbusch, Wolfgang. *Tastes of Paradise: A Social History of Spices, Stimulants, and Intoxicants*. Translated by David Jacobson. New York: Vintage Books, 1993.

Starhawk. *Dreaming the Dark: Magic, Sex and Politics*. Boston: Beacon Press, 1982. See especially appendix A, "The Burning Times: Notes on a Crucial Period of History."

Theodoropoulos, David I. *Invasion Biology: Critique of a Pseudoscience*. Blythe, CA: Avvar Books, 2003.

Organizations and Other Resources

American Medical Marijuana Association
www.americanmarijuana.org

Drug Policy Alliance
70 West 36th Street, 16th Floor
New York, NY 10018
(212) 613-8020
www.drugpolicy.org

Drug Reform Coordination Network
1623 Connecticut Avenue NW, 3rd Floor
Washington, DC 20009
(202) 293-8340
www.stopthedrugwar.org

Hemp Industries Association
PO Box 1080
Occidental, CA 95465
(707) 874-3648
www.thehia.org

Marijuana Policy Project
PO Box 77492
Washington, DC 20013
www.mpp.org

National Organization for the Reform of
    Marijuana Laws
1600 K Street NW, Suite 501
Washington, DC 20006-2832
(202) 483-5500
www.norml.org

The No White List Coalition
www.geocities.com/nowhitelist

The Sentencing Project
514 Tenth Street NW, Suite 1000
Washington, DC 20004
(202) 628-0871
www.sentencingproject.org

United Plant Savers
PO Box 400
East Barre, VT 05649
(802) 476-6467
www.unitedplantsavers.org

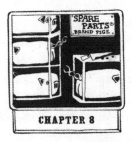

CHAPTER 8

Vegetarian Ethics and Humane Meat

I love meat. The smell of it cooking can fill me with desire, and I find its juicy, rich flavor uniquely satisfying. At the same time, everything I see, hear, or read about standard commercial factory farming and slaughtering fills me with disgust. I hold great respect for the ideals that people seek to put into practice through vegetarianism.

Vegetarianism is the original manifestation of food activism. Since ancient times vegetarians have sought to embody ideals that they see as making the world a kinder, gentler place. A small minority of people throughout history—mostly inspired by religious ideals—have eschewed animal flesh, among them Buddhists, Hindus, Jains, Roman Catholic Trappist monks, and Essenes, an ancient Jewish sect. Historically vegetarianism has been a practice of asceticism: a rejection of material pleasure and an embrace of universal compassion. In more recent times vegetarianism has largely been motivated by political and ethical ideas, as well as the pursuit of good health, as we shall explore below.

I was a half-hearted vegetarian for a couple of years, even vegan (avoiding not only meat but all animal products) for a little while, based on the abstract idea that animal fats are unhealthy, which I no longer believe to be true. When I tried being vegan, I found myself dreaming about eggs. I could find no virtue in denying my desires. I now understand that many nutrients are soluble only in fats, and animal fats can be vehicles of rich nourishment. Of course, much depends upon how the animals are raised, and also upon how you integrate them into your diet.

Animals raised factory-style, pumped up with antibiotics and growth hormones and fed the by-products of chemical agriculture, contain high levels of toxicity that have become concentrated up the food chain. They are also often treated cruelly and live in deplorable conditions. A friend who attends a state agriculture school was in a livestock class that required students to perform acts of unnecessary violence such as dehorning mature bulls, rather than the alternative procedure of cauterization in infancy, which involves far less pain and suffering. Students' concerns about animal welfare were dismissed by the professor with "Don't go PETA on me" (PETA being the animal-rights direct-action group People for the Ethical Treatment of Animals). "The industrial farm is said to have been patterned on the factory production line," writes Wendell Berry "In practice, it looks more like a concentration camp."[1]

Where the meat comes from and how the animals lived are factors that figure into my eating decisions. I am grateful to be meeting farmers everywhere who are talking about the ethics that guide their animal raising and slaughtering practices. I appreciate that they are reflecting upon these difficult questions, trying to learn what exactly it means to breed and kill animals in a conscientious way. Animal-rights activists may consider "humane meat" to be an oxymoron, but for many of us seeking to satisfy our nutritional needs while upholding values of simple decency, humane meat is instead an ideal to strive for and support.

Factory-Farming Horrors

The lives and the deaths of animals in mass production are ugly, and the more I learn about them, the less I want to eat factory-farmed meat, eggs, and dairy. Food labels and ads often depict contented animals outdoors, presumably on small family farms. In reality, the lives of the animals whose meat, milk, and eggs are found in supermarkets and most restaurants are anything but pastoral; they live in cruel confinement in unhealthy conditions and are pushed—by technological means such as genetically engineered growth hormones—to produce beyond their natural limits.

The markets for meat and other animal products, like the markets for other foods, have been steadily concentrated in fewer and fewer hands. Four firms control 80 percent of the cattle market, and five firms control 63 percent of the hog market.[2] A branch of the U.S, Department of Agriculture (USDA), the Packers and Stockyards Program, is charged with monitoring the meat industry and taking action to remedy price collusion and other anticompetitive behavior. But government watchdogs often turn out to have strong allegiance to the industries they are theoretically supposed to be regulating; according to an internal audit by USDA's inspector general, the program has failed to investigate such behavior and has not filed a single administrative complaint for anticompetitive behavior in the meat or poultry industry since 1999.[3]

In addition to horizontal concentration, which limits competition among processors and leaves farmers with few large buyers, the meat-processing industries are concentrating vertically, with the major firms controlling every aspect of production, from breeding and raising the animals to slaughtering and processing their meat. In vertically integrated production, the corporate-owned animals are farmed out (as it were) by contract to feedlot farms; the animals are "passed along from stage to stage, but ownership never changes and neither does the location of the decision-making," reports the U.S. National Farmers Union. "Starting with the intellectual property rights that governments give to the biotechnology firms, the food product always remains the property of a firm or cluster of firms."[4]

How could mass production of animal products be anything but ugly? The gruesome realities of the industry that delivers cheap animal products to the supermarket are kept far from public view, but every so often a new sensational exposé captures public attention. In 2003 Virgil Butler started an online blog following his firing by Tyson Foods, the world's largest poultry processor, from the job he had held for ten years at poultry processing plants in Arkansas. Butler's graphic accounts of his job "have electrified animal-rights activists around the globe," according to the *Los Angeles Times*.[5] Here is an excerpt from his blog:

Here come the birds through the stunner into the killing machine. It's time to get busy. You can expect to have to catch every fifth one or so, many that are not stunned. Remember, they come at you 182–186 per minute. There is blood everywhere, in the 3' x 3' x 20' trough beneath the machine, on your face, your neck, your arms, all down your apron. You are covered in it. Sometimes you have to wash off the clots of blood, without taking your eyes off the line lest one slip by, which they will. . . .

The sheer amount of killing and blood can really get to you after awhile, especially if you can't just shut down all emotion completely and turn into a robot zombie of death. You feel like part of a big death machine. Pretty much treated that way as well. Sometimes weird thoughts will enter your head. It's just you and the dying chickens. The surreal feelings grow into such a horror of the barbaric nature of your behavior.

You are murdering helpless birds by the thousands (75,000 to 90,000 a night). You are a killer. You can't really talk to anyone about this. The guys at work will think you are soft. Family and friends don't want to know about this. It makes them uncomfortable and unsure of what to say or how to act. They can even look at you a little weird. Some don't want much else to do with you when they know what you do for a living. You are a killer.

Out of desperation you send your mind elsewhere so that you don't end up like those guys that lose it. Like the guy that fell on his knees praying to God for forgiveness. Or the guy they hauled off to the mental hospital that kept having nightmares that chickens were after him. I've had those, too. (Shudder) Very creepy. You find something else to dwell on to try to remove yourself from the situation. To keep your mind from drowning in all those hundreds of gallons of blood you see. Most people who work this room and work in the hanging cage use some sort of stimulant to keep up the pace and some sort of mellowing substance to escape reality. . . .

You shut down all emotions eventually. You just can't care about anything. Because if you care about something, it opens the gate to all those bad feelings that you can't afford to feel and still do your job. You have bills to pay. You have to eat. But,

you don't want chicken. You have to be really hungry to eat
that. You know what goes into every bite. All the horror and
negativity. All the brutality. Concentrated into every bite. . . .
Welcome to the nightmare I escaped.[6]

The graphic recounting of horrors such as these can have a strong
impact. One hundred years ago Upton Sinclair scandalized readers and
catalyzed regulatory reform of the meatpacking industry with his best-
selling novel *The Jungle* (1906), which exposed practices in the slaughterhouses of Chicago's stockyards—at the time the biggest animal-processing
district in the world.

> It was all so very businesslike that one watched it fascinated. It
> was porkmaking by machinery, porkmaking by applied mathe-
> matics. . . . The carcass hog was scooped out of the vat by
> machinery, and then it fell to the second floor, passing on the
> way through a wonderful machine with numerous scrapers,
> which adjusted themselves to the size and shape of the animal,
> and sent it out at the other end with nearly all of its bristles
> removed. It was then again strung up by machinery, and sent
> upon another trolley ride; this time passing between two lines
> of men, who sat upon a raised platform, each doing a certain
> single thing to the carcass as it came to him. One scraped the
> outside of a leg; another scraped the inside of the same leg.
> One with a swift stroke cut the throat; another with two swift
> strokes severed the head, which fell to the floor and vanished
> through a hole. Another made a slit down the body; a second
> opened the body wider; a third with a saw cut the breastbone;
> a fourth loosened the entrails; a fifth pulled them out—and
> they also slid through a hole in the floor. There were men to
> scrape each side and men to scrape the back; there were men
> to clean the carcass inside, to trim it and wash it. Looking down
> this room, one saw, creeping slowly, a line of dangling hogs a
> hundred yards in length; and for every yard there was a man,
> working as if a demon were after him. At the end of this hog's
> progress every inch of the carcass had been gone over several
> times; and then it was rolled into the chilling room, where it

stayed for twenty-four hours, and where a stranger might lose himself in a forest of freezing hogs.[7]

The same Chicago stockyard that Sinclair described, known as the "disassembly line," is widely credited as having been Henry Ford's inspiration for the automobile assembly line.

As if factory-style death wasn't gruesome enough, the *lives* of animals raised en masse are generally cruel and horrible. In the egg industry, for example, freshly hatched male chicks, who will bear no eggs, are literally thrown into garbage bags to suffocate; chickens' beaks are routinely cut off; and egg-laying hens are crowded into cages where they cannot open their wings or turn around. To produce veal, calves are shut in tight stalls so they cannot exercise their muscles, which would toughen their tender flesh; they are fed a diet designed to induce anemia and keep their flesh white; and they are deprived of water and sunlight. Foie gras is a pâté made from the swollen and fatty livers of geese force-fed huge quantities of high-fat food. Eating meat requires death, yes, but not torture.

It's hard for me to imagine how the mass production of flesh could be anything other than horrible. Car manufacturing may lend itself to factory production, but factory-farming of animals inevitably leads to cruelty and disease. Mass-produced animal foods are almost always diseased. Animals are fed constant subtherapeutic doses of antibiotics to encourage more rapid weight gain and to ward off some of the diseases that are common in the overcrowded conditions in which they are made to live. This practice in turn encourages the evolution of antibiotic-resistant diseases in both animals and people. The recombinant bovine growth hormone used to stimulate milk production (see page 164) creates udder infections and pus-filled milk that requires pasteurization. It's safe to assume that factory-farmed eggs carry salmonella. The ever-expanding scale of farming, concentrating unprecedented populations of animals in close proximity, gives rise to zoonotic (jumping from animal species to humans) diseases such as bovine spongiform encephalopathy (BSE, or mad cow disease) and avian flu.

After the first wave of mad cow disease in Britain, but before the first case was reported in the United States, former rancher Howard Lyman went on a crusade to warn U.S. consumers that the industry practice of feeding cows to cows made a mad cow outbreak in the United States inevitable. Lyman appeared on Oprah Winfrey's TV show in April 1996 as part of a panel discussion on food safety. When Lyman described the practice of feeding cows to cows, Oprah expressed revulsion and stated, "It has just stopped me cold from eating another burger!"

The day after the show aired, the beef futures market plummeted. Industry analysts referred to this as the "Oprah crash." Oprah invited industry representatives to debate Lyman on her show, which they declined, but she gave them ten minutes anyway to make their case. Subsequently a group of Texas cattlemen filed a suit against Oprah and Lyman under Texas's False Disparagement of Perishable Food Products Act. Texas and at least twelve other states (Alabama, Arizona, Colorado, Florida, Georgia, Idaho, Louisiana, Mississippi, North Dakota, Ohio, Oklahoma, and South Dakota) have enacted such laws to protect their agricultural industries from economic damage caused by unfounded media reports disparaging their practices or products.

The charges against Oprah and Lyman were dismissed, but food disparagement laws have had a chilling effect on meaningful public debate, because media outlets want to protect themselves from lawsuits. Public discussion of important issues—not only mad cow disease but questions about the safety of genetically modified foods—become legal minefields because of food disparagement laws. "Lawsuits like this stifle speech about matters that have implications for the health and welfare of every American consumer," reflects Lyman. "At a time when threats to food safety are arguably greater than ever—threats exacerbated by intense confinement conditions that abet the spread of disease, and by controversial feeding practices—we need a free and open discussion about these matters."[8]

Meanwhile, Lyman's predictions about mad cow disease have come true, and the industry has been forced to abandon the practice of feeding cows to cows. Lyman believes that mad cow disease is much more widespread than has been reported and that its symptoms in humans are not being recognized. Thirty-six countries have banned imports of U.S. beef after cases of mad cow here; their fear of importing the disease has been compounded by USDA attempts to cover up new cases and international criticism of the agency's monitoring methods.[9]

The USDA's latest plan for monitoring and controlling emerging epidemics among farm animals is the National Animal Identification

System (NAIS). This program would require that every farm animal in the United States be registered with the USDA and assigned a fifteen-digit federal identification number. Every animal would be implanted with a unique radio-frequency tag, so that its whereabouts can be monitored in a single centralized database. "Sounds like Animal Farm meets Big Brother," observes journalist Amanda Griscom Little.[10]

The NAIS has been extremely unpopular with small farmers, and it is opposed by a grassroots groundswell. The plan was developed in consultation with the meat industry's trade association and contains provisions for owners of large herds of animals that are bought, moved, and slaughtered together (the model in the largest vertically integrated livestock firms) to identify an entire herd with a single ID number. This means that the program will be more burdensome and costly for small farms, which will have to tag each animal, than for large ones, which will be able to tag groups en masse. "It's horribly insidious," says Lynn Miller, editor of *Small Farmer's Journal*. "The USDA is poised to push us off our farms."[11] Ironically, this factory-farm loophole will further reinforce economies of scale and encourage even greater concentrations of livestock, the very conditions that gave rise to the disease epidemics that the program is ostensibly designed to control.

Varieties of Vegetarian Volition

The realities of factory-farmed meat make a compelling case for vegetarianism, though people are motivated to become vegetarians by many different concerns. A number of people I've talked to about it just always felt a visceral revulsion toward meat and stopped eating it, even as children, as best they could. Many vegetarians stop eating meat for more ideological reasons. Religious beliefs have inspired vegetarians for thousands of years. Reincarnation, for instance, suggests that the same souls incarnate as animals and as humans, raising the possibility that the animal you are eating was your grandmother or some other beloved soul. Many different ideals, from renunciations of the pleasures of the body to expressions of compassion toward all living creatures, lead spiritual adherents to reject animal flesh.

Animal welfare is another ancient motivation for vegetarianism. Can we not refrain from murdering our fellow beings? This question has often been linked to the human tendency toward violence, and philosophies of pacifism and nonviolence have also long inspired vegetarians. "For as long as men massacre animals, they will kill each other," the vegetarian Greek philosopher and mathematician Pythagoras is said to have observed.[12] As if to illustrate Pythagoras's point, during the rise and spread of Christianity many vegetarian sects were attacked as heretical. According to the British Vegetarian Society, "These non-violent vegetarian ascetics were painted as fanatical deviants, feared, loathed, and frequently persecuted by the established church."[13] Pythagorean ideals of peaceful coexistence with animals reemerged during the Enlightenment and were embraced by several different Christian movements of the nineteenth century. Until the past century, in fact, vegetarians were often referred to as Pythagoreans.

Promoting a more equitable usage of natural resources is another important motivation for many vegetarians. A watershed book that helped catalyze the contemporary vegetarian movement is Frances Moore Lappé's 1971 *Diet for a Small Planet*. This book drew connections between the persistence of world hunger and the practice of feeding grain to livestock. Each pound of beef, reported Lappé, required twenty-one pounds of high-quality grain that could otherwise nourish people directly.[14] But a resource allocation analysis does not necessarily lead to the conclusion that vegetarianism is more ethical than eating meat. Animals are healthier on pasture than on grain, and they can graze on marginal land where intensive crops would not be possible. When Alisa Smith and J. B. MacKinnon began their year on the Hundred-Mile Diet (see page 27), they had been vegetarian for fifteen years. Facing a paucity of locally grown vegetable protein sources, they realized, "The most readily available protein sources are all animal-based: fish and shellfish, eggs, dairy, meat. It is increasingly clear that local, sustainable eating is not always going to be vegetarian."[15]

Related to resource allocation issues, yet distinct, is concern about the ecological impacts of large-scale farming, ranging from the deforestation of the Amazon rain forest to create grazing land to the dramatic air and water toxicity associated with concentrated animal feeding operations. Large-scale factory farms concentrate the wastes of huge numbers of animals in small areas, creating noxious odors, contaminating drinking water sources, killing fish populations, encouraging antibiotic-resistant bacteria, and endangering human health. In California's San Joaquin Valley, one of the U.S. regions with the worst air quality, local pollution-control officials say that more smog-producing gases are produced by the region's rapidly growing dairy industry—with an unprecedented concentration of 2.5 million dairy cows—than by either automobiles or pesticides.[16]

Yet another inspiration for vegetarianism comes from a feminist critique of meat eating, which draws parallels between the processes of domination and domestication of both animals and women. "The same societal influences create these oppressive systems and the only way for all to be free is to connect the issues of oppression," states a flyer from Feminists for Animal Rights. My friends at the Bloodroot Collective—whose café in Bridgeport, Connecticut, founded in 1977, is still thriving—wrote in their 1980 cookbook *The Political Palate*:

> Our food is vegetarian because we are feminists. We are opposed to the exploitation, domination, and destruction which come from factory farming and the hunter with the gun. We oppose the keeping and killing of animals for the pleasure of the palate just as we oppose men controlling abortion or sterilization. We won't be part of the torture and killing of animals.[17]

The feminist-vegetarian critique has been elaborated by Carol J. Adams in two volumes, *The Sexual Politics of Meat* (1990) and *The Pornography of Meat* (2003). "Objectification permits an oppressor to view another being as an object," writes Adams. "The oppressor then violates this being by object-like treatment: e.g., the rape of women that denies women freedom to say no, or the butchering of animals that converts animals from living breathing beings into dead objects."[18] Adams describes meat eating as a "mirror and representation of patriarchal values" and "the re-inscription of male power at every meal."[19]

For most people political ideals such as feminism, pacifism, concern about world hunger, fairness, animal welfare, and the state of the earth are all too abstract to motivate such radical behavioral change as becoming a vegetarian. Ultimately more compelling than all these noble impulses, the biggest motivation for vegetarianism (at least in

North America) seems to be personal health. Specific reasons vary: to reduce the risk of heart disease; to avoid exposure to growth hormones, antibiotics, and chemical and radioactive toxicities that concentrate in animal fats; to lose weight; to reduce the risk of cancer; to remedy digestive disorders; to feel lighter; or all of the above.

The earliest proponents of vegetarianism in the United States promoted it as a means of improving both spiritual and physical health through personal purification. Sylvester Graham was a temperance lecturer for the Bible Christian Church beginning in 1830. Graham likened meat eating to drinking alcohol; he warned that each activity was excessively stimulating and advocated abstinence from both, as well as various other forms of dietary purification, including the use of whole-wheat flour (which became widely known as graham flour; crackers made of this flour are still known as graham crackers).

Despite this historical association of vegetarianism with health and purification, through the 1970s the established health professions mostly took the position that a vegetarian diet was nutritionally deficient. This attitude changed somewhat during the 1980s and 1990s, when U.S. culture became obsessed with fat and "low-fat" became the most popular food-marketing strategy. Today's nutrition authorities have advocated not so much a switch to vegetarianism as moderation in the consumption of meat and other animal products and the substitution of leaner types of meat for fatty ones.

The low-fat trend is an outgrowth of a theory called the lipid hypothesis. This theory was first proposed in the 1950s to explain the more than tripling of U.S. death rates from heart disease between 1900 and 1950. The lipid hypothesis blamed heart disease on saturated animal fats and cholesterol. This idea gained widespread support, and by 1984 it had emerged as the prevailing view concerning the cause of coronary heart disease. Animal fats were officially demonized, and as a repercussion, vegetarianism received greater legitimacy than ever before.

Unfortunately, the consensus that developed in support of the lipid hypothesis was based upon an interpretation of the data with a key misunderstanding: the measurements of dietary fat intake that supported the lipid hypothesis failed to distinguish between saturated animal fats and trans fats from hydrogenated vegetable oils.[20] Now that trans fats are recognized as the most dangerous fats, all the data that had supported the lipid hypothesis look completely different. Dr. George Mann, one of the researchers whose 1950s research supported the lipid hypothesis, but whose research since—a long-term study monitoring the diet and heart health of sixteen thousand people—contradicts it, refers to the lipid hypothesis as "the greatest scam in the history of medicine,"[21] perpetuated by "reasons of pride, profit, and prejudice."[22]

Saturated animal fats are important vehicles of nourishment. Traditional cultures everywhere have enjoyed diets rich in saturated fats without concurrent high incidences of heart disease. The original question that the lipid hypothesis set out to answer—what was causing the dramatic rise in coronary heart disease—is more accurately answered by the *replacement* of traditional animal fats such as butter and lard with hydrogenated vegetable oils such as margarine and shortening.

Slowly the lipid hypothesis is losing support. In 2006 researchers announced the results of an eight-year study of the diets of forty-nine thousand women. "The largest study ever to ask whether a low-fat diet reduces the risk of getting cancer or heart disease has found that the diet has no effect," reported the *New York Times*.[23] "Eventually our government and medical experts will have to be forced to issue revised policies on saturated fat, just as they finally have had to admit that trans fats are dangerous," predict Dr. Mary G. Enig and Sally Fallon.[24]

Meanwhile, the lipid hypothesis prevails in medical practice, unquestioned by most medical doctors and nutritionists, despite the fact that reducing fat consumption has done nothing to decrease the incidence of coronary heart disease. "Low-fat" continues to be a hugely popular strategy for marketing ridiculously overprocessed foods. And because of the continuing misconception that animal fats are inherently unhealthy, many people today—vegetarians and meat eaters alike—consider vegetarianism to be a categorically healthier diet than one that includes meat.

Is a vegetarian diet healthier? Sure, a varied diet of chemical-free plant-source foods is much healthier than factory meat and potatoes. However, general comparisons are difficult because some vegetarians subsist on junky processed foods, and some meat eaters eat moderate quantities of good-quality meat in tandem with varied vegetable food.

For many people, vegetarian identity and practice are fluid over the course of a lifetime. In the cultural demographics I have encountered in my life, a significant proportion of people, perhaps a quarter, perhaps a third, have experimented, at least briefly, with a vegetarian diet. When you experiment, you learn things. Some people become committed lifelong vegetarians—and more power to them! Most of us gradually return to various degrees of omnivorousness and postvegetarianism, following our body's cravings, as well as our culture's path of least resistance.

The communal kitchen at Short Mountain, which I share with twenty or more people on an ongoing basis, has gone through dramatic changes in its relationship with meat over the years that I have lived here. It has never been a vegetarian kitchen (that I know of), but it has existed in the context of a somewhat vegetarian subcultural milieu. When I first arrived here in 1993, meat was an infrequent periodic event; the occasional goat or chickens we slaughtered, venison from neighbors, and fish a couple of times a year were testament to our nondogmatic culture. Meat preparation was always somewhat controversial, though, less because of individuals' ethical concerns about meat than because of the practicalities of preparing it in our kitchen. Some people preferred not to be subjected to the aromas of cooking meat; others were unhappy with how meat was handled, expressing concern over protocol, hygiene, and contamination.

My own meat cravings became much more pronounced as my body rebuilt after the period of nausea and wasting I recounted in chapter 6. As I found myself seeking out meat, I realized that I would rather be eating meat I knew something about than the random factory flesh so readily available through constant convenience consumerism. I heard about a farm nearby, called Peaceful Pastures, that offered organic meat from pastured, conscientiously raised animals in a CSA-style plan, and I proposed that Short Mountain buy a share. Our consensus process wasn't ready to agree to such a radical change. The vegetarians were not eager to encourage more meat preparation, and many folks, including meat eaters, felt that we needed to work out acceptable storage, preparation, and hygiene protocols first.

Nevertheless, more and more meat started appearing in our kitchen. Our neighbors saw how greatly appreciated meat was and brought it to our weekly potlucks. Some potlucks were almost all meat, much to the frustration of our vegetarian minority and the embarrassment of those of us wishing for our community to remain vegetarian-friendly. When our friend J. started a similar CSA-style farm-share program, offering meat from animals he raised, this time we agreed to buy a share. Being supportive friends trumped the reservations about meat, which persist.

We've never quite implemented any systematic meat preparation protocols. At one point we considered building a separate meat kitchen, but nothing ever came of it. At various moments, specific cutting boards have been set aside for meat preparation. Some of us have become (I think) more aware about meat storage and hygiene. But still, it's meat, and it's greasy and smelly, and some folks would rather not be around it. There remains an undercurrent of disgruntled resignation for the vegetarian minority around meat in our kitchen.

I wish to honor the vegetarians in my life and vegetarians everywhere. I greatly admire the ideals that inspire them. Vegetarianism is a logical choice given the ugly facts about factory-farmed meat; by extension, this logic leads to veganism because factory-farmed milk and eggs are no better for your body, the welfare of animals, or the earth than factory-farmed meat.

Vegetarians, especially vegans, have few nutritious choices in mainstream culture and frequently find themselves mocked and attacked. I've met some dogmatic vegetarians, but far more frequently I have witnessed carnivores project judgment and hostility upon vegetarians. As a group I regard vegetarians as an oppressed minority who deserve more respect and better food choices. We can all—even meat eaters and postvegetarians—be vegetarian allies, as well as nourish ourselves, by preparing delicious foods that celebrate fresh vegetables. And certainly vegetarian food need not be an inferior culinary experience.

Recipe: Tabbouleh

Ingredients (enough for eight to twelve servings)
1 cup bulgur wheat
1 1/2 cups lemon juice (about six big lemons) and/or vinegar, brine, or other flavorful liquid
1/2 cup olive oil
2 cucumbers, diced

2 tomatoes and/or sweet peppers, diced
1 bunch parsley, chopped
1 bunch mint, chopped
1 bunch scallions or chives, chopped
1 carrot, grated
Salt and pepper to taste

I especially love tabbouleh in the summertime, when cucumbers and tomatoes are fresh and herbs abound, but this is a lovely dish to enjoy any time of year, with whatever vegetables you have. This tabbouleh is rich and flavorful, in contrast to many tabboulehs, which I find bland and uninteresting. My mother taught me how to make tabbouleh right. Her secret was to marinate the bulgur overnight in lemon juice and olive oil to plump it up, rather than cooking it in water. Bulgur is already-cooked wheat that is dried and cracked, and it does not need to be cooked. Each grain of bulgur swells with the flavors of lemon juice and olive oil, which can be augmented by other fruit juices, wine, vinegar, pickle or kimchi brine, sauerkraut juice, or water.

Once the bulgur has absorbed the liquids and plumped up, add vegetables. Substitute other vegetables, by all means! Try grated radishes or turnips, summer squash, garlic scapes, or nasturtium flowers. Use lots of colors and make the tabbouleh beautiful. Mix ingredients together thoroughly and add salt and pepper to taste. The longer all the ingredients marinate together, the more delicious the tabbouleh will become. If cultured with brine or other live-culture elements, it will ferment and become even tastier. Enjoy the tabbouleh for days.

Blood on Your Hands

"We are other creatures rearranged," reflects philosopher Alan Watts, "for biological existence continues only through the mutual slaughter and ingestion of its various species. I exist solely through membership in this perfectly weird arrangement of beings that flourish by chewing each other up."[25] Breatharians, mythical mystics meditating upon mountaintops, opt out of this arrangement altogether. Fruitarians eat only the fruits produced by plants, which does not require the plant to be harmed—eating a carrot kills a plant and eating a leaf of lettuce harms a plant. The ethic of harmlessness can be taken to extremes, and yet even the breath of a breatharian brings death to countless microscopic life forms floating in the air. Actions people take attempting to live without taking other lives are, according to Watts, "a ritual gesture of reverence for life which in no way alters the fact that we live by killing."[26]

Eating meat obviously requires a life to be taken. Drinking milk and eating eggs do as well, for the continued production of these animal products depends upon breeding; only female offspring are capable of producing milk or eggs, and something must become of the males. In the not-so-distant past, and still in many places, animal slaughters were performed by someone in the family or perhaps a local butcher. This taking of life was frequently ritualized; in any case it served as a visible reminder of where meat comes from. Killing and butchering animals integrated meat eaters into the cycles of life and death. There was no way to avoid acknowledging the taking of the animal's life, no euphemisms or extruded boneless flesh to obscure the dirty deed.

Today we sequester the ugly realities of slaughter and butchering behind closed doors where most of us do not have to see it, hear it, or smell it. Slaughterhouses have a hard time finding workers. "We're desperate," reports a slaughterhouse human resources director. "Because even though we pay a very decent wage, the working conditions are terrible. It's not a job that normal people want anymore. It's just very tough."[27] Outside the slaughterhouse doors we are in heavy denial, completely divorced from the source of our meat. Slaughtering an animal is a powerful way to take responsibility for eating meat and to place oneself honestly in the intertwined cycles of life and death.

There are animal lovers who are also meat eaters and who have devoted themselves to the humane and ethical breeding, raising, and slaughter of animals. Shana Kresmer-Harris, whom I met at the Sequatchie Valley Institute's Food for Life gathering, told me that she became a vegetarian as a child after helping her older sister raise a cow as part of a 4-H program. She was appalled when she learned that their beloved pet cow was to be slaughtered and refused to eat it or any meat at all after that. She was a vegetarian for years, until she was pregnant, when she found herself with intense cravings for meat. "If I was going to eat meat, I should at least be able to slaughter the animals," she reasoned, and she has been raising, slaughtering, and butchering animals for meat ever since.

"This is a culture that doesn't deal well with death," observes Shana. "In order to have more life, we need death. That's the way life really is." We create elaborate institutions—slaughterhouses and funeral homes—staffed by experts to handle death on our behalf. We shelter ourselves from the experience and realities of death, while popular culture feeds our resulting fixation with ever more graphic simulations of violence. If you want meat you can feel good about, try raising an animal and slaughtering it. Shana talks about her "contract" with her animals. She sees it as her responsibility to keep them safer and better fed than they would be in the wild, and when she kills them, she feels she owes them "a swift death, with as little fear around it as possible."

The problem is that—for the vast majority of us who have grown up without learning how to kill swiftly by watching people around us slaughter animals—a swift kill doesn't necessarily come easily. My friend Mark Shipley writes of his first goat slaughter: "Cutting the throat I wound up slicing into the hand of the guy who was instructing me, sending him to the hospital and . . . the goat undoubtly suffered more than it should have. But I learned a great bit, about humility, patience, and judgement. I have been pensive."[28]

The first slaughter I was part of was agonizing because we didn't know what we were doing. I was in Cameroon, in central Africa, in 1985, traveling with my friend Todd. We were staying in a small town in the northeast of the country, called Yagoua, in the home of a friend who was in the Peace Corps there. She was out of town for a few days and we had her house to ourselves. At the local market, the only way chicken was sold was alive. In the absence of refrigeration, meat must be slaughtered and then quickly eaten (unless it is to be cured). In our travels Todd and I had been eating mostly prepared food from street vendors, but here we were with a kitchen, so we decided to do some cooking for ourselves.

We bought our bird and named him Horace. We kept Horace as a pet for a day or two before slaughtering him. We flipped a coin to see who would do the deed and it fell upon Todd. Todd had watched people kill chickens by jerking their necks to snap the spine. It looked so straightforward when he watched women doing it who had done it that way their whole lives, but he quickly learned that the technique was not so easy. Todd injured Horace but did not kill him. Horace was bleeding and squawking, trying desperately to escape. Here our memories diverge. Todd recalls that he grabbed Horace's neck, and fueled by adrenaline, pulled his whole head off, spraying blood everywhere. I recall running into the house for a cleaver, and Todd finally killing Horace with that, spraying blood everywhere. Whichever version really transpired—isn't memory funny?—at the hands of inexperienced incompetents Horace died a prolonged and fearful death.

This was not the only clumsy slaughter I have witnessed. Like any skill, killing has a learning curve. The most dramatic slaughter I have seen was when some friends of mine killed a pig they had raised, Cracklin' Rose. They had some kind of gun that used pressurized air rather than a gunpowder explosion to propel a small bullet. One member of the slaughter team, Lucky, was skeptical about the air gun, so he sharpened his knife just in case. The buildup to the shooting was intense, as it always is, at least for me. We all knew the outcome we were gathered for—the slaughter of a live pig named Rosie, that we would then be butchering into meat that we would eat—but the actual act of pulling the trigger is definitely the dramatic climax of the event. The air gun was quiet compared to a conventional gun; this had been one of the appeals of this method. But following the muffled sound of firing, the pig neither collapsed nor reacted in any other way. The tiny pellet had shot through the pig's brain without the pig even noticing. The pig was still standing there, alive, with a small trickle of blood dripping from her head.

Lucky switched to Plan B. He unsheathed his knife, grabbed the pig's collar, and wrestled her to the ground. By this time she was definitely reacting, squealing, and struggling. Time seemed to slow as Lucky slashed Rose's throat once, not reaching the artery (buried fairly deep in a pig) but causing her to struggle even more strenuously to get out of his grip. Lucky realized the first cut had not killed her and slashed at her throat again. As the blood began to gush out, Rose continued to struggle, until finally she collapsed dead in Lucky's bloodied arms. As we all breathed a collective sigh of relief that this agonizing, drawn-out death was over, Lucky began to sob. He had summoned the courage to finish the job that needed to be finished, but it left him emotionally spent.

I recount these stories not to suggest that killing is best left to experienced professionals, but rather to acknowledge that it requires skills that we need to relearn. I have developed some competence at slaughtering chickens by decapitation with a hatchet, which I sharpen each time. And I am happy to report that my friends' next pig slaughter went much more smoothly. They encourage folks who are interested to come help butcher the animals, making their farm quite literally community-supported, integrating the broader community into the farm and the realities of animal slaughter. Butchering a pig takes a village. People in many different cultural traditions have approached this communally. Once the pig is dead, it takes a number of people, or a big machine, to move its huge body around. It must be dipped in a tub of hot water to loosen its coarse bristles, and every inch of its skin must then be scraped to remove them. Then there's plenty of sawing, cutting, curing, and smoking to do. It's quite a production!

Like other aspects of food production, the grassroots must reclaim animal slaughtering and butchering. Hiding death behind the closed doors of factory slaughterhouses—the only places where meat to be sold may legally be slaughtered—is a denial of reality that keeps us from experiencing and fully understanding the cycles of life of which we are part. I think that becoming more directly involved in the taking of life is ultimately a form of taking responsibility.

I'm very curious about hunting and its place in political ideology. Hunting has been championed by the political right as part of its glorification of guns and the right to bear arms. In the cultural divide that separates the red states from the blue states, hunting is a wedge issue. In general, I find guns scary. I've never shot a gun. I feel menaced and intimidated by people who wield them, and I have no interest in being around them. Guns as a fetish I find very creepy, as I do "canned hunting," in which animals in captivity are hunted, and any hunting defined primarily as a sport, which is most hunting in the United States.

Yet the use of guns by people to hunt for food seems very sensible to me. It seems vastly more ethical to eat animals from the wild than domesticated animals. Bringing animals into the world for our pleasure and keeping them in captivity is a far crueler practice than the act of killing them. In many regards hunted game seems like the most ethical, as well as the healthiest, form of meat you can eat. "I used a rifle to opt out of an insane system," wrote Richard Manning in *Harper's*, describing hunting for elk. "I killed, but then so did you when you bought that package of burger, even when you bought that package of tofu burger. I killed, then the rest of those elk went on, as did the grasses, the birds, the trees, the coyotes, mountain lions, and bugs, the fundamental productivity of an intact natural system, all of it went on."[29]

Sometimes I think about learning to shoot a gun and sitting among the unfenced vegetables one dawn awaiting a deer nibbling away at some plant I've been cultivating. *Go ahead, Bambi, make my day!* The problem for me is that I don't think I could actually pull the trigger. But my cowardice in no way removes the blood stains from my omnivore hands.

Humane Meat

For most people, including those of us who have experimented with vegetarianism and found our way back to meat, the issues surrounding meat are not all black and white. Farm animals, even though they are destined for slaughter, can be allowed to live decent lives. Animals can be kept in confinement or they can be given space to graze, and many farmers are doing what they can to enable their animals to live and die in ways that are less cruel and more considerate.

But you can't know that from a label. Labels such as "organic," "free range," "grass fed," and "cruelty free" can obscure decidedly unwholesome practices. For instance, many "free-range" chickens never see the light of day and are free to range only within an enclosed space, and the rules for "organic" meat allow farmers to feed their animals nonorganic feed under certain circumstances. Unregulated buzzwords such as "cruelty free" tell you much less than a visit to the farm to see for yourself. "Nothing to hide," writes Virginia farmer Joel Salatin. "That's the moniker of a farm-friendly producer."[30]

The first requirement for meat to be "humane" is that the animals have to live well. They cannot be confined in a cage or a stall. They must be given ample opportunity to interact with the environment and move around. Many people are starting to recognize that this is an issue not only of consideration toward the animals but of the quality of food. The eggs from chickens that have had the opportunity to roam and eat greens and bugs are much higher in omega-3 fatty acids and other important nutrients than the eggs of chickens fed only grain, and their yolks reflect this richness in their color, which is deep orange rather than pale yellow. Likewise, meat and milk from grass-fed animals are much more nutritious than the meat and milk of animals fed exclusively grains. (Humans, too, are much healthier if we graze on raw greens rather than consuming a primarily grain-based diet.) And, of course, animals with the freedom to wander and forage tend to be more content.

Although assigning human emotions such as contentment to animal behavior is a bit of a projection, animals thriving in their environment often do show it. This is how some neighbors of mine, the Sanders family of the Top of the World Farm in Westpoint, Tennessee, describe the animals whose meat they are direct-marketing: "We feed our pigs only on pasture, corn, kitchen scraps, and acorns. They are raised in the sunlit outdoors, on pasture and in the woods, free to roam and dance in the wind. (Yes, the legends are true. Pigs do dance in the wind before a storm. We've seen them with our own eyes, and laughed out loud.)"

Another nearby farm, Sequatchie Cove Farm, is raising obscure heritage breeds of pigs, such as Ossabaw pigs, originally brought to the Western Hemisphere by Columbus and preserved by isolation on Ossabaw Island off the coast of Georgia. "Pigs traditionally have had little direct management," says Bill Keener, the biodynamic farmer who is raising them. "So this year we have given them the full range of the farm to forage for their food. If you have been out hiking around you might have come across them cracking hickory nuts, acorns, or walnuts down on the river or in the woods vacuum-cleaning up the persimmons."

The other major distinguishing factor for humane meat is how the animals are killed. Animals can be slaughtered with trauma, violence, and anonymity or calmly and quickly, with gratitude, tenderness, and even love. Intent and spirit can be as important as technique. Shana Kresmer-Harris describes herself as "very psychically and emotionally connected" to her animals; this keeps her "from thinking of them as part of the machine." She, like many people who raise animals on a small scale, prefers to slaughter the animals herself, precisely so they are not fed into a slaughter machine.

One farm I've visited is structured as a meat, dairy, and egg CSA. By

Everything I Want to Do Is Illegal

I want to dress my beef and pork on the farm where I've coddled and raised it. But zoning laws prohibit slaughterhouses on agricultural land. For crying out loud, what makes more holistic sense than to put abattoirs where the animals are? But no, in the wisdom of Western disconnected thinking, abattoirs are massive centralized facilities visited daily by a steady stream of tractor trailers and illegal alien workers. But what about dressing a couple of animals a year in the backyard? How can that be compared to a ConAgra or Tyson facility? In the eyes of the government, the two are one and the same. Every T-bone steak has to be wrapped in a half-million dollar facility so that it can be sold to your neighbor. The fact that I can do it on my own farm more cleanly, more responsibly, more humanely, more efficiently, and in a more environmentally friendly manner doesn't matter to the government agents who walk around with big badges on their jackets and wheelbarrow-sized regulations tucked under their arms.

OK, so I take my animals and load them onto a trailer for the first time in their life to send them up the already clogged interstate to the abattoir to await their appointed hour with a shed full of animals of dubious extraction. They are dressed by people wearing long coats with deep pockets with whom I cannot even communicate. The carcasses hang in a cooler alongside others that were not similarly cared for in life. After the animals are processed, I return to the facility hoping to retrieve my meat. When I return home to sell these delectable packages, the county zoning ordinance says that this is a manufactured product because it exited

selling shares in the farm, the owners are able to distribute the meat from the animals they slaughter and butcher there to shareholders, rather than selling it. Though the farm's facilities are fairly basic, the farmer is meticulous about hygiene. Luckily the farm has thus far remained "under the radar" of regulatory agencies, because unfortunately a farm's cleanliness means nothing to the law.

Rather than being based upon objective, quantifiable bacteriological standards, U.S. laws require slaughtering to take place in a finite number of state-of-the-art USDA-approved facilities. Laws prohibit

By Joel Salatin

the farm and was reimported as a value-added product, thereby throwing our farm into the Wal-Mart category, another prohibition in agricultural areas. Just so you understand this, remember that an on-farm abattoir was illegal, so I took the animals to a legal abattoir, but now the selling of said products in an on-farm store is illegal.

Our whole culture suffers from an industrial food system that has made every part disconnected from the rest. Smelly and dirty farms are supposed to be in one place, away from people, who snuggle smugly in their cul-de-sacs and have not a clue about the out-of-sight out-of-mind atrocities being committed to their dinner before it arrives in microwaveable, four-color-labeled, plastic pack-

aging. Industrial abattoirs need to be located in a not-in-my-backyard place to sequester noxious odors and sights. Finally, the retail store must be located in a commercial district surrounded by lots of pave-ment, handicapped access, public toilets and whatever else must be required to get food to people. The notion that animals can be raised, processed, packaged, and sold in a model that offends nei-ther our eyes nor noses cannot even register on the average bureaucrat's radar screen—or, more importantly, on the radar of the average consumer advocacy organization. Besides, all these single-use megalithic structures are good for the gross domestic product. Anything else is illegal.

Excerpted from "Everything I Want to Do Is Illegal," *Acres USA*, vol. 33, no. 9 (September 2003). Used by permission.

the sale of meat that has not been slaughtered in USDA facilities. The outcry a century ago after Upton Sinclair exposed conditions in factory slaughterhouses led to a regulatory system that, ironically and per-versely, requires animals to be slaughtered in factory slaughterhouses. Factory farming and factory slaughter created sanitation problems; the regulations adopted to address those problems outlawed on-farm slaughter and tightened regulation of factory slaughterhouses. There is no recognition in the law that animals may be safely and hygienically slaughtered and butchered on the farms where they lived their lives, as small farmers have done for the entire history of domestication. Small farms are bound, inappropriately, by the same rules that govern concentrated animal feeding operations consisting of tens of thousands of animals.

The one exception to the USDA slaughterhouse requirement is for on-farm poultry sales. In most places small farms may sell, directly from the farm, chicken and other fowl they have slaughtered on the farm. Even so, there are numerous reports of inspectors harassing farmers who slaughter poultry on-farm and trying to shut down their farms. After a visit from the U.S. Food Safety and Inspection Service, Joel Salatin sent some of his chickens to a laboratory for testing, along with some supermarket chickens, and the bacterial counts of the supermarket chickens were twenty-five times higher than those of his chickens. "It didn't matter that our chickens were twenty-five times cleaner," writes Salatin in his book *Holy Cows and Hog Heaven*. "Guess what? They had no thresholds! They had no empirical scientific standards! All they had was a subjective notion that open-air processing was inherently unclean, end of discussion."[31]

The Tennessee farm, Peaceful Pastures, received an unannounced visit from a team of federal and state agriculture inspectors in March 2002. "Their sole intent appeared to be shutting down our every operation," recounts farmer Jenny Drake. After nearly a year of investigations, allegations, intimidation, and legal expense, during which no formal notices were ever issued by the government agencies,[32] Drake decided life would be easier utilizing a USDA-approved slaughtering facility for the chickens. She tried to be positive about this development and continued to focus on issues related to the well-being of the animals:

> On one hand this is a good thing as it will completely open up the restaurant and retail markets for our birds. It will also cease this particular, senseless battle with Big Brother. On the other hand, I hate to lose control of the processing, and now there are people out of a good paying, seasonal, part time job. We also do not know if we will be able to get back the pet food components (gumbo, heads, feet) as the USDA restricts what you may retrieve from inspected animals. We will research the

options and institute whatever measures are necessary to minimize the stress on the birds during hauling. Our current
thinking is to drive at night and arrive well before sunrise; the
birds would nap throughout the journey.[33]

Even going to a slaughterhouse is not necessarily sufficient. U.S.
law makes a distinction between USDA slaughterhouses with on-site
inspectors and smaller state-regulated custom slaughterhouses that
slaughter animals and butcher meat for hunters and institutional use,
but not for resale. Meat for resale must go through the USDA facilities. There have been prosecutions over the sale of meat from custom
slaughterhouses. Diane and Mike Hartman, who own Mom's Dairy in
Gibbons, Minnesota, were arrested in 2004 for selling—directly from
their farm—meat they had raised and had had slaughtered at a custom
slaughterhouse rather than at a USDA facility. Even though no consumer complaints were ever filed against them, tests on the meat
found it to be perfectly safe, and the Minnesota constitution specifically guarantees farmers the right to sell the products of their farms,
the Hartmans were convicted in 2005. They say they chose the slaughterhouse *because* it was small and they felt more secure that their animals would not be mixed up with others.[34] The laws under which they
were convicted are designed for the needs of mass production. They
do not allow for the somewhat different logic that can make more
sense for a small-scale operation wishing to retain some control over
the process.

In the long, inscrutable, anonymous food chain of the supermarket,
we're trusting mass producers, mass marketers, and mass regulators.
The mass scale makes for mass risks. In the course of my research I
learned that the FDA has been permitting meat packers to use carbon
monoxide in sealed packaging to preserve the fresh color of the meat,
disguising age and spoilage. This practice, banned by the European
Union as deceptive and unsafe, is defended by the industry's American
Meat Institute Foundation because it keeps meat looking presentable
for longer in supermarket coolers.[35] "It all comes down to a matter of
who we will trust," writes Joel Salatin. "Anyone who believes the government watchdog agencies have no political agenda and are trust-
worthy is living with their head in the sand."[36]

I am not encouraging anyone to buy meat from unknown or unaccountable sources. But I am encouraging you to think about whom you trust to safeguard your food: an unhealthy and cruel system of mass slaughter or small farmers trying to do better. Take the time to get to know farmers, visit farms, and even observe, or participate in, on-farm slaughters. Then even the products of an unregulated slaughter will not be unknown.

Recipe: Bone Broth

An important aspect of producing humane meat is honoring the animal whose life has been taken by making use of every part of it. In our culture we have become accustomed to eating only the musculature of animals and discarding the bones, fat, organs, and other parts or having them diverted before the meat reaches us into various industries that make use of meat by-products. Traditional meat-eating cultures have always incorporated all parts of the animals they ate into their cuisines, appreciating the dense nutrients found in other parts of the animals' bodies.

Organ meats are especially rich in vitamins and iron, thanks to the specialized functions of different organs in the body. Bone marrow contributes its own unique functional nutrients, including the omega-3 fatty acid DHA, which is essential for organ development. In China, bone marrow broth is called "longevity soup," according to Paul Pitchford in *Healing with Whole Foods*.[37] Bones and cartilage are also rich sources of mineral electrolytes as well as collagen, which breaks down into thickening gelatin, aids digestion, and has been used to relieve many chronic disorders.

This recipe is for a stock made from meat, including poultry; refer to the recipe for gefilte fish (page 153) to read about how to prepare fish stock. Make stock from whatever kind of bones are leftover after you eat meat. If you tend to generate just a few bones at a time, you can collect them in a bag in the freezer and make stock once you've accumulated a bunch. Bones alone contain nutrients and give body to the stock, but they do not have much flavor, so include some meaty bones in the stock for flavor. Roast the meat and bones before adding them to the stock pot for maximum flavor. Be sure to get the drippings into the stock by adding a little boiling water to the roasting pan after the meat and bones are done cooking and using a spoon to mix the drippings into the water.

Place the bones, meat, and drippings into a stockpot. Large bones that have become brittle from roasting should be broken to release marrow into the stock. Add vegetables if you like, including onions (with their skins), garlic, celery, parsley, mushrooms (including tough stems), carrots and other root vegetables, and even seaweed. Cover everything in the pot with cold water and add a tablespoon or two of vinegar. (The acidity of the vinegar helps extract minerals and other bone nutrients.)

Slowly heat the stock until it reaches a boil. As it heats, scum will collect on the surface. Skim it off with a spoon and discard. Lower the heat to a gentle simmer and cook for at least six hours, or for up to three days for full gelatin extraction. Uncover the pot for some of the cooking time so the stock will reduce, but when leaving the pot unattended, it's safer to keep it covered. Add water if the stock level gets low. After cooking, strain out the solids, skim off the excess fat (if desired), and salt to taste.

Stock can be sublimely satisfying. When I sip on rich stock, it fills a deep craving, and my body feels like a sponge absorbing warm, fatty, savory nutrient goodness. Stock can be enjoyed as a simple broth; used as a starting point for any kind of soup, stew, or sauce; or frozen for future use. "Stock is everything in cooking," said the renowned French chef Auguste Escoffier. "Without it nothing can be done."[38]

Recipe: Souse

Souse is made from the head of a pig. Another name for it is head cheese, though it is not cheeselike in any way, except that it joins together small bits (of meat) into a loaf shape. Head cheese sounds scary, and the idea of it makes many people squeamish, but the flavor of souse is supersweet and inviting. It reminds me of something between meat loaf and pâté. I don't know where you'll find a pig's head, but this is a recipe for when you do. You can eat very well on what people trim away from a carcass as they prepare the "choice" cuts. I learned how to make souse after I helped my friends J. and S. slaughter and butcher Jack and Diane, two pigs they had raised. At the end of the slaughtering day I took the disembodied heads home and consulted a few of my favorite books: Pat Katz's *Craft of the Country Cook* and Carla Emery's *Encyclopedia of Country Living*. I also called my friend Judy Fabri, a walking encyclopedia of country living, who talked me through her method.

Judy's method was simplest: boil the whole head. The other books went on about what a delicate flavor and texture the brain has, so I did the work of removing the brain, which involved sawing through the skull. My friend Lapis walked into the kitchen as I was sawing a head in half. "You're always doing something controversial," he announced, shaking his head. Indeed, the fact that I was doing this project at all drove River away (I offered to do it outside, but he didn't want to be anywhere near it) and caused a bit of a stir. I removed the brains, rinsed them in cold water, boiled them for half an hour to "set" them, then fried them and served them as an hors d'oeuvre before dinner. Brains have a unique creamy texture that a few of us really got into, but most people's horror at the *idea* of eating brains overshadowed the actual flavor of the dish.

I also removed the eyeballs, as several recipes directed. I imagined eyeballs as delicate, like little fragile balloons filled with liquid, so I initially approached my task with caution and gentleness. But soon I was using force: I slipped a small dessert spoon behind the eye to pry it out of its socket, then grabbed the very solid eye with my hand and used a knife to cut it away from the muscles holding in place. I'm not recounting these graphic details to gross you out. This is part of the reality of the meat most of us love to eat, and it's good to get real.

Before you start, remove any remaining bristles from the head. It's easier to singe them off with a flame than to scrape them from a disembodied head. Then place the head and any other meat scraps in a stockpot and cover with water. Add vinegar to help extract collagen and minerals from the bones and cartilage. Season with salt, peppercorns, hot chili peppers, sage, and any other seasonings you like, and gently boil for at least six hours, or until the flesh falls away from the bones (but boiling for even longer is better). Skim off any scum that rises to the surface in the initial period of boiling. If you're leaving the stock boiling for long periods, keep it covered, but if you're checking on it regularly, let it boil uncovered so the stock will reduce.

After boiling, strain the stock through a colander to separate the liquid from the solids. Once the solids cool, pick through them with your fingers and separate out the meat from the fat and bones. "Keep whatever you can pick that feels soft," advises Judy. You can keep strips of skin and gristle to chew on—or not. There's lots of meat in a head. Once you have picked off all the meat, discard the bones and the fat (or save the fat to render into lard).

Next, skim the fat off the stock. Fat rises to the top and can be gently removed using a ladle. Transfer the fat to a can, where it will solidify; you can use it in cooking. This stock is rich in collagen, and it too should solidify when cooled. Cool a spoonful, and if it fails to solidify, boil it down further to thicken it.

Souse can be mostly meat, like a meat loaf, with a small amount of stock added to hold it together, or it can be made with a greater proportion of stock as more of a gelatinous aspic, with bits of meat floating in it. Heat however much of the stock you want to use. Add the picked-off meat to it, simmer for about fifteen minutes, and then season to taste. Transfer the mixture to loaf pans, spread it evenly, and chill it in the refrigerator to set it. Use the extra stock for soups or stews.

Souse may be enjoyed sliced and cold on bread or crackers with mustard and horseradish, or it can be sliced and fried. Closely related to souse is a Pennsylvania specialty called scrapple. To make it, simply add some cornmeal to the stock to set with the meat.

Action and Information Resources

Books

Adams, Carol J. *The Pornography of Meat.* New York: Continuum, 2003.

————. *The Sexual Politics of Meat: A Feminist-Vegetarian Critical Theory.* New York: Continuum, 1990.

Bloodroot Collective. *The Political Palate: A Feminist Vegetarian Cookbook.* Bridgeport, CT: Sanguinaria, 1980.

E. G. Smith Collective. *Animal Ingredients A to Z.* Oakland, CA: AK Press, 2004.

Emery, Carla. *Encyclopedia of Country Living.* 9th ed. Seattle: Sasquatch Books, 1999.

Henderson, Fergus. *The Whole Beast: Nose to Tail Eating.* New York: Ecco, 2004.

Katz, Pat. *The Craft of the Country Cook.* Point Roberts, WA: Hartley and Marks, 1988.

Kneidel, Sally and Kneidel, Sara Kate. *Veggie Revolution: Smart Choices for a Healthy Body and Healthy Planet.* Golden, CO: Fulcrum Publishing, 2005.

Lappé, Frances Moore. *Diet for a Small Planet.* New York: Ballantine Books, 1971.

Midkiff, Ken. *The Meat You Eat: How Corporate Farming Has Endangered America's Food Supply.* New York: St. Martin's Press, 2004.

Rifkin, Jeremy. *Beyond Beef: The Rise and Fall of the Cattle Culture.* New York: Dutton, 1992.

Robbins John. *Diet for a New America.* Walpole, NH: Stillpoint, 1987.

Salatin, Joel. *Holy Cows and Hog Heaven: The Food Buyer's Guide to Farm Friendly Food.* Swoope, VA: Polyface, 2004.

Sinclair, Upton. *The Jungle.* New York: Signet Classics, 1906.

Spencer, Colin. *The Heretic's Feast: A History of Vegetarianism.* Lebanon, NH: University Press of New England, 1995.

Vallianatos, Evaggelos. *This Land Is Their Land: How Corporate Farms Threaten the World.* Monroe, ME: Common Courage Press, 2006.

Films

The Meatrix 1 and *2.* Free Range Graphics, 2003 and 2006; two-minute Internet flash videos available at www.themeatrix.com.

Organizations and Other Resources

American Vegan Society
PO Box 369
Malaga, NJ 08328
(856) 694-2887
www.americanvegan.org

Animal Welfare Institute
Animals in Agriculture Program
PO Box 3650
Washington, DC 20027
(703) 836-4300
www.awionline.org

Beyond Vegetarianism: Transcending Outdated Dogmas
www.beyondveg.com

Eat Wild: Clearinghouse for Information about Pasture-based Farming
29428 129th Avenue SW
Vashon, WA 98070
www.eatwild.com

Global Resource Action Center for the
Environment (GRACE) Factory Farm
Project
215 Lexington Avenue, #1001
New York, NY 10016
(212) 726-9161
www.factoryfarm.org

Dr. Temple Grandin
www.grandin.com
*This Web site, posted by a professor of
animal science at Colorado State
University, offers information about
techniques for humane slaughter.*

Heifer Project International
PO Box 8058
Little Rock, AR 72203
(800) 422-0474
www.heifer.org

Humane Slaughter Association
The Old School
Brewhouse Hill
Wheathampstead
Herts AL4 8AN
United Kingdom
44 (0)1582 831919
www.hsa.org.uk

International Vegetarian Union
www.ivu.org

Keep Antibiotics Working Coalition
PO Box 14590
Chicago, IL 60614
(773) 525-4952
www.keepantibioticsworking.com
*Dedicated to eliminating a major cause
of microbial antibiotic resistance: the
inappropriate use of antibiotics in food
animals.*

NoNAIS.org (and related Web sites)
www.nonais.org
www.stopanimalid.org
www.noanimalid.com
www.libertyark.net

North American Vegetarian Society
PO Box 72
Dolgeville, NY 13329
(518) 568-7970
www.navs-online.org

People for the Ethical Treatment of
Animals
501 Front Street
Norfolk, VA 23510
(757) 622-PETA
www.peta-online.org

Vegan Action
PO Box 4353
Berkeley, CA 94704
(510) 548-7377
www.vegan.org

Vegetarian Resource Group
PO Box 1463
Baltimore, MD 21203
(410) 366-VEGE
www.vrg.org

Vegetarian Society
Parkdale
Dunham Road, Altrincham
Cheshire WA14 4QG
United Kingdom
0161 925 2000
www.vegsoc.org

Virgil Butler Blog
www.cyberactivist.blogspot.com

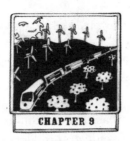

CHAPTER 9

Feral Foragers:
Scavenging and Recycling
Food Resources

Scarcity is a central pillar of our economic and social structure. Without the threat of it, what would motivate all the hard work and sacrifice? The global players tell us that without the intensifying advancement of economies of scale, monocrop specialization, chemical pesticides and herbicides, and genetic engineering, there could never possibly be enough food for the mass of humanity to survive.

To cite a classic example, Richard Nixon's secretary of agriculture, Earl Butz, pronounced thirty-some years ago that "before we go back to an organic agriculture in this country, somebody must decide which fifty million Americans we are going to let starve or go hungry."[1] Similarly, in today's debates over biotechnology those who oppose genetically modified crops are often accused of standing in the way of progress that could alleviate hunger, malnutrition, and poverty. Hunger is the ultimate unquestionable justification, and it has been used to manipulate all sorts of political debates.

But are hunger, malnutrition, and poverty really caused by an overall shortage of food resources? I am inclined to believe that there is plenty of food growing around the world for everyone to be adequately fed. Hunger is not caused by insufficient total resources but rather by the uneven distribution of those resources. "While hunger is real, scarcity is an illusion," write Frances Moore Lappé and Joseph Collins.[2]

Even with all the "improvements" in agriculture, hunger continues to be widespread. After a brief period of reduction in the estimated numbers of hungry people around the world, the United Nations Food and Agriculture Organization now reports that hunger is on the rise, with 852 million people "chronically hungry" and five million children dying from hunger every year.[3] Even within the United States the population of the hungry is expanding. U.S. Department of Agriculture statistics counted 38.2 million people in 2004—about thirteen percent of the total population—in households suffering from hunger and food insecurity, up from thirty-one million in 1999.[4]

Yet in spite of the fact that so many people in the United States are hungry, an incredible quantity of food gets discarded. Timothy Jones, an anthropologist at the University of Arizona who spent ten years picking through trash and measuring food loss, concludes that nearly half the U.S. food supply goes to waste. Waste begins in the field, where an average of 12 percent of U.S. crops are plowed under, often unharvested for economic reasons. The greatest sources of wasted food are retailers and consumers; both regularly overstock and end up discarding perishable items. Food retailers in the United States throw away $30 to $40 billion worth of food each year, and households toss out 14 percent of the food they purchase. Jones estimates that an average family of four discards $590 worth of groceries per year, adding up to $43 billion for U.S. households as a group. Altogether $100 billion worth of food, half the U.S. supply, goes to waste.[5] Many activists are tapping into this colossal waste stream, rescuing food in order to redistribute it, as well as utilizing food that is beyond edibility as resources for fuel and fertilizer.

Tapping into the Waste Stream

In keeping with the simple truth of the slogan "Reduce, reuse, recycle," the place to start is reducing waste in our own lives. Waste is not inevitable; we create it. Each of us can reduce waste by being realistic about how much to buy and prepare, storing leftovers conscientiously, making creative use of them, and composting organic materials. We can also avoid overly packaged foods. Packaging accounted for 31.7 percent of the municipal solid waste generated in the United States in 2003, according to the Environmental Protection Agency.[6]

Beyond minimizing waste, many creative scavengers go out in search of waste to reuse and recycle through transformative magic. While this chapter focuses on food reclamation efforts, activists everywhere are applying similar creativity to other related waste streams. For example, Julia Christensen has undertaken an exciting project called *How Communities Are Re-Using the Big Box*, in which she is documenting creative reuses of massive "big box" retail stores that often become obsolete in just a few years and move to even bigger spaces.

Food reclamation projects are organized in many different ways and at many varied scales. Sometimes it's just someone with his or her eyes open who notices unharvested crops and gathers them. This is called gleaning. Common law recognizes the ancient right of people to come onto fields after harvest and take what they can find. My neighbor Krista harvests excess berries and other fruit from all our neighbors to put up for winter. Other friends, Buck and Greg, scope out fruit wherever they drive and turn their roadside gleaning into wines, meads, and brandies. These accomplished spinners and fiber artists have also gleaned vast quantities of cotton, which they manually deseed and transform into gorgeous garments. And many other people I know and have written about in these pages are accomplished gleaners.

People have also joined together in many different places to collect discarded food and get it into the hands and mouths of people who need it. Food Not Bombs (FNB) is a decentralized but extremely widespread grassroots movement—"a revolutionary mutual-aid community" in the words of the Detroit group—of people engaging in food redistribution efforts. The movement started in 1981 in Boston and Cambridge, Massachusetts, with a group of friends who were active in campaigns against nuclear weapons and power. The name Food Not Bombs evolved from a stencil they used to spray-paint on sidewalks at the exits of supermarkets: "Money for food, not for bombs." The activists first used "Food Not Bombs" as the name of their group in an action, originally conceptualized as street

Food Not Bombs logo.

theater, in which they served free food and created a soup line outside the Federal Reserve Bank in Boston in March 1981, as the stockholders of the First National Bank of Boston (a major investor in nuclear power) met inside:

> As nuclear power protesters, we wanted to do street theater that would remind people of a 1930s-style soup kitchen, to highlight the waste of valuable resources on capital-intensive projects such as nuclear power while many people in this country went hungry and homeless. At first, we thought we would have actors play the homeless, but then we realized we could get people who actually were homeless to participate. . . . We collected day-old bread from a bakery and some fruit and vegetables from the local co-op on the morning of the stockholders' meeting and cooked a huge pot of soup. We set up a table at the Federal Reserve Building, and to our surprise, over one hundred people showed up for a meal.[7]

Once the group learned how easy it was to collect surplus food, and what tremendous demand there was for it, they started collecting and serving food regularly. With the surplus perishables of a food co-op, a local tofu manufacturer, a bakery, and eventually more enterprises, the original FNB collective distributed food every other day to shelters in Boston's South End neighborhood. They also became a regular fixture serving food at protest events and began to inspire activists in other places, including San Francisco and Washington, D.C., to do similarly.

FNB unites protest with service and has a very down-to-earth appeal. "It will take imagination and work to create a world without bombs," explain C. T. Lawrence Butler and Keith McHenry, of the original FNB collective, in their book *Food Not Bombs*:

> Food Not Bombs recognizes our part as providing sustenance for people at demonstrations and events so that they can continue participating in the long-term struggle against militarism. We also make bringing our message to other progressive movements part of our mission. We attend other organizations' events and support coalition-building whenever possible. We

work against the perspective of scarcity that causes many
people to fear cooperation among groups. They believe they
must keep apart to preserve their resources, so we try to
encourage feelings of abundance and the recognition that if we
cooperate together, all become stronger.

Being at the center of the action with our food is part of our
vision. Sometimes we organize the event; sometimes we provide food at other organizations' events. Providing food is more
than just a good idea. It is a necessity. Either the movement can
seek food services from the outside and be dependent on businesses that may not be progressive, or we can provide for ourselves. Clearly, it is Food Not Bombs' position that providing
for our own basic needs, in ways that comprehensively support
the movement, is far more empowering. We have provided
food at long-term, direct actions, such as the annual Peace
Encampment sponsored by the American Peace Test at the
Nevada Nuclear Weapons Test Site; to tent cities that highlight
homelessness and hunger in San Francisco, Boston, New York,
and Washington, D.C.; and for the regular feeding of the
homeless in highly visible locations throughout the country.[8]

The San Francisco FNB group began serving food in Golden Gate
Park every week. After three months without incident, one day in
August 1988 they received a visit from police, who told them they could
no longer serve food there. The group decided to defy the police and
continue serving food to the city's hungry and homeless. The following
Monday, when the group set up their free food in the same spot, they
were surrounded by lines of riot police, and nine servers were arrested.
This brought FNB tremendous publicity and solidarity. "Arresting
FNB members proved to be a major political miscalculation on the part
of City Hall and an enormous break for FNB," according to one
account. "People being arrested for sharing free food made the head-
lines and greatly expanded interest in the group."[9] As FNB's support
grew, the San Francisco police stubbornly persisted, and arrests of
FNB activists there continued on and off for a decade; by 1997 there
had been over a thousand arrests, which spurred action and inspired
FNB groups far and wide.

The grassroots spread of FNB has been accomplished primarily through decentralized underground media: word of mouth, flyers, zines, the Internet, and punk music. One of the lessons drawn by FNB in the San Francisco experience is never to apply for a permit, for just

The Revolution Needs No Permit

By C. T. Lawrence Butler and Keith McHenry

Sometimes people argue that it makes the city happy if you get a permit so they know you are using some city sidewalk or park. You give them the name of the organization, its mailing address, and a phone number, and they give you a permit. If the permit policy is really that simple, you might look into it, but avoid giving the identity of your group until you know for sure.

Case in point: on July 11, 1988, after serving for several months without city interference, the San Francisco Food Not Bombs group wrote a simple, one-page permit request to the Recreation and Parks Department at the suggestion of some community organizers. This unfortunately alerted the government to the meal distribution program, and gave it an opportunity to deny us a permit. It then used this as an excuse to harass the food table and arrest volunteers.

Although the government may create reasons for denying you a permit, you should not be intimidated. Make it clear that you are willing to adopt any proposal that will make your operation safer and more successful, but also that you will not agree to any demand making it impossible for you to continue your operation. Even after long hours of meeting with government officials, hard-earned permits can be revoked at any moment. From the government's point of view, a permit is something it can take away whenever it wants. (Remember Indian treaties?) Because of this, we strongly recommended that you *not* contact the local government. The revolution needs no permit.

Excerpted from *Food Not Bombs* (Tucson, AZ: See Sharp Press, 1992, revised 2000). Used by permission.

prior to the start of the arrests the San Francisco group had requested a permit from the city. Butler and McHenry recommend to fledgling FNB chapters, "The revolution needs no permit."

"Food Not Bombs is one of the fastest-growing revolutionary movements active today and is gaining momentum," proclaims a FNB flyer. "There are hundreds of autonomous chapters sharing free vegetarian food with hungry people and protesting war and poverty throughout the Americas, Europe, Asia, and Australia." Indeed, I've encountered FNB groups myself at protest events for the past decade, and I've gotten to know FNB folks in several different cities.

Some of the FNB collectives have endured over time; others were fleeting, short-lived experiments by young people trying to do something positive in the world. My friend Socket, who was in FNB in Northampton, Massachusetts, while in college and then later in Oakland, California, calls FNB "gateway activism." By that, I understand he/she (Socket likes to cross between the two and mostly resides somewhere in between) to mean that FNB is an accessible, easy-to-plug-into form of activism with tangible rewards that is often a port of entry through which people find their way into other activist projects.

FNB groups use many different methods for obtaining food surpluses, among them picking through supermarket dumpsters, which are generally a dependable source. Socket joined me one night for an outing of dumpster-diving with Derrick, a Nashville FNB friend whose passion for dumpster-diving for food is exceeded only by his passion for dumpster-diving for fashions. The Nashville FNB group generally hits the dumpsters Friday and Saturday nights and serves meals Saturday and Sunday afternoons. I've been a lifelong trash picker and compost rescuer, so the concept of digging through a dumpster and eating food from it is not intrinsically troubling to me. However, my preconceived notion of what our haul would be was lots of junk, such as stale packaged dougnuts. This was because I have heard some dumpster divers pride themselves on their "freegan" or "opportunivore" adaptability.

What shocked me as we made our rounds was how much perfectly fine produce we found. Everything in the store must look perfect. Anything with the slightest blemish, or even approaching the prime it will soon be beyond, gets tossed. The biggest supermarket chains use compacting dumpsters, and some of them even spray bleach into the dumpsters as a deterrent to dumpster-divers. Dumpster-divers learn through experience where the best dumpsters are.

We wore headlamp-style flashlights so we could see in the dark and have our hands free. Our first stop was Food Lion, where Derrick climbed up into the dumpster and started handing things down to Socket and me. The first item was portobello mushrooms! We rejected some that were smelly, but most were still fine. Then red, yellow, and orange bell peppers, radishes, platters of precut vegetable crudités, cauliflowers, and something I had never seen before, individually plastic-wrapped "Potatoh!"s. In a second dumpster at the same store we found bagels, pitas, and sandwich rolls. In just this one stop we had found plenty of reasonably wholesome food to feed ourselves for days.

But we weren't feeding ourselves; we were gathering food for a group effort to cook enough food for about thirty-five people in a plaza in downtown Nashville. Our next stop was the Dollar General Market. I was on my guard here because I noticed a police car as we turned into the empty parking lot, and I imagined that dumpster-diving was technically illegal. Derrick says he's been stopped and questioned a few times by police as he's dumpster-dived, but he's never been arrested. This dumpster turned out to be our tropical paradise, with lovely ripe pineapples and key limes, as well as cantaloupes and tomatoes. And the police didn't follow us in.

Our next stop was a local produce market. Here I got so excited by what I could see that I jumped into the dumpster myself. Right there on top were jalapeños, tomatillos, and big Italian eggplants. As I excavated deeper, beneath layers of broken-down cardboard boxes and food in various stages of decay, I unearthed scallions, cilantro, grapes, zucchini, and slender curvy Asian eggplants. When I was ready to document our bounty—still in the dumpster—I realized that I had lost my notebook in there. So I had to dig around again until I found it. We then visited another Food Lion, where we found cookies, canisters of pressurized whipped cream, ricotta cheese, bags of precut stir-fry vegetables, and more pineapples and portobello mushrooms. Our last stop, at a discount supermarket called Aldi, yielded more cauliflowers, apples, peppers, onions, and a couple of bags of powdered mini donuts, which Derrick considers a sign of good luck.

Dumpster-diving has attracted many committed devotees. Dumpster-divers take great satisfaction from meeting their needs and desires out of other people's waste, and these resourceful scavengers help support thriving subcultures everywhere. "After years of dumpster-diving, it came to be expected that each dumpster score would top the previous, and that there was in fact nothing the dumpster wouldn't provide," writes the anonymous author of *Evasion*.[10]

A zine called *dumpsterland*, by a self-proclaimed hobo puppeteer named Dave, contained some excellent dumpster-diving tips:

> Get out the yellow pages. Yes, it's true! All great dumpsters lie within that precious resource. Every store and every distributor makes waste. Some may be harder to get at, some impossible, but this is where you begin. . . .
>
> Most frustration with dumpster-diving comes from hitting them on trash pickup days. . . . Go search it out on Wednesday and Saturday, after closing time. If that doesn't do much go on Monday and Thursday. Don't give up! . . .
>
> Scratch below the surface. The top layer of any dumpster is rarely indicative of what treasures are buried within. Get in there! Root around! Move those top bags aside, dammit. Do you want to buy potatoes or do you want them for free? . . .
>
> The subtle nuances will come to you. Don't ever forget to leave the area around the dumpster as clean or cleaner than you found it. Also, untie bags rather than rip them open if you can. . . .
>
> As an aside, dumpsters are not sustainable. Throwing away food, clothing, building materials, and everything else imaginable is nasty business, utterly repulsive and sinister. I dumpster-dive because it exists.[11]

Dumpsters are not the only sources of food waste. Often, recyclers can make connections with food businesses to collect their unwanted food and take it *before* it enters the waste stream. For example, every week my fellow communard Sister Soami collects huge garbage bags full of day-old bread at an upscale Nashville bakery and spends a day dropping off loaves for all our neighbors—like a sourdough Santa.

And, of course, people who work in food businesses everywhere take home excess production, imperfect seconds, or what they can get away with. My friend Ed brings home fish from the dock where he works unloading freshly caught fish from boats and preparing them for auction. Ed's daughter Caity works in a bakery and brings home all sorts of delectable pastries, cakes, and cookies that are no longer fresh enough to sell after the first day. Ideally food gets rescued, diverted, or liberated *before* it gets thrown into a dumpster.

In Asheville, North Carolina, friends of mine are part of what one of them describes as "community-supported activism." This is a loose network of individuals and organizations who pick up the discarded food generated by a thriving, large health-food supermarket and distribute it widely. The participants all emphasize that the key to maintaining such food pickup relationships is consistency and reliability. Their distribution network has received huge quantities of fine food, including cases of frozen organic meat products just past their expiration dates but still frozen, never thawed, and perfectly delicious.

FNB—for reasons of both ideology and food safety—has generally remained in the realm of vegetarian food; perhaps cheese sometimes, but generally no meat. The Asheville distribution network crosses the line into frozen meats. But pulling meat, thawed for who knows how long, out of a dumpster sounds just too sketchy for most people. Which brings us to our next topic: dead animals from the road.

Roadkill Radicals

If you pay attention and look at the road while driving (or, even more so, while walking or biking), you will inevitably encounter roadkill. Animals moving across the landscape are often unavoidable prey at fifty-five miles per hour. Little systematic counting has been done, but extrapolating from data collected by road crews in Ohio, one analysis estimates there are an average of more than one hundred million roadkill victims in the United States each year.[12] Dr. Splatt, the pseudonym of a high-school science teacher who for thirteen years has organized students around New England to participate in a roadkill census, comes up with a very similar estimate of 250,000 animals killed by cars in the United States on an average day.[13] Some people see food in these unfortunate victims of our car culture and regularly pick roadkill up off the road to take home and eat.

A few passionate souls I have encountered eat roadkill almost every day. My neighbors Casper and Pixey bring roadkill stews to our potlucks. For a while they did their frying in grease rendered from a roadkill bear they came across in the mountains. On one of my friends Terra and Natalie's visits, they had strips of roadkill venisons splayed across their dashboard drying into jerky.

When I first met Terra, she was vegan. Then she and her boyfriend Ursus—who has the word *vegan* tattooed onto his shin—discovered roadkill and quickly became roadkill carnivores. In her zine, *The Feral Forager*, Terra explains how they came to start eating roadkill:

> Our first feral feast of roadkill was on spring equinox of 2002. That past winter we had experimented with skinning and tanning, using a possum and a raccoon we had found on the roadside. . . . On spring equinox we were driving in the suburbs of a large southeastern city and spotted a fox dead on the roadside. Our first thought was what a great fur it would make. We scraped it up (it wasn't very mangled at all) and took it to our friends' house downtown, and Ursus skinned it in the backyard while our friends assisted. When it was all done and hanging gutless and skinless from a tree, it was like some collective epiphany: why not eat it? There was a great firepit there and several willing "freegans," along with a few pretty hardcore vegans (including Ursus) who raised no protest. After a couple hours on a spit, the grey fox was edible. I guess it was something about the start of a new season—it was almost ritualistic, without trying to make it so. Some stood by and watched while four or five of us feasted on the fox. Ursus, a hardcore vegan, was perhaps the most voracious. There was something primal about his eating—like a wild man caged for years eating only bagels and bananas. Ursus tanned the skin and later wore it around his neck like a scarf.[14]

Terra, Ursus, Natalie, and other members of the Wildroots Collective in western North Carolina now eat roadkill nearly every day, have a good supply put away in a freezer, and have tried dozens of different species of animals found dead on roadsides.

The Wildroots folks have become enthusiastic promoters of roadkill and work hard to spread information and skills to empower other people to tap into this huge available food supply. Members of the collective do a good bit of traveling on the do-it-yourself skillsharing circuit, teaching people how to judge the edibility of a dead animal on the road and guiding them through the experience of skinning and cleaning a small animal. At the 2005 Food For Life gathering at the Sequatchie Valley Institute/Moonshadow, one of the most memorable events was the hands-on roadkill workshop, in which we learned about the cleaning, skinning, and butchering of roadkill animals. The Wildroots folks brought a roadkill groundhog with them, and our friend Justin, another roadkill enthusiast, brought a squirrel he had found on his bike ride to the gathering. (The more slowly you travel, the more you notice not only roadkill but all sorts of roadside harvesting possibilities.)

People enthusiastically took front-row seats to see these animals get skinned. Some people shuddered in horror, had to look away, or other-wise expressed their squeamishness. But most people watched quietly, fascinated, as Natalie coached Dylan, a previously uninitiated thirteen-year-old (there with his family) through the skinning of the squirrel, and Jenny and Justin skinned the groundhog. Direct experiential edu-cation like this can be transformative. Laurel Luddite wrote about her first roadkill butchering experience, "The responsibility made me nervous at first. As I cut I began to feel confident that not only could I butcher this deer, but I could also fulfill my need for food whenever I saw some lying by the side of the road."[15]

Roadkill has been a source of food for poor people since there have been cars. In American culture eating roadkill generally has a pejora-tive classist connotation, epitomizing ignorant hillbilly behavior. Now Wildroots and other enthusiasts are embracing roadkill with a political ideology, rejecting the values of consumer culture by "transforming dis-honored victims of the petroleum age into food which nourishes, and clothing which warms."[16] Beyond ideology, they are spreading practical information and skills to empower people.

Terra's zine, *The Feral Forager*, offers a basic primer for safely eating roadkill:

Picking up roadkill is a good way to get fresh, wild, totally free-range and organic meat for absolutely free. When you find the roadkill you should try to determine if it is edible or not. If you saw the animal get hit then it's obviously fit to eat (although you may have to put it out of its misery). If the critter is flattened into a pancake in the middle of the highway then it's probably best to leave it. Most of the time (not always), good ones will be sitting off the road or in a median where [they aren't] constantly being pulverized.

Sometimes it can be hard to determine how fresh a carcass is. A lot of factors can contribute to how fast the meat spoils, especially temperature. Obviously, roadkill will stay fresher longer in colder weather and spoil faster in warmer weather. It's best to go case by case and follow your instincts. Here are some considerations to help you decide:

- If it is covered in flies or maggots or other insects it's probably no good.
- If it smells like rotting flesh it's probably spoiled, although it is common for dead animals' bowels to release excrement or gas upon impact or when you move the carcass.
- If its eyes are clouded over white it's probably not too fresh (though likely still edible).
- If there are fleas on the animal there's a good chance it's still edible.
- If it's completely mangled, it's probably not worth the effort.

Rigor mortis (when the animal stiffens) sets in pretty quickly. Most of the animals we've eaten have been stiff. There's no reason to assume the animal is spoiled just because it's stiff. . . .

Potential Risks of Eating Roadkill: One of the most severe risks of roadkill is rabies. In order to assure your safety from this deadly serious brain inflammation, you may want to use rubber gloves when gutting and skinning any warm-blooded animal (warm blooded as in mammals and birds, not in regard to blood temperature). If you don't feel the need to exercise this absolute caution, at least make sure you don't have any open wounds on your hands or skin that touches the animal. Roadkill is usually safe from rabies because it dies quickly when the animal dies. Also, rabies will cook out of the carcass. Generally speaking, boiling the animal first (rather than just grilling it) is a good idea, especially if it's a notorious rabies carrier (like raccoons, skunks, and foxes).[17]

Wild Food Scavenging

Roadkill meat is just one element of a broader wild-foods foraging-gathering ethic that many food activists embrace. "If everyone simply stopped to take advantage of the most obvious and abundant wild foods growing a hundred yards back from the roadside on his or her way home from work," writes Gary Paul Nabhan, "I'm sure that radical changes in our society's entire perception of foods and their costs would follow."[18] I touched briefly upon the topic of weed eating in the recipe for chickweed pesto in chapter 1 (see page 34), but I cannot reiterate strongly enough that many wild plants—both indigenous natives and introduced plants that have naturalized—are more densely nutritious than the cultivated plants for which they are usually weeded out. They are adapted to the environment, hardy, and self-sufficient—all qualities we need. Also, because so many different plants are edible, regular foragers eat a far greater variety of plants—each with unique phytochemical elements—than people who rely exclusively on cultivated crops.

The reasons why people forage for wild food go beyond sustenance. Many activists I meet view foraging as a path toward liberation from corporate groceries, the grind of a nine-to-five job, and other trappings of civilization. "In our own quests to develop these skills we have come to realize that we are like infants," the members of the Wildroots Collective reflect. "Instead of learning skills essential to living, such as crafting tools from earthen materials, skinning animals, making clothes, identifying and preparing wild food and medicinal plants, our educations have trained us to be good little participants in a global capitalist system, alienated from our survival, dependent on the technological-industrial, resource-extracting, land-gobbling, animal-enslaving, indigenous-culture-destroying machine."[19]

Perhaps the most passionate forager I have crossed paths with is Fritz, a punky young transgendered traveler who searches for wild foods everywhere he goes—and finds them. Fritz always impresses me with not only his knowledge of wild edibles, but also his persistence in harvesting and processing them, which are the limiting factors for many people in the know. I fondly recall Fritz disappearing into the woods here one spring afternoon and returning with a full basket of tiny toothwort roots, which he painstakingly grated into a potent, delicious, horseradish-like sauce. Another foraging role model in my life is an old Japanese man I met in the Kauai rain forest when I was on a solo backpacking adventure in Hawaii long ago. He claimed to have lived in the forest for years on wild food and hikers' excess provisions. I shared some of my food with him, and he pointed out to me the leaves of sweet potato, a perennial plant in that climate offering abundant fresh greens. Both the man and the sweet potatoes were domesticates gone feral.

Empower yourself by expanding your awareness of wild foods. "The average American can identify three hundred corporate logos but only about seventeen plants," observes Food Not Lawns founder Heather Flores (also known as Heather Humus). "This is pathetic. There are thirty thousand edible plant species known to humans."[20] Books can sometimes help you identify edibles, but nothing compares to getting out with someone experienced. My earliest edible plant walks were as a kid, with my cousin David, armed with a copy of Euell Gibbons's *Stalking the Wild Asparagus*. We never did find any asparagus, but we did find wild grapes. Years later I went on weed walks in New York's Central Park with my friend Judith. Her enthusiasm for what she introduced to me as "plant allies" was infectious, and I started knowing some common weeds, eating them, and getting to know more.

I tend to be very adventurous about tasting plants I don't know; my rule of thumb is that it's okay to taste unknown plants (though not fungi) so long as you experiment slowly. Smell before you taste. Taste just a tiny bit. Chew it well, mix it with saliva, and see how it feels in your mouth. If it tastes unpleasant or you start reacting in some strange way, spit it out and don't eat any more. If it feels okay in your mouth, swallow. Wait a little while. Taste some more, if you want, but never eat a lot on a first encounter. See how it sits with you and come back for more tomorrow.

Wild Mushrooms: A Taste of Enchantment

What do you get when you cross the *Iron Chef* with *Fear Factor* and *Survivor*? You get most Americans' view of eating wild mushrooms. Fungilliterati notwithstanding, of the ten thousand species of mushrooms identified in North America, maybe twelve are known to be lethal. But before you cast caution to the wind, know that some of these deadly dozen are quite common. The "destroying angel" and the "death cap" are responsible for nearly all mushroom-induced fatalities. So although there certainly are deadly mushrooms out there, there are very few to watch out for. Once you know what to look for, these are as easy to pick out as carrots from cauliflower.

What about mushrooms that won't kill you but will make you wish you were dead? There are a few of these as well. However, the vast majority of "poisonous" mushrooms merely cause mild to severe stomach upset. Granted, this is enough to make some of us not want to ever eat wild mushrooms again. Out of ten thousand species identified in North America, only 250 are known to be more or less toxic. Of these, only twenty are common.

What about the other 9,750? As far as we know, they're harmless. But then again, we don't know everything. That's where you come in.

Actually, it's perfectly safe to

Many knowledgeable teachers are taking up the activist work of spreading important wild-foods wisdom through grassroots experiential education. My teaching partner Frank Cook—together we have taught many fermentation and wild food foraging workshops—is deeply devoted to walking the land and meeting the plants wherever he goes. He frequently organizes plant walks and enjoys helping people break through what he calls "the green wall" that prevents them from getting to know plants and exploring their world. My friend Crazy Owl is another irrepressible spirit who loves to share his considerable plant foraging knowledge, inviting all who will come to join him on walks into "the enchanted forest."

Teachers are everywhere. In New York City Steve Brill has been

By Alan Muskat

touch or smell nearly every wild mushroom, including the deadly ones. You'll find that mushrooms can smell like seafood, chlorine, cucumbers, vinyl, almonds, anise, marzipan, maple syrup, ink, garlic, dog mess, and raw potatoes—and most of these are edible. In fact, most mycophagists (that's mushroom-eaters) agree that at least two hundred types of wild mushrooms are worth eating.

Most of us would be quite content with a basketful of morels, chanterelles, porcini, meadow mushrooms (the "wild portabello"), matsutake, or chicken-of-the-woods. But many more varieties are edible, medicinal, or both. Each is as nutritious as it is delicious, and many can be found growing wild in most of North America—maybe even in your own woods or backyard, where shopping is a pleasure.

At nature's supermarket, the produce is always local, organic, fresh, and free. This is one place where you get what you don't pay for. Learn to gather your own; you'll be glad so few people do!

Excerpted from *Wild Mushrooms: A Taste of Enchantment*, 4th ed. (Asheville, NC: self-published, 2004). Used by permission.

leading wild-food foraging walks in city parks since 1982. He became notorious in 1986 after he was arrested for the crime of harvesting dandelions. Reported the Associated Press:

> Two park rangers disguised as nature-lovers used marked bills, a surveillance camera and walkie-talkie to get the goods on the bespectacled botanist who calls himself "Wildman." . . . Brill insisted he's not a criminal. "We take only renewable resources," he said. "We pick maybe one dandelion weed out of hundreds of thousands that are mowed down. I'm just trying to get people into nature, to show them they can touch things, and smell things and taste them."[21]

Brill is still leading wild-food walks—more than ninety in 2005 alone—all around the New York metropolitan area. Chances are someone near you is leading foraging walks, or perhaps your calling is to become such a guide.

Foraging knowledge is not limited to plants. There is a huge movement of mycology hobbyists who organize mushroom walks and fungus forays in their areas. My friend Alan Muskat, self-described "mythic mycologist and epicure of the obscure," has long experience harvesting edible and medicinal mushrooms. He sometimes sells wild mushrooms to restaurants, and for years he has led classes and walks. He has also written and self-published a book, *Wild Mushrooms: A Taste of Enchantment*, to help people get started. He advises foragers not to be overly goal-oriented: "Don't go in the woods just to fill your basket. Like life, mushroom hunting is a great exercise in non-attachment, in letting go of expectations, because you never know what you will or won't find."[22]

Another whole realm of exciting foraging exploration is entomophagy, or the use of insects as food. Insects are plentiful in most places, and though our culture has generally made eating insects taboo, many people around the world regularly eat insects for sustenance. Some foraging activists are learning and sharing this knowledge. The more diversified our foraging skills, the more we will find to eat on any given outing.

An extreme perspective on foraging presents it as a wholesale rejection of agriculture. The anonymous author of the zine *Beyond Agriculture* invites readers to join the "ongoing Feral Jihad against Agriculture."[23] Euell Gibbons, in his 1966 book *Stalking the Healthful Herbs*, writes, "We would be better off nutritionally if we threw away the crops we so laboriously raise in our fields and gardens and ate the weeds that grow with no encouragement from us."[24] In 1988 John Zerzan, a prominent voice in recent "anarcho-primitive" literature, published in the anarchist newspaper *Fifth Estate* an essay titled "Agriculture—Essence of Civilization," which has been much referred to since. "Agriculture is the birth of production," writes Zerzan. "The land itself becomes an instrument of production and the planet's species its objects. Wild or tame, weeds or crops speak of that duality that cripples the soul of our being, ushering in, relatively quickly, the despotism, war and impoverishment of high civilization over the great length of that earlier oneness with nature."[25] Zerzan and others advocate not for a return to smaller-scale, more sustainable farming but rather forgoing agriculture as we know it and reintegrating as hunter-gatherers. Some descriptive phrases I've heard to describe this reintegration process are "going feral" and "rewilding."

Personally, I don't think this is an either/or choice. We need both more foraging of wild plants *and* more local cultivation; they are not inherently in conflict. Some visionary idealists see opportunities for foraging and cultivation to synthesize and complement one another. After all, the origins of farming involved simply encouraging the proliferation of wild edibles, and holistic models of gardening, such as permaculture, seek such integration. One compelling philosophy of living and eating is called "paradise gardening," an intensified form foraging that has been articulated, practiced, and promoted by a North Carolina man named Joe Hollis.

> Paradise gardening is a way of life which serves to maintain the garden, and is in turn maintained by it. . . . Like any other creature, we *are* our niche. . . . Our goal is to "naturalize" ourselves in the environment. This will involve changing ourselves and changing the environment: convergence toward a "fit." . . . The process of Paradise Gardening involves . . . the (re)integration of needs: not to the market for food, the spa for exercise, the doctor for healing, theatre for entertainment, school for learning, studio to create, church for inspiration, etc., but to the garden for all these *at the same time*. Enriching the garden by naturalizing useful and beautiful species and learning to incorporate them into our lives. We begin, of course, with the present and potential natural vegetation, to which may be added species introductions from similar areas worldwide; then slight modifications of the environment—micro-habitat enhancement—and the resultant possibilities for new species: a palette of plants, a cornucopia never available to previous generations.[26]

Hollis emphasizes important differences between paradise gardening and agriculture as we know it: "Our addiction to annual species and disturbed habitats has put us at odds with the main thrust of the biosphere (and ourselves)." As an alternative, he suggests greater reliance on perennials, which grow and produce more each year without requiring the soil to be touched. Hollis also emphasizes urgency: "We live during a narrow 'window of opportunity.' Having

Insects: A Forgotten Delicacy

Most people in North America will quiver at the thought of eating bugs. In fact even some survival guides mention eating bugs as "the unthinkable." But in spite of this blatant specieism, everyone (including the strictest vegan) who's ever eaten anything has unintentionally eaten millions of insects.

Insects are in fact a very nutritious food source. They are high in fat, protein, and many other vitamins, including B12. That is part of the reason why indigenous people around the world seek out these abundant food sources. . . . For those of us modern feral folk who have gotten past the mental block of cultural conditioning, we have discovered that insects are not only nutritious but can also be very tasty. But don't go out eating everything you see—some are poisonous or can cause allergies. . . . Here is a list of edible bugs that I have tried and how you can prepare them:

Grasshoppers and Crickets: If you have the patience to catch them! Like all hard-shelled insects you should cook them to kill any parasites, and you may want to remove the wings and legs. I have found they are best roasted in a pan or over a fire shish-kebob style. (Kill them first if you can, and they can hop around even with their heads off.) They are surprisingly tasty and filling—they taste something like popcorn. Crickets are incredibly high in calcium and potassium.

Ants and Their Eggs: One of the best wilderness foods I have ever eaten! The large black carpenter ants are the choice ones to go for. All ant eggs are edible and can be eaten raw or cooked. The carpenter ant's eggs taste a lot like grains when boiled, and taste like eggs when roasted. I hear that small ant eggs can be eaten raw and taste like couscous, but the only time I tried this it tasted like a come, at least, to a realization that a revolutionary shift of consciousness and lifestyle is required, we find that we have only a few generations to do it in, before it will be too late."

By Terra

hundred ants biting my tongue (there were live ants on the eggs too). If you're cooking the eggs you can add the ants right in there with them. I wouldn't suggest eating fire ants, but then again I've never tried to, and the chemical that causes the burning sensation may cook out (let us know if you try this).

Rolly Pollies, or Pill Bugs: Rolly Pollies are actually a crustacean and not an insect (just think of them as land shrimp). They can be roasted whole and taste a little like popcorn.

Grubs (Beetle Larvae): All beetle larvae can be eaten raw; they taste kind of fishy. They can be added to soups, stews, and stir-fries. They can also be roasted, after which these little fat-filled protein snacks taste a lot like pop-corn.

Snails and Slugs (Escargot): Snails can be shelled (throw them in boiling water first) and sautéed with garlic (wild or cultivated), or added to soups. Slugs probably present the biggest challenge getting over the mental block. They can be prepared like snails only you don't have to shell them.

Earthworms: These subterranean squirmers are packed with soil minerals and microorganisms that simply can't be substituted in our modern vegan diets. They can be eaten alive, added to stews, or dried in the sun on a hot rock, and then ground into a very nutritious flour, which can be used as a soup thickener, or cut with other flours and used in flatbreads or other baking.

For more information check out www.food-insects.com.

Excerpted from *The Feral Forager*, a self-published zine, available from Wildroots at www.wildroots.org/ff.php. Used by permission.

Recipe: Burdock and Stinging Nettles

My own paradise garden of mutual naturalization has two plants I want to share here: burdock and stinging nettles. Both are Eurasian weeds, introduced species where I live (though there are native stinging nettles species in this region), but they adapt easily and are self-perpetuating with barely any encouragement. And both are delicious seasonal foods with important nourishing and tonifying properties.

Burdock (*Arctium lappa*) is one of my favorite plants to eat. The root has a sweet, earthy flavor and crunchy texture that I enjoy raw, fermented, or cooked. Burdock is a biennial, meaning that its life cycle takes two years, and it doesn't go to seed until the second year. The first-year plants, low to the ground with large, hairy leaves but no tall central stalks yet, have the more tender, delicious, and flavorful roots. Harvest them in the fall or early in the spring to take advantage of the energy they have stored in their roots. Burdock plants typically grow in groups; when I harvest, I always leave at least one plant in each group to grow the second year, go to seed, and perpetuate more burdock.

The distinction between weeds and cultivated plants need not be sharp; a small amount of cultivation can do wonders to encourage a weed you like. I walk around each fall spreading mature burdock seeds—which grow in burrs that stick like Velcro to hair, clothes, pets, and anything else (hence the name *bur*dock)—to create new stands of burdock around our land, especially in marginal, uncultivated areas. Whenever I want to harvest burdock I go to one of these stands with a strong shovel to dig first-year roots.

I like to eat raw burdock root whole, like a carrot, skin and all. Burdock root sliced lengthwise into strips makes a great filling for nori rolls; the root is a common ingredient in Japanese cuisine, in which it is known as *gobo*. Burdock roots can be shredded into slaws, krauts, and kimchis or sliced (on the diagonal is my favorite) for stir-frying, oven-roasting, boiling into soup stock with other vegetables, or brewing into medicinal teas or herbal elixir meads (see page 117).

Herbals often refer to burdock as a blood purifier that tonifies the liver and kidneys and is helpful for treating skin ailments such as eczema and psoriasis. "The dynamics of burdock root's detoxicant functions are interesting," writes Peter Holmes in *The Energetics of*

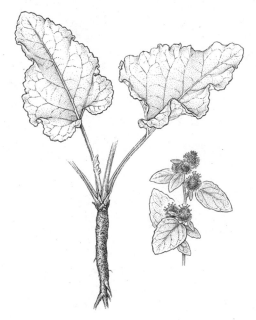

Burdock. ©Bobbi Angell. Used by permission.

Western Herbs. "The root specifically retrieves toxins from the connective tissue and shunts them into the bloodstream."[27]

Stinging nettles (*Urtica dioica*) is another common weed that I love to eat and drink. My herbalist friend Judith got me hooked on nettles tea while I still lived in New York. There, I drank dark green infusions of dried nettle leaves that I bought, which tasted like concentrated chlorophyll and left me feeling green and radiant.

When I planted a small patch of nettles a dozen years ago, it was somewhat controversial. Some of the folks I live with worried that the weed would spread and become an invader in our gardens. What makes nettles potentially problematic is that the plant is covered with sharp stingers that leave a tingling sensation in the skin. Seeking to assuage the worries of a nettles invasion, I carefully chose a spot from which the nettles could not easily spread, a marginal space between our barn and the driveway. After a dozen years, the patch has become dense with nettles and has rounded the corner of the barn; however, it has not spread much beyond. Each spring, as new growth emerges from the nettles patch, we give it room by cutting back the dead growth from the year before. This is all the cultivation that the perennial nettles patch requires.

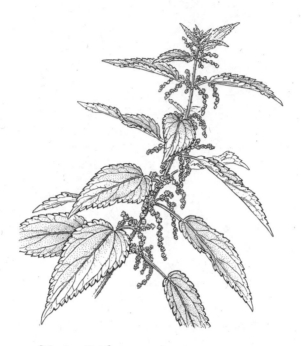

Stinging Nettles. ©Bobbi Angell. Used by permission.

It's best to harvest nettles in the spring, before the plant goes to seed, which alters its chemical composition. My method is to use scissors to cut the stalks, with a bowl in my other hand to catch the falling stalks and leaves. I mostly avoid touching them, though I find that I can brush against the nettles without being stung as long as I'm careful about moving toward the growing tip, *with* the stingers; only if I brush past the plant in the opposite direction, against the stingers, do I get stung.

The stings are not so bad. They are quite stimulating, actually, and one traditional way of using nettles as medicine is urtification, or flogging with the plant to deliberately sting an area of the skin and thereby deliver the nettles' medicine directly to that area. "Urtification creates an intense physical and energetic stimulus to capillaries/circulation, nerves/meridians, muscle fibers, lymphatic flow, and cellular metabolism, combined with multiple surface injections (like a vaccination) of a fluid containing, among other things, histamines, acetylcholine, and formic acid," writes herbalist Susun Weed.[28] People use urtification to treat arthritis, sore muscles, and localized inflammations, as well as recreationally. Regular eating or drinking of nettles nourishes the blood; tonifies the kidneys, lungs, and digestive system; relieves fatigue; helps regulate metabolism and adrenal function; drains fluid congestion; and makes hair strong. "Our doctors and pharmacists are ashamed of fetching such a common weed from behind the fences and including it in their formulas," wrote the German physician-herbalist Hieronymus Bock in 1532, "even though in both cookery and medicine it has proven its mighty, impressive effects."[29]

The nettles' stingers are deactivated by heat, so I steam nettle leaves before eating them. They are delicious when simply steamed, or they can be added to soups, casseroles, pestos, or pâtés. To infuse nettles into a strong tonic beverage, it is best to dry the leaves first. Harvest the stalks and either hang them from a string or spread them out on a screen in a hot, dry spot out of direct sunlight (which can degrade nutrients). Once they are crisp and dry, you can crush the leaves and store them in a sealed glass jar to use as needed. To infuse, place a handful of nettles in a Mason jar, then pour boiled water over them to fill the jar. Seal the jar and leave it to infuse for several hours, until it cools to room temperature, by which point the contents will be a deep, dark green. Strain out the plant material and enjoy this "green milk," which can be stored in the refrigerator.

Recycling Used Cooking Oil into Fuel

With the expected coming scarcity of fossil fuels and the ever-escalating costs of securing dwindling petroleum resources, there is much activity around the world focused on creating biofuel alternatives. The most widely used biofuel in the United States currently is ethanol, an alcohol fermented and distilled from corn that is typically mixed with gasoline. Any carbohydrate can be similarly fermented, and projects are under way around the world fermenting abundant carbohydrates into ethanol. Brazil has undertaken an especially ambitious ethanol program, fermenting it from sugarcane. Twenty-five percent ethanol fuel is now standard in Brazil (compared to 2 to 10 percent "gasohol" blends available in some parts of the United States); new cars are now being manufactured in Brazil that can run on 100 percent ethanol, and Brazilians are even exporting ethanol to Asia.

The other major form of automotive biofuel is biodiesel, which can be made from vegetable oil or animal fat. The engines invented by Rudolf Diesel in 1892 were originally conceptualized as having the flexibility to run on virtually any fuel, including whale oil and vegetable oils. "Motive power can be produced by the agricultural transformation of the heat of the sun," Diesel said.[30] George Washington Carver experimented with peanut oil in diesel engines, but until recently there was little exploration of biofuels for diesel engines, mostly because petroleum-based fuels were so cheap, and refiners could sell one of their by-products as diesel fuel. But shifting economic and environmental realities since the 1970s have spurred interest in biodiesel research, and today biodiesel is being produced from many different "feedstocks," most prominently rapeseed (canola, used widely in Europe), sunflower, soybean (the favorite in the United States), and palm oils.

Biofuel production is great, and I'm glad government and industry are directing resources to alternative fuels. Many big vehicle fleets are running on biodiesel blends, including some in the military, the postal service, school districts, and municipalities. Minnesota became the first state to require that biodiesel be blended into all diesel fuel sold there, at a 2 percent level (marketed as "B2"), and the federal government has begun offering tax incentives to encourage more biodiesel blends. "Biodiesel has buzz," observes North Carolina biodiesel activist Lyle Estill:

> In the commercial fuel sector it has buzz as a lubricity additive to petroleum diesel. In the clean air crowd it has buzz for its reduced emissions. In agricultural circles it is talked about as a new cash crop. Academia is excited because biodiesel is a frontier, full of unknowns. There is plenty of ground-breaking research still to be done on how to make fuel from soy or algae or flies that feed on hog waste. Biodiesel has buzz with the peaceniks because there is "No War Required" to obtain it. It has traction with those on the Right side of the political spectrum because it can be "Made in America."[31]

But fuel from soybeans and corn and sugarcane also means more monoculture, more genetically modified acreage, and more agrochemicals. In their institutionalized forms, biofuels really aren't especially eco-friendly at all, and they mostly benefit large corporate grain processors, most prominently Archer Daniels Midland.

Biofuels, like anything in mass production, are far removed from our daily experience, in the same abstract netherworld as petroleum itself—or for that matter food or any of the conveniences of our consumer society. And since we started this chapter with a discussion of hunger, with millions starving and food scarcity the dominant paradigm, how can we justify using precious food resources for fuel? "Definitely there is a danger that the competition can hit food security and food availability," worries Gustavo Best of the United Nations Food and Agriculture Organization.[32] Biofuels are an alternative to petroleum, not a panacea.

One form of biofuel is especially exciting because it does not require redirecting *any* edible food or agricultural resources. Biodiesel activists around the world are collecting a messy, smelly, difficult-to-dispose-of, abundant waste material—used fry oil, of which U.S. food industries produce more than three billion gallons per year[33]—and converting it into fuel. Community biodiesel operations recycling used cooking oil are shining examples of sustainability. This grassroots network is rapidly expanding and inspiring me and many others to want to become part of it.

Fry oil, or any feedstock oil, requires a bit of processing to turn it into biodiesel, specifically a chemical reaction called transesterification, which separates the viscous glycerin from the oil, enabling it flow at cooler temperatures. To accomplish this, wood alcohol (methanol) and a chemical catalyst (lye or caustic soda) are mixed together into methoxide and then added to the oil. The oil is a triglyceride—three fatty-acid chains joined with glycerine. The alcohol joins with the fatty-acid chains to form alkyl esters (biodiesel), freeing the glycerin, which is responsible for the viscosity of the oil. The glycerin, which separates out, becomes a by-product of the process that can be composted and has many potential applications as yet to be fully developed.

Diesel engines can also run on straight vegetable oil (SVO), once solid particles are filtered out and any water is removed; however, for the viscous vegetable oil to flow and combust steadily, it must be warm. So typically people who run on SVO convert their engines to dual-tank fuel systems, using a more refined fuel (biodiesel or petroleum diesel) to warm the SVO before switching to SVO as the fuel source, and then switching back a few minutes before stopping, so the fuel lines don't get clogged when they cool down. These are hassles that most people prefer not to have to worry about. Running on processed biodiesel generally requires only minor changes to the automobile.

People in many different places are learning how to process waste cooking oil into biodiesel. It involves a bit of chemistry and a bit of plumbing, and many impassioned activists are totally geeking out on this accessible and appropriate technology. Maria "Mark" Alovert is one of the do-it-yourself biodiesel pioneers; she has designed many backyard setups, has traveled widely teaching workshops, and has written and self-published the *Biodiesel Homebrew Guide* as well as many articles posted online on the finer points of small-scale biodiesel production. She is not alone; free exchange of information has characterized the grassroots biodiesel movement. Reflects Mark, "Due to the rise of infosharing on the Internet, there has been, in the last seven to eight years, a boom in the number of people making their own biodiesel, experimenting with equipment and techniques, and sharing their experiences over Internet forums and Web sites."[34] Collectives or co-ops of various shapes and sizes recycling local waste oil into fuel have sprouted up in communities around the world, and the movement is spreading fast.

Lyle Estill, one of the founders of Piedmont Biofuels, a 150-member biodiesel co-op in Pittsboro, North Carolina, made his first batch of biodiesel in 2002 after he first learned of the existence of this technology, tried to locate some to buy, and discovered that it was not commercially available in his state. He and a friend made that first batch in a blender, following the directions in Joshua Tickell's book *From the Fryer to the Fuel Tank*. "Anyone can make biodiesel in a blender," says Lyle. "The problem is scaling up the process to make more meaningful quantities of fuel."[35]

As he pondered this problem, Lyle spotted a flyer hanging on a bulletin board in a local café, with a headline inquiring, "Think Fuel from Vegetable Oil Is Impossible?" The flyer advertised a course on biofuels at nearby Central Carolina Community College, in which Lyle promptly enrolled. The course was taught by two instructors, Rachel Burton and Leif Forer, who had limited experience but great enthusiasm. "What intrigued me was that these two were about to embark on the creation of a large-scale biodiesel processor and were willing to take the class with them," recounts Lyle. "Lack of knowledge, experience, or resources did not dampen their spirits a bit."[36]

Three years later, when I visited Piedmont Biofuels in 2005, their first experiments had morphed into a thriving co-op providing fuel to 150 members. Members can pump ready-made 100 percent biodiesel (referred to as "B100") at five different pumping locations or use shared equipment for do-it-yourself production. And the co-op is in the midst of expanding its scale, recycling an abandoned chemical plant into a biodiesel factory capable of turning out twenty thousand gallons of biodiesel a week, for a million gallons a year. The Piedmont Biofuels activists are at the forefront of the biodiesel revolution, empowering themselves and others with simple creative technology, tapping into a huge waste stream, and producing fuel for people in their community.

Automotive power is not the only way that fry oil can be recycled as fuel. A Boston-area restaurant, Deluxe Town Diner in Watertown, Massachusetts, is reusing the thirty to forty gallons of vegetable oil it goes through each week in its fryers to heat the restaurant. "Why should we drain the planet's resources by burning up expensive heating oil when we have our own supply of oil right here in the restaurant?" asks owner Don Levy.[37]

I'm inspired, and I want to help recycle used fry oil into fuel where I live. As this book has been in production, I've been working with a group of friends to start processing biodiesel here on our land. We've been assembling materials, collecting used oil from local restaurants, visiting other biodiesel processing operations, reading, and asking lots of questions. This movement is spread by nuts-and-bolts skillsharing. By the time you're reading this, I expect to be one of several folks around here driving around on biodiesel, spewing exhaust that smells like doughnuts.

Composting and Humanure

No discussion of rescuing food from the waste stream would be complete without some reference to compost. Composting is the ultimate (and the original) recycling process. It is an everyday miracle, a beautiful metamorphosis to witness, and an indispensable link in the ongoing cycle of life and death and fermentation. J. I. Rodale's *Encyclopedia of Organic Gardening*, like many accounts, waxes poetic: "In the soft, warm bosom of a decaying compost heap, a transformation from life to death and back again is taking place."[38] This transformation is the basis of soil fertility and an obvious strategy for dealing with food waste.

Food comprises an estimated 12 to 16 percent of U.S. waste, according to various estimates.[39] What is shocking to me is that more of this waste stream is not diverted at the source, before it becomes waste, into compost, which would quickly transform it into a valuable resource. Instead it becomes a burden, piling up in landfills, being incinerated into air pollution, or floating on trash barges in the sea, with no clear destination.

For urban dwellers without any land, composting may seem impossible. When we lived in a fourteenth-story apartment in New York City, my roommates and I tried an enclosed anaerobic (oxygen-free) composting system in a covered plastic garbage container in our apartment. What a disaster! We learned that anaerobic composting stinks. Composters generally seek to create conditions that favor aerobic bacteria. After we finally acknowledged what a disgusting, smelly mess it was, we had to somehow get rid of it. We snuck the hefty anaerobic stink bomb out of the building in the middle of the night, lugged it a block away, and left it in a construction dumpster. Later, when I moved downtown where there was more of a community gardening scene, I would walk my food scraps ten blocks to add them to a garden's compost pile. It was important to me, as a gesture.

You can choose whether you generate waste or appropriately channel resources. Compost is an important effort to make if you seek to minimize waste and contribute materially to the cycle of life. You can find a garden with a compost pile you can add to, or, with even just a tiny bit of outdoor space, a balcony, or roof access, you can compost in stacked milk crates. Alternate layers of kitchen scraps with layers of grass cuttings, leaves, or other dry plant material as you fill the crate. After you fill a crate pile another on top of it; remove finished compost from the bottom. Worm-bin coffee tables are another strategy for apartment composting, according to Cleo Woelfle-Erskine, editor of *Urban Wilds: Gardeners' Stories of the Struggle for Land and Justice.*[40]

Some people go out and collect organic waste to compost. Heather Flores, founder of Food Not Lawns, reports that in her hometown of Eugene, Oregon, "we cruise the back doors of the stores and cafés in town and pick up their vegetable waste for compost piles."[41] In Nashville, Tennessee, a community gardening group called Earth Matters organizes an annual "Leaf-Lift," collecting homeowners' bagged fallen leaves in autumn and composting them, along with food scraps and other organic wastes, in massive sculptural forms.

A few forward-looking cities, first in Europe in the 1990s, and now in the United States, have begun municipal programs for composting food scraps. San Francisco distributes green plastic "biobins" in which households and businesses can collect food scraps; haulers collect the scraps on a designated schedule and bring them to commercial composting operations outside the city. The mature compost is sold as fertilizer to northern California vineyards and marketed as "Four-Course Compost." The program has reduced municipal landfill input by 19 percent; it has expanded into the East Bay, and activists in other cities are promoting similar models.[42] Even if we can't convince local policymakers to embrace composting, we all can find ways of composting our own scraps and encourage our friends to join us. Composting recycles: it recovers the food as a resource and rescues it from the fate of becoming a burden, part of the waste stream.

When we examine the waste stream in its entirety, another huge share of it is food in its postdigested state: excrement. Manure need not be treated as waste. Many types of animal manure have been used to heat and generate energy, and just like food scraps, manure can be rapidly transformed into soil-building humus through composting. "One organism's excrement is another's food," observes Joseph Jenkins, the author of the cult classic *The Humanure Handbook*. "Everything is recycled in natural systems, thereby eliminating waste."[43]

We humans each produce an average of about three hundred

pounds of shit per year.[44] In our contemporary culture, we treat shit as unspeakable and flush it away to make it disappear instantly. Personally, I like to talk about shit. When I feel completely reborn by a particularly satisfying movement, I like to share my enthusiasm. If a friend is sick and experiencing changes in shit texture or consistency, I like to hear about that, too. For me it's about claiming the body and all its functions without shame. I also like to talk about sex and symptoms of illness, and I even enjoy the odors that bodies give off. What is the benefit of pretending our bodies do not do these things? Who do we think we are fooling? It is a manifestation of the same disconnection from the earth that has happened with our food. We must face our shit, embrace our bodies, and feel our connection to the earth.

In our effort make our excrement disappear, we create huge problems. Each time we flush away our poop or piss, with it go an average of 3.3 gallons of water per flush, and each of us flushes an average of 5.2 times a day.[45] Our daily flushes alone consume more water than the total daily water supply in many regions of the world. The typical person in the United States flushes 6,263 gallons of potable water down the toilet each year, adding up to 1.75 *trillion* gallons per year for the United States as a whole. "We defecate into water, usually purified drinking water," writes Joseph Jenkins. "After polluting the water with our excrement, we flush the polluted water 'away,' meaning we probably don't know where it goes, nor do we care."[46] Wherever it goes, those gallons of water are now sewer-flavored, shit and piss and other bodily fluids mixed with detergents and paints and solvents and whatever else gets poured down drains and storm sewer systems. Reclaiming that water requires the use of more chemicals and elaborate, expensive processing. "The solution is to stop fouling our water," writes Jenkins, "not to find new ways to clean it up."[47] (For more on water activism, see chapter 10.)

Historically people have recycled their excrement into soil by various techniques, some very successful at eliminating pathogens, others less so. *The Humanure Handbook* explains in simple terms techniques for thermophilic (high-temperature) composting of humanure, in which a mix of feces, sawdust, grass clippings, and vegetable scraps encourage heat-generating organisms to do their thing and thereby kill intestinal pathogens and quickly break the materials down into rich humus. Observes Jenkins: "*Humanure*, unlike *human waste*, is not waste at all—it is an organic resource material rich in soil nutrients. Humanure originated from the soil and can be quite readily returned to the soil."[48]

In some parts of the United States extremely rigid regulations prohibit the use of composting toilets. Friends of mine with land in Vermont, where they camp and host group events, have been forced to rent portable chemical toilets rather than create composting toilet systems. The fear behind regulations like this is that human excrement not composted correctly has the potential to pollute groundwater. "A review of composting toilet laws is both interesting and disconcerting," notes Jenkins, citing nonsensical, almost superstitious laws, "apparently written by people who are either lacking in knowledge and understanding, or are fecophobic, or, most likely, all of the above."[49] Jenkins advises:

> When researching the laws, look into those that regulate backyard composting (if any), because that's what you're doing. . . . It's not sewage disposal, garbage disposal, or plumbing, or anything like that. If you look into *those* laws you may become overwhelmed and confused.[50]

As with any legal question, Jenkins says, "the semantics are important and not trivial."

Each of us has a choice as to whether to treat this daily production of our bodies as toxic waste or as a resource. At the community where I live we have no sewage hookup, no septic system, no porta-potties, just outhouses and pits in the ground. We compost all our shit. As each deposit is made, it is covered with sawdust. Twice a year we empty our central four-seater and leave the partially composted excrement in a huge pile for a year to break down. Then we use it to fertilize our fruit trees.

Emptying the shitter is a humbling experience, an hour of digging in deep shit and hauling it in wheelbarrows. What amazes me every time is how quickly the shit breaks down. The top layer is still recognizable as shit, but once you get below the surface to the stuff that's begun to decompose, the shit and other materials become one, transformed into worm-rich humus with no visual or olfactory likeness to shit.

Reduce, reuse, recycle. Live this ethic fully. Eat it, wear it, drive it, live in it, create it. Become more connected to the cycles of life and encourage other people to join you. Extricate yourself from constant convenience consumerism and strive to eliminate waste. Make scavenging, foraging, and recycling a way of life.

Action and Information Resources

Books

Alovert, Maria "Mark." *Biodiesel Homebrew Guide*. 10th ed. Self-published, 2005. Available online at www.localb100.com.

Brill, Steve. *Identifying and Harvesting Edible and Medicinal Plants in Wild (and Not So Wild) Places*. New York: Harper, 1994

Butler, C. T. Lawrence, and Keith McHenry. *Food Not Bombs*. Tucson, AZ: See Sharp Press, 2000.

DeFoliart, Gene R. *The Human Use of Insects as a Food Resource: A Bibliographic Account in Progress*. Self-published, 2003. Available online at www.food-insects.com.

Diamond, Jared. *Guns, Germs, and Steel: The Fates of Human Societies*. New York: W. W. Norton, 1999.

Estill, Lyle. *Biodiesel Power: The Passion, the People, and the Politics of the Next Renewable Fuel*. Gabriola Island, BC: New Society, 2005.

Flores, Heather C. *Food Not Lawns: How to Turn Your Lawn into a Garden and Your Neighborhood into a Community*. White River Junction, VT: Chelsea Green, 2006.

Gibbons, Euell. *Stalking the Healthful Herbs*. Chambersburg, PA: Alan C. Hood, 1966.

———. *Stalking the Wild Asparagus*. Chambersburg, PA: Alan C. Hood, 1962.

Gordon, David George. *The Eat-a-Bug Cookbook*. Berkeley, CA: Ten Speed Press, 1998.

Handerson, Robert K. *The Neighborhood Forager: A Guide for the Wild Food Gourmet*. White River Junction, VT: Chelsea Green, 2000.

Hart, Robert. *Forest Gardening: Cultivating an Edible Landscape*. White River Junction, VT: Chelsea Green, 1996.

Hoffman, John. *The Art and Science of Dumpster Diving*. Port Townsend, WA: Loompanics, 1993.

Jacke, Dave, with Eric Toensmeier. *Edible Forest Gardens*. 2 vols. White River Junction, VT: Chelsea Green, 2005.

Jenkins, Joseph. *The Humanure Handbook*. 3rd ed. Grove City, PA: Joseph Jenkins, 2005.

Johnson, Lorraine, and Mark Cullen. *Real Dirt: The Complete Guide to Backyard, Balcony & Apartment Composting*. Toronto: Penguin Books of Canada, 1992.

Lappé, Frances Moore, and Joseph Collins, with Cary Fowler. *Food First: Beyond the Myth of Scarcity*. New York: Ballantine, 1977.

Lappé, Frances Moore, Joseph Collins, and David Kinley. *Aid as Obstacle: Twenty Questions about Our Foreign Aid and the Hungry*. San Francisco: Food First, 1980.

Luddite, Laurel, and Skunkly Munkly. *Fire and Ice*. Apeshit Press, 2004.

Menzel, Peter, and Faith D'Aluisio. *Man Eating Bugs: The Art and Science of Eating Insects*. Berkeley, CA: Ten Speed Press, 1998.

Muskat, Alan. *Wild Mushrooms: A Taste of Enchantment*. 4th ed. Asheville, NC: self-published, 2004. Available online at www.alanmuskat.com.

Niehaus, Theodore F. *A Field Guide to Pacific States Wildflowers*. New York: Houghton Mifflin, 1998.

Pahl, Greg. *Biodiesel: Growing a New Energy Economy*. White River Junction, VT: Chelsea Green, 2005.

Peterson, Lee Allen. *A Field Guide to Edible Wild Plants: Eastern and Central North America*. New York: Houghton Mifflin, 1999.

Tickell, Joshua. *Biodiesel America: How to Achieve Energy Security, Free America from Middle-East Oil Dependence and Make Money Growing Fuel*. Tallahassee, FL: Tickell Energy Consulting, 2006.

———. *From the Fryer to the Fuel Tank*. Tallahassee, FL: Tickell Energy Consulting, 2000.

Weed, Susun S. *Wise Woman Herbal: Healing Wise*. Woodstock, NY: Ash Tree, 1989.

Periodicals

Food Insects Newsletter
333 Leon Johnson Hall
Montana State University
Bozeman, MT 59717-0302
www.hollowtop.com/finl_html/finl.html

Biodiesel Cyberinformation
Collaborative Biodiesel Tutorial
www.biodieselcommunity.org

Journey to Forever Online Biofuels Library
www.journeytoforever.org/biofuel_library.html

LocalB100.com
www.localb100.com

Films

Fat of the Land. Lardcar, 1995; www.lardcar.com.

The Gleaners and I. Directed by Agnès Varda. Zeitgeist Films, 2001; www.zeitgeistfilms.com.

Organizations and Other Resources

Big Box Reuse
www.bigboxreuse.com

Food Not Bombs
PO Box 744
Tucson, AZ 85702
(520) 770-0575
www.foodnotbombs.net

Food Not Lawns
31139 Lanes Turn Road
Coburg, OR 97408
www.foodnotlawns.com

Joe Hollis
Mountain Gardens
Shuford Creek Road
Burnsville, NC 28714
(828) 675-5664
www.mountaingardensherbs.com

International Food Policy Research Institute
2033 K Street NW
Washington, DC 20006-1002
(202) 862-5600
www.ifpri.org

Piedmont Biofuels
PO Box 661
Pittsboro, NC 27312
(919) 321-8260
www.biofuels.coop

Sequatchie Valley Institute/Moonshadow
1233 Cartwright Loop
Whitwell, TN 37397
(423) 949-5922
www.svionline.org

Wildroots Collective
PO Box 1485
Asheville, NC 28801
(866) 460-2945
www.wildroots.org

CHAPTER 10

Water:
Source of All Life

There is no way we can consider all the political issues revolving around the food we eat without talking about water. As basic and central as food is to our well-being, water is more so. Our bodies are 70 percent water. Humans can survive for weeks without food, but without water we can survive only a few days at most. And without water, there is no food.

Life began in water and radiated out onto land from shore. Human settlements followed the same pattern, with the oldest and largest cities located on the confluence of waterways. Access to water has always driven patterns of migration and settlement, not only for humans but for life in virtually all its manifestations. Mass social organization is possible only through the accumulation of water resources and the creation of infrastructure to distribute them. Whoever controls water has power and social control. Safeguarding and providing water to people has been one of the important functions of the state, especially in densely populated areas. Yet in the realm of water, today the state as an institution is in retreat, abdicating its traditional functions to private corporations.

Where does your water come from? Knowing the answer to this question is a step toward awareness and empowerment. Get to know your watershed and learn about the source of the water that comes out of your tap. As with food, if we blindly trust authorities to safeguard our supply, it may not be so safe.

Protecting the Water Commons

Water is a precious and dwindling resource that desperately needs protection. Agriculture accounts for the majority of the water humans use. According to the United Nations Educational, Scientific and Cultural Organization (UNESCO), 70 percent of water usage worldwide is agricultural, mostly for irrigation.[1] Using "conventional" input-intensive methods, it takes as much as 250 gallons of water to produce a pound of corn and 8,500 gallons to produce a pound of grain-fed beef.[2] Irrigation systems are often inefficient, with the majority of the water evaporating or running off the field, carrying with it agricultural chemicals into surface water supplies. Irrigation also alters soil conditions, eroding precious topsoil and depositing salts, which accumulate and eventually render the land inhospitable to plant life.

Agriculture doesn't have to use so much water. Traditional, locally bred plant varieties and animal breeds have been adapted to local water patterns through selection over time, exhibiting qualities such as drought tolerance, which enable them to produce even without regular watering. However, high yields from "improved" hybrid seeds depend upon a considerable and consistent supply of water.

In many regions, water demand is met by pumping underground water supplies (known as groundwater, in contrast to surface supplies, such as water from rivers, lakes, and reservoirs). Most of the food produced in the Great Plains of the United States is irrigated with water from the Ogallala aquifer, a single vast underground system spanning eight states. The problem is that the aquifer is being drained much faster than it's being replenished. In the past fifty years the aquifer has lost over a third of its volume, and each year another foot and half of water is pumped from it,[3] though the recharge rate from surface water seepage is just half an inch per year.[4] Food produced using water from such a slowly renewing source is doubly unsustainable, using up not only fossil fuel for agricultural chemicals and transportation but also water supplies that have accumulated over millennia and that will take many generations to replenish.

As underground water levels are depleted, surface lakes and rivers often disappear. In coastal areas, excessive groundwater pumping can lead to seawater seeping into drinking water supplies. UNESCO warns that drawing on groundwater supplies "unavoidably results in depleting the storage and has unfavourable consequences."[5] Nevertheless, it is common practice. Groundwater is the source of about 25 percent of the water supply, both in the United States and globally.[6]

"The world is incurring a vast water deficit, one that is largely invisible, historically recent, and growing fast," summarizes the Earth Policy Institute's Lester R. Brown.[7] In our property system, any scarce resource becomes a commodity. Water is "one of the great business opportunities," states *Fortune* magazine. "The dollars at stake are huge . . . Water promises to be to the twenty-first century what oil was to the twentieth."[8] Indeed, speculators have begun to trade in water "futures" just as they do any other commodity.

Policymakers proclaim that market forces will lead to more rational use of water. The World Bank, as part of its overall program of encouraging governments to divest themselves of services and industries, has aggressively promoted privatization of public water infrastructure since the 1990s, promising better water services through market efficiency and private investment. Yet those water systems that have been privatized have consistently seen higher consumer prices and disappointing levels of infrastructure investment. "What has now become clear is that the major multinational water corporations have no intention of making a significant contribution to the capital needed to ensure access to clean and affordable water," concludes a study by the U.S. consumer watchdog group Public Citizen. "The rhetoric of private sector financing is a myth."[9]

Atlanta, Georgia, is the biggest American city to have privatized its water system. In 1998 the city signed a twenty-year, $428 million contract with a subsidiary of Suez, one of the global giants of the water services industry, to operate its water system. Once Suez took over, the company realized that it had underestimated the amount of work needed to maintain the system and demanded an additional $80 million from the city.

Atlanta's mayor refused, because the whole reason the city had contracted out water services was to save money. Suez laid off half the water system's employees and tried to get extra money out of the city, for example by billing routine maintenance work to the city as "capital repairs." Maintenance was neglected, while water and sewer rates increased. Worst of all, water quality suffered, with frequent discolorations and boil-water advisories. Though the water services industry had hoped the Atlanta experience would open up the U.S. market to them, in 2003 Atlanta officials terminated the contract. Chris New, Atlanta's deputy water commissioner, said, "My biggest concern is a lot of people have lost confidence in the water itself.[10]

The government of Bolivia, in debt and heavily dependent upon World Bank loans, heeded the bank's advice to privatize water; in 1999 Bolivia awarded a forty-year contract to a subsidiary of the Bechtel Corporation for water services to Cochabamba, a city of more than six hundred thousand people. In this case, to meet the budget shortfall, water price increases went into effect immediately, with rates as much as tripling. The people of Cochabamba were shocked and angered by the dramatic rate increase. There was a four-day general strike, followed by escalating street protests. The Bolivian military took over the city and banned demonstrations. In the ensuing protests military forces injured 175 people and killed an unarmed seventeen-year-old. Government officials offered to roll back the rate increases, but the opposition leaders demanded that the contract be terminated. The Bolivian president did so, just six months into the contract. Bechtel responded by filing (but later withdrew) a $25 million lawsuit against Bolivia to compensate for "lost future profits."[11]

Another whole realm of water privatization is bottled water. In the United States bottled water sales more than tripled in the 1990s and continue to climb. In 2005 sales of bottled water in the United States approached $10 billion.[12] Global bottled-water sales were $100 billion in 2004, according to the Earth Policy Institute.[13]

One problem with this trend is that if the people who can afford to buy bottled water are drinking primarily that, the constituency for tap water is reduced, and by extension, for public investment in water systems. If the $100 billion being spent worldwide each year on bottled water were being invested in public water-supply systems, water quality and access would improve markedly. "A major shift to bottled water could undermine funding for tap water protection, raising serious equity issues for the poor," warns the Natural Resources Defense Council (NRDC). "The long-term solution to our water woes is to fix our tap water so it is safe for everyone, and tastes and smells good."[14]

Another big problem with bottled water is the plastic packaging. The 6 billion gallons of bottled water that were sold in the United States in 2002 required 1.5 million tons of plastic. And around thirty million plastic water bottles are discarded each day, piling up on landfills.[15] Obtaining the essential daily sustenance of water from disposable plastic containers is totally unsustainable behavior.

However, it is sustainable as a business opportunity. The corporations that dominate this rapidly growing industry are all household names from the food industry: Nestlé, PepsiCo, Coca-Cola, and Danone (the French-based manufacturer of Dannon yogurt). The water these corporations bottle as well as use in other beverages all comes from somewhere, and communities around the world are engaged in battles with water bottlers to keep them from extracting this precious resource.

Nestlé's niche is springwater, and the company has been buying up springs around the United States. Wisconsin activists succeeded in legal efforts to prevent Nestlé from pumping water at two different springs in that state. In Red Boiling Springs, Tennessee (where my friend Jeff Poppen, the CSA farmer featured in chapter 1, lives), Nestlé started pumping and bottling local water in 2003, with the help of a $1 million job-creation grant from the U.S. Department of Commerce. The promised local jobs never materialized, but the water extraction did.[16]

In Maine Nestlé acquired Poland Springs and other nearby sources, then sharply increased the volume of water being extracted. A local group has proposed that the state impose a water extraction fee of three cents per 20-ounce water container to fund a "Maine Water Dividend Trust." The activists' initial effort to place the proposal on the ballot as a voter referendum failed, but they continue working to build grass-roots support for the initiative.

Not all bottled water flows from springs. Sometimes it is taken directly from municipal taps or from polluted groundwater supplies. The NRDC analyzed 103 brands of bottled water in 1999 and found that a third of them had "significant" bacterial or chemical contamination. The NRDC's legal analysis found that the U.S. Food and Drug

Administration's regulation of bottled water is minimal and full of loopholes, "weaker in many ways than [Environmental Protection Agency] rules that apply to big city tap water. . . . While much tap water is indeed risky, having compared available data we conclude that there is no assurance that bottled water is any safer than tap water."[17]

In some cases, particularly in dry regions, the pumping of water from underground aquifers has dried up wells and other traditional water sources. Residents of several different towns in India have risen up against Coca-Cola bottling plants for their draining of local aquifers and polluting of local waters and land. In Kala Dera, Rajasthan, Coke's state-of-the-art groundwater extraction resulted in a dramatic reduction of the water table. After only six years of the plant's operation, fifty nearby villages reported water shortages as wells dried up. Many of these villages formed "struggle committees," and together they brought together two thousand people to march on the plant in 2004 to demand that the water extraction stop. "Drive away Coca-Cola, save the water!" is their rallying cry. An Indian government hydrogeologist warns that continued extraction will lead to deterioration of water quality and ecological repercussions such as rising surface temperatures and an increased likelihood of earthquakes, caused by the earth's upper crust drying up.[18]

The people around Kala Dera move forward with their struggle inspired by the success of activists in Plachimada, in the Indian state of Kerala. Residents there have maintained a constant vigil at the gates of the local Coca-Cola bottling plant since April 2002, protesting similar water shortages there resulting from groundwater pumping. The state government shut down the bottling plant, on a temporary basis, during a drought emergency in March 2004, but the local village council, or *panchayat*, has refused to allow the plant to reopen, and Kerala state pollution officials have ordered Coke to pipe water to communities where water supplies have been lost. In addition to depleting water resources, this plant was distributing its solid waste to local farmers as "fertilizer." Testing revealed cadmium and lead in the fertilizer, meaning that the land it had been spread on was contaminated with heavy metals; the state has since ordered Coke to stop distributing its toxic waste to farmers.[19]

These water and waste struggles in India have been bolstered by international solidarity. In the United States and Europe, college students are boycotting Coke and organizing campaigns to kick Coke off campuses. I believe that a boycott of Coca-Cola is a fine idea, but I think that boycott should extend to *all* global corporate food. It's not like drinking Pepsi is a more sustainable alternative.

Wherever we live, we must acknowledge our dependence on the flow of water and honor and protect the sources that sustain us. Those sources are the source of all life, a common heritage that must remain

The Cochabamba Declaration
December 8, 2000

Here, in this city which has been an inspiration to the world for its retaking of that right through civil action, courage, and sacrifice standing as heroes and heroines against corporate, institutional, and governmental abuse, and trade agreements which destroy that right, in use of our freedom and dignity, we declare the following:

For the right to life, for the respect of nature and the uses and traditions of our ancestors and our peoples, for all time the following shall be declared as inviolable rights with regard to the uses of water given us by the earth:

1. Water belongs to the earth and all species and is sacred to life, therefore, the world's water must be conserved, reclaimed, and protected for all future generations and its natural patterns respected.

2. Water is a fundamental human right and a public trust to be guarded by all levels of government, therefore, it should not be commodified, privatized or traded for commercial purposes. These rights must be enshrined at all levels of government. In particular, an international treaty must ensure these principles are noncontrovertable.

3. Water is best protected by local communities and citizens who must be respected as equal partners with governments in the protection and regulation of water. Peoples of the earth are the only vehicle to promote earth democracy and save water.

Adopted by the participants in the conference, "Water: Globalization, Privatization, and the Search for Alternatives," in Cochabamba, Bolivia, December 8, 2000.

in the public domain. Water is a biological necessity, recycling endlessly, and our bodies are part of its cycle. Water transcends commodification, just as the earth does. We are of it, so how can it be our property?

Clean Water Activism

Rather than cherishing and honoring water as the precious life-giving substance that it is, our profit-driven culture squanders it and pollutes it, without regard for long-term consequences. Major sources of water pollution include toxic industrial waste, agricultural chemicals, and feces. Some waste flows directly into waterways; in other cases it enters sewer systems, where "sludge" is filtered out and the water is treated with "purifying chemicals" (an oxymoron) before being released back into surface water supplies.

One purifying chemical often added to water, chlorine, has been hailed as the greatest public health achievement of the twentieth century, preventing the spread of infectious disease through public water supplies. Chlorination is a cost-effective means of killing waterborne bacteria. But chlorine has some distinctly unhealthy drawbacks. Chlorine reacts with organic compounds, which are especially prevalent in water from surface sources such as lakes and reservoirs, to form compounds called organochlorines or trihalomethanes, known in the lingo of the water purification industry as disinfection by-products. These compounds have been linked to an increased incidence of cancers, as well as birth defects, asthma, decreased fertility and sperm counts, and other human health problems.[20]

Arguably, an increased risk of certain diseases is well justified by the tremendous public health benefits of chlorination. But it's important to understand that chemically purified water involves tradeoffs. We lose something for what we gain, and it would be far better not to contaminate the water in the first place. And chlorination isn't the only or the best way to make contaminated water potable, though it is the cheapest. Many other methods, among them safer chemicals, ionization with copper or silver, ultraviolet light, reverse osmosis, and, of course, filtration, offer water purification alternatives.

Another chemical widespread in municipal water systems is fluoride.

Before it became known for preventing cavities, fluoride was considered an industrial pollutant. Fluoride is a toxic by-product of many industrial processes, including the production of aluminum, and high levels of fluoride exposure have been linked to many different human health problems.

Not dentists but rather aluminum industry scientists first proposed water fluoridation as a strategy for cavity control. In 1945, with fluoride emissions at an all-time high due to heightened wartime production, the federal government started its first water fluoridation experiment in Grand Rapids, Michigan, intended to be a fifteen-year study. With this pilot program barely under way, a full-on water fluoridation campaign emerged. Edward L. Bernays, often referred to as the father of public relations, orchestrated it at the behest of Oscar Ewing, the long-time lawyer for Alcoa (a major aluminum manufacturer) who was appointed in 1947 to head the federal agency overseeing the Public Health Service (PHS).[21]

Bernays was remarkably successful at giving fluoride the image of being safe and effective for cavity prevention, without substantive evidence. The Michigan study was aborted, and PHS officially endorsed water fluoridation in 1950. Since then two-thirds of U.S. water systems have been fluoridated.[22] Unfortunately, despite the wholesome image, there are growing questions about both fluoride's effectiveness and its safety. Critics charge that the chemical's cavity-prevention qualities have been overstated, and that water fluoridation is a cause of many different bone problems, including defective development, fractures, bone and joint cancers, and arthritis, as well as lowered IQ levels, neurotoxicity, and thyroid and pineal gland problems. One of the major groups crusading against water fluoridation is the union that represents scientists employed by the Environmental Protection Agency (EPA). Union members, who have reported political pressure to arrive at predetermined conclusions, call for "an immediate halt to the use of the nation's drinking water reservoirs as disposal sites for toxic waste."[23]

Water supplies everywhere benefit from informed activists demanding clean water. In some places river cleanup campaigns have achieved remarkable successes, for instance with the Hudson River in New York. But rivers are not cleaned up overnight; this work requires dedication, organization, follow-through, and perseverance. Passionate water lovers in every region are engaged in clean water campaigns, investigating the inflows and outflows within particular watersheds, drawing attention to major polluters, promoting water conservation, and organizing to demand enforcement of clean water laws.

One fierce voice demanding clean water has been that of Diane Wilson, a fourth-generation Texas shrimper and mother of five who has doggedly challenged various powerful industries polluting the Gulf of Mexico. "I've got four generations in one town," explains Diane. "That's why I battle here."[24] Diane became concerned about water quality in 1989, after a shrimper she knew who was suffering from cancer showed her a newspaper article on the EPA's Toxic Release Inventory, which named their home, Calhoun County, Texas, as the most toxic county in the nation. That single article propelled her into a life of activism. As she tells the story:

> I was extremely inexperienced—I've always been on the bay all my life. I've dealt with water and the elements and the tides and the fish—but I never ever would've considered myself an environmentalist.
>
> So all I did was call for a meeting, and I had such repercussions from this county, from the political structure—from just calling a meeting, and it just puzzled me. I didn't know what was going on, I was naïve, all I knew was those numbers that were in the paper. I got the bank president, the county commissioner, the mayor, I got economic development and city secretaries, all down at the fish house. I was suddenly getting all this hate—it was bizarre. I couldn't figure out why would they care—I was just a woman down in Seadrift calling a meeting. They didn't want me to have the meeting, they just wanted me to forget it and be a good citizen and stop causing problems. I had my meeting, and was promptly attacked by probably a dozen mayors, chambers of commerce, and businesses. They believed that just questioning industry, the corporations, was going to cause an economic problem.[25]

Undaunted, Diane started asking lots of questions. She learned about all the major chemical and plastic manufacturers that dump toxic waste into the Gulf of Mexico, and she focused her efforts on organizing people to oppose a huge polyvinyl chloride (PVC) factory expansion proposed by Formosa Plastics, a notorious polluter. While fighting the permit Formosa was in the process of seeking from the EPA, she recounts:

> Just by a fluke, I was talking to the EPA attorney one day and she thought she was talking to Formosa's attorney (we're both named Diane), so she started talking to me about the discharge and what they were putting in the water. I found out that the process didn't matter, the EPA had allowed them to go ahead and start discharging like they were going to get a permit anyway, so it was like a little game they were playing with me and the only one they hadn't told was the public.
>
> When I realized that the law didn't matter, that they were going to do what they were going to do and the federal government was going to work along with them, I was so outraged. I thought something had to be done to make people realize exactly what this meant, because most people don't think about it—it's like losing part of your civil rights. So it dawned on me to sink my shrimp boat, because I knew that action would force someone to look at it—it's kind of like a farmer saying he's going to burn his farm. That was a painful decision because I truly loved that boat, I had been shrimping on it a very long time, but I believe sometimes when you appeal to a higher law you have to be willing to go out there.

Diane sank her boat right atop Formosa's discharge pipe out in the bay. When the Coast Guard arrived, "they said I was a terrorist on the high seas." But the resulting publicity compelled Formosa to agree to a plan for zero discharge by recycling all its waste.

Diane Wilson is an activist who has demonstrated that a single individual's actions can make a big difference. "People have to be willing to get out there and do more than write a letter," she exhorts. "It's when people put themselves on the line, when you get face to face with your corporations and your politicians, when you have a sit-in in their office, they see you." Diane regards fear as the major reason why more people don't engage in direct action. "By just doing actions where we put ourselves up against our fears, you conquer that fear and it makes you stronger," she says. "We need to be bold and imaginative and brave. We've got to be heroes."[26]

Infrastructure Awareness

Most of us growing up in cities and suburbs with elaborate water infrastructures never really have to think much about the flow of water. Civil engineers think about it for us. This infrastructure is certainly convenient, and it facilitates population density. But it also cuts off the mass of us from intimate awareness of the constant flow of this centrally important element. Knowing the source of our water, and protecting that source, is part of interaction with the land.

At this point in the manuscript my editor, Ben Watson, inserted a Post-it note: "The source of my water here in Francestown, New Hampshire, is literally just up the road from me, and we have a volunteer, democratically elected Village Water Company. It makes us proud to know that we and our neighbors maintain this source and ensure its quality and distribution, and it makes us all aware of land use decisions and impact on environmental quality." Indeed, true democracy grows out of peoples' intimate relationships with the land and the elements.

In our life at Short Mountain, maintaining our own infrastructure by periodically walking a half mile up the mountain to our spring is part of keeping the water flowing. The water drips out of some rocks in the mountainside. We catch the small flow with a short length of guttering, loosely attached to the rocks. Often in big storms the gutter gets knocked down. That's why we have to go check it every so often. From the gutter, our dependable trickle flows into a fifty-five-gallon drum, from which a half mile of black plastic pipe carries it downhill (the direction water likes to flow) to a series of cisterns and into our kitchen and bathhouse. When the cisterns overflow, the trickle continues down the hollow into streambeds that flow into the Stones River and eventually feed the Mississippi and empty into the Gulf of Mexico. We are diverting a portion of it for our use, but the water continues its inevitable descent.

Thanks to the permaculture movement and groups like the Greywater Guerillas in the San Francisco Bay Area and the Desert Harvesters in Tucson, Arizona, much exciting activism is happening to help empower people to better understand and make the most of natural water flows. The more rainwater we can collect, the more water we will have available to use (without mining precious underground supplies), to flow through us and sustain us through periods of drought. Another strategy for water conservation is to collect and reuse graywater, which is wastewater containing soap and biological residues but not contaminated with feces or toxic chemicals. Graywater reclamation is an exciting emerging field with great potential for diverting wastewater, reusing it in gardens, and returning it to the ground, where it can percolate through the filtering earth back into groundwater reserves, rather than being mixed with feces and toxic chemicals so that it requires more extensive purification at sewage treatment facilities.

Minimizing what you draw from the public water system and what you send back into the sewer system is a form of taking responsibility. Reduce, reuse, recycle. "If we catch this [rain]water and use it in our homes and gardens, we step outside the destructive cycle of dammed rivers and depleted aquifers," write the Greywater Guerillas. "In the same way that composting creates rich soil from trash, water catchment and greywater cycling create opportunities for growth in barren places."[27]

We must all cultivate greater awareness of water and its flows so the grassroots can reclaim community control of this vital resource from the corporations, just as we are struggling to do with food. Each of us must find hope and inspiration to reconnect with the rhythms of the natural world and work toward a brighter future.

Recipe: Drink More Water

Consume water to flush your body, not the toilet! In our toxic world, abundant water flowing through our bodies helps cleanse our blood and tissues. "Insufficient water consumption causes toxicity of the body as well as constipation, tension, tightness, overeating, dryness, and kidney damage," warns nutritionist Paul Pitchford.[28]

Invest in a good home water filter, if you can, so you can be sure your water is free of chemical and bacterial contamination. Filtration systems vary in their effectiveness, and the cheapest home systems, unfortunately, are not very effective. Remember that drinking coffee, tea, soda, beer, or orange juice is not the same as drinking water. The other beverages are made of water, but they contain additional ingredients that require our bodies to have more water in order to process them. For every cup of other beverages that you drink, drink a glass of water. If you feel tired, weak, stressed, or constipated, or have a headache, drink more water. Learn to love the flavor and texture of your water; become a water connoisseur with a passionate interest in protecting your watershed.

Action and Information Resources

Books

Barlow, Maude, and Tony Clarke. *Blue Gold: The Fight to Stop the Corporate Theft of the World's Water*. New York: The New Press, 2002.

Black, Maggie. *The No-Nonsense Guide to Water*. Oxford, UK: New Internationalist, 2004.

Brown, Lester R. *Outgrowing the Earth: The Food Security Challenge in an Age of Falling Water Tables and Rising Temperatures*. Washington, DC: Earth Policy Institute, 2004.

Glennon, Robert. *Water Follies: Groundwater Pumping and the Fate of America's Fresh Waters*. Washington, DC: Island Press, 2002.

Greywater Guerillas. *Guide to Water*. Self-published, 2001.

Lancaster, Brad. *Rainwater Harvesting for Drylands*. Tucson, AZ: Rainsource Press, 2006.

Reisner, Marc. *Cadillac Desert: The American West and Its Disappearing Water*. New York: Penguin, 1993.

Roddick, Anita, with Brooke Shelby Biggs. *Troubled Water: Saints, Sinners, Truths and Lies about the Global Water Crisis*. Chichester, West Sussex, UK: Anita Roddick Books, 2004.

Shiva, Vandana. *Water Wars: Privatization, Pollution, and Profit*. Cambridge, MA: South End Press, 2002.

Wilson, Diane. *An Unreasonable Woman: A True Story of Shrimpers, Politicos, Polluters, and the Fight for Seadrift, Texas*. White River Junction, VT: Chelsea Green, 2005.

Woelfle-Erskine, Cleo, and Laura Allen. *Dam Nation: Dispatches from the Water Underground*. Brooklyn: Soft Skull Press, 2006.

Film

Thirst. Directed by Alan Snitow and Deborah Kaufman. PBS, 2004; www.thirstthemovie.org.

Organizations and Other Resources

American Rivers
1101 14th Street NW, Suite 1400
Washington, DC 20005
(202) 347-7550
www.americanrivers.org

America's Wetland
PO Box 44249
Baton Rouge, LA 70804-4249
(866) 4WETLAND
www.americaswetland.com

Coosa River Basin Initiative
408 Broad Street
Rome, GA 30161
(706) 232-2724
www.coosa.org

Corporate Accountability International
46 Plympton Street
Boston, MA 02118
(617) 695-2525
www.stopcorporateabuse.org

Desert Harvesters
(520) 882-9443
www.desertharvesters.org

Earth Policy Institute
1350 Connecticut Avenue NW, Suite 403
Washington, DC 20036
(202) 496.9290
www.earth-policy.org

EnviroLink Network
PO Box 8102
Pittsburgh, PA 15217
www.envirolink.org

Environmental Justice Coalition for Water
654 13th Street
Oakland, CA 94612
(510) 286-8400
www.ejcw.org

Greywater Guerillas
PO Box 3831
Oakland, CA 94609

Hudson River Sloop Clearwater
112 Little Market Street
Poughkeepsie, NY 12601
(845) 454-7673
www.clearwater.org

Hudson River Watch
www.hudsonwatch.net

India Resource Center
www.indiaresource.org

International Rivers Network
1847 Berkeley Way
Berkeley, CA 94703
(510) 848-1155
www.irn.org

Maine's Water Dividend Trust
PO Box 52
Fryeburg, ME 04037
(207) 935-2971
www.waterdividendtrust.com

Natural Resources Defense Council
40 West 20th Street
New York, NY 10011
(212) 727-2700
www.nrdc.org

Ogallala Commons
PO Box 245
Nazareth, TX 79063
(806) 938-2529
www.ogallalacommons.org

Public Citizen
Water for All Campaign
215 Pennsylvania Avenue SE
Washington, DC 20003
(202) 546-4996
www.citizen.org/cmep/water/

Rainwater Harvesting
www.rainwaterharvesting.org

Riverkeeper
828 South Broadway
Tarrytown, NY 10591
(800) 21-RIVER
www.riverkeeper.org

Sierra Club
Water Privatization Task Force
85 Second Street, 2nd Floor
San Francisco, CA 94105
(415) 977-5500
www.sierraclub.org/cac/water/

Sweetwater Alliance
PO Box 44173
Detroit, MI 48244
www.waterissweet.org

Tennessee Clean Water Network
706 Walnut Street
Knoxville, TN 37902
(865) 522-7007
www.tcwn.org

United Nations Educational, Scientific
and Cultural Organization
Water Portal
www.unesco.org/water

U.S. Environmental Protection Agency
Local Drinking Water Information
www.epa.gov/safewater/dwinfo.htm

The Water Page
www.thewaterpage.com

World Health Organization
Water, Sanitation, and Health
www.who.int/water_sanitation_health/ind
ex.html

World Water Council
www.worldwatercouncil.org

Epilogue

Bringing Food Back to Earth

Throughout this book I have reiterated the urgency of becoming more connected to the sources of our food and water. I have reported on some movements that I see happening, and I have tried to weave these movements together into a coherent analysis. In order to thrive, we must reclaim simple sustenance as an activity we are more directly engaged in, interacting with other organisms in our midst.

The future is scary. Climate change, chemical pollution, radioactive pollution, genetic pollution . . . need I go on? Current trends give rise to widespread despair. These bleak realities of how we have been degrading our earth and squandering our precious resources make me lose hope—sometimes. I also despair over the widening gulf between rich and poor, and over unjust wars that I fear will be avenged against the children I love. At least my basic needs are met, though. I have plenty of water and food, a comfortable home, and no crushing debt. My despair is about the future, and meanwhile life goes on.

For many people, despair is in the here and now. Around the world, one group of people living precariously close to the edge are farmers. The "Green Revolution" seduced farmers to abandon traditional agricultural practices for "improved" high-input methods, with promises of dramatic increases in yields and productivity. The high-tech seeds, chemicals, and irrigation all cost money, though, so farmers everywhere got caught in a spiraling cycle of debt and dependence.

For astonishing numbers of farmers, despair has led to suicide. India in particular has had a huge epidemic of farmer suicides. Vandana Shiva reports that twenty thousand farmers committed suicide in India between 1998 and 2000.[1] Some five thousand farmer suicides have been recorded since the late 1990s in a single southern state, Andhra Pradesh.[2] The typical method is to drink pesticides. According to an

Indian reporter who has visited and documented hundreds of families in which farmers have killed themselves, "The suicides are a symptom of vast agrarian distress."[3]

Suicide is a way out for struggling farmers in other places, too. An analysis of U.S. suicide data from 1980 to 1985, a period of great crisis for farmers, found that farmers had higher suicide rates than a control group; the analysis also identified a relationship between suicide rates and farm economic conditions.[4] The widow of a New Zealand farmer who hung himself in 2001 attributed her husband's death to the epidemic of mad cow disease: "It was a very real illness brought on by the BSE crisis and the gradual decline of the farming industry. It hit him very badly. Farmers have been under an incredible level of stress and what they are going through now must be soul-destroying."[5]

Our first task is to overcome despair and not allow it to swallow us up. We must try to find hope, believe in the future, be willing to move forward, and reinvent change. "There is, in many indigenous teachings, a great optimism for the potential to make positive change," concludes Winona LaDuke. "Change *will* come. As always, it is just a matter of who determines what that change will be."[6]

The act of suicide can be an expression of desperation and escape—or a grand gesture of defiance to inspire change. One farmer who killed himself on the world stage, sacrificing his life to draw attention to the plight of farmers everywhere, was Kyung-Hae Lee, former president of the Korean Advanced Farmers Federation. Lee stabbed himself in the chest, beneath a banner reading "WTO Kills Farmers," outside a World Trade Organization (WTO) meeting in Cancun, Mexico, on September 10, 2003.

Lee's words in a Korean farmers' publication a few months before his suicide seem in retrospect to explain his action: "Human beings are in an endangered situation," he wrote. "Uncontrolled multinational corporations and a small number of big WTO members' officials are leading an undesirable globalization [that is] inhumane, environment-distorting, farmer-killing, and undemocratic. It should be stopped immediately."[7]

In order to heed Lee's message and stop the earth-killing machine of corporate global food, we must strengthen and build movements for more sustainable, localized, healthy food. The people I've met, who have inspired me to write this book, offer abundant evidence that small, localized underground food movements are happening everywhere. Join them and broaden their vision.

All the other chapters of this book include recipes, mostly because I wanted to keep all this information and ranting grounded in the pleasures of the palate. I love sharing my ideas about food, but it is ironic to me that part of this process has been creating recipes that people follow, because I hardly ever follow recipes. I often consult recipes, typically checking several different sources, but then I end up ignoring them, varying the ingredients, using what's around, and learning from my experiments. That's what I like for people to do with my recipes.

Recipes offer step-by-step instruction, and some people want that very badly. Beyond food, people love recipes for health, wealth, spiritual well-being, sexual prowess, and a better world. I'm afraid that in the end I have no easy-to-follow recipe to offer my readers for how we can go about taking back community control of our food and water and, more broadly, our power and our dignity. There are no easy formulaic answers.

But as we search for answers, and allies, we can get our hands dirty working the soil and growing some of our own food. We can get to know farmers and support local markets. We can get to know plants, learn to save seeds, and learn how to heal our bodies and our souls. These activities ground us in the earth, and out of them grow health, abundance, community, and dreams of a better future.

Notes

Introduction

1. Vandana Shiva, *Tomorrow's Biodiversity* (New York: Thames and Hudson, 2000), 45.
2. Farm and Farm-Related Employment Data Set, www.ers.usda.gov/Data/FarmandRelatedEmployment/ (U.S. Department of Agriculture, Economic Research Service, for the year 2002; accessed May 1, 2006).

Chapter 1

1. Frances Moore Lappé, "Food, Farming, and Democracy," *The Journal of Gastronomy* 5, no. 2 (Summer–Autumn, 1989), quoted in Betty Fussell, *The Story of Corn* (New York: North Point Press, 1992), 162.
2. *Agriculture Fact Book 2000* (Washington, DC: U.S. Department of Agriculture Office of Communications, 2000), 21.
3. Truth about Trade and Technology, "Borlaug: Biotech Critical to Feeding Growing, Hungry World" (October 20, 2005), www.truthabouttrade.org/article.asp?id=4625.
4. Wendell Berry, "Think Little," in *A Continous Harmony: Essays Cultural and Agricultural* (New York: Harcourt Brace Jovanovich, 1974), 80.
5. U.S. Department of Agriculture Economic Research Service, "Food CPI, Prices, and Expenditures: Food Expenditures by Families and Individuals as a Share of Personal Disposable Income" (table 7), www.ers.usda.gov/Briefing/CPIFoodAndExpenditures/Data/table7.htm.
6. "Food Checkout Week," *Cannon Courier*, February 9, 2006, 1.
7. Marion Nestle, *Food Politics: How the Food Industry Influences Nutrition and Health* (Berkeley: University of California Press, 2003), 18
8. "True Cost Revolution," *Adbusters* 44 (November–December 2002), 75.
9. Rich Pirog and Andrew Benjamin, *Checking the Food Odometer: Comparing Food Miles for Local versus Conventional Produce Sales to Iowa Institutions* (Ames, IA: Leopold Center for Sustainable Agriculture, 2003), 5.
10. World Trade Organization, "Trade Liberalisation Statistics," http://gatt.org/trastat_e.html.
11. Alberto Jerardo, "The U.S. Ag Trade Balance . . . More Than Just a Number," *Amber Waves* (February 2004), www.ers.usda.gov/amberwaves/February04/Features/USTradeBalance.htm.
12. Choy Leng Young, "Great Pacific Northwest Salmon and Crab Being Sent to China to Be Filleted and De-Shelled before Arriving on U.S. Tables," *Bloomberg News*, July 16, 2005, as published in *The Agribusiness Examiner* 414 (October 8, 2005).
13. Barbara Kingsolver, "Lily's Chickens," in *Small Wonder* (New York: Perennial, 2002), 115.

14. Deborah Barndt, *Tangled Roots: Women, Work, and Globalization on the Tomato Trail* (Lanham, MD: Rowman & Littlefield, 2002), 198.

15. Environmental Working Group, "Farm Subsidy Database," (November 2005 Update), www.ewg.org/farm.findings.php.

16. Editorial, "Cow Politics," *New York Times*, October 27, 2005.

17. Vandana Shiva, quoted in Patrick Herman, *Food for Thought: Towards a Future for Farming*, translated, adapted, and updated by Richard Kuper (Sterling, VA: Pluto Press), 2003, xiii.

18. *Rigged Rules and Double Standards: Trade, Globalization, and the Fight against Poverty* (Oxford: Oxfam International, 2002), 22.

19. Andrew Maykuth, "Aid Hurting African Farmers: Free-trade Measures, Meant to Help, Drain Ghana's Economy," *Philadelphia Inquirer*, June 30, 2005, A1.

20. Carlo Petrini, opening speech at Terra Madre, October 20, 2004.

21. U.S. Department of Agriculture, Agriculture Marketing Service, "Farmers Market Growth," www.ams.usda.gov/farmersmarkets/FarmersMarketGrowth.htm.

22. Jeff Poppen, "An Article Written about Our CSA in the Fall of 2003," (self-published, 2003).

23. Robyn Van En Center for Community-Supported Agriculture Online CSA Directory, available online at www.csacenter.org.

24. U.S. Department of Agriculture, *2002 Census of Agriculture* (Washington DC: USDA National Agricultural Statistics Service, 2005), 8.

25. Ben Watson, *Cider, Hard and Sweet* (Woodstock, VT: The Countryman Press, 1999),

26. "U.S. Soft Drink Sales Up Slightly in 2004, Beverage Marketing Corporation Reports," news release from Beverage Marketing Corporation, March 14, 2005, www.beveragemarketing.com/news2uu.htm.

27. This warning label was found on both raw milk and raw apple cider in Maine, 2004.

28. Felipe Fernández-Armesto, *Food: A History* (London: McMillan, 2001), 243.

29. Guy Debord, "Hunger Reducer," ("Abat-faim"), *Encyclopedie des Nuisances* 5 (November 1985), translated from the French by NOT BORED! (August 2004), www.notbored.org/abat-faim.html.

30. Vandana Shiva, "A Tribute to the Earth's Caretakers," speech at Terra Madre (October 2004), www.terramadre2004.org/eng/discorsi/pdf/Vandana_Shiva_ENG.pdf.

31. Brian Tokar, "Agribusiness, Biotechnology and War," *Z Magazine* 15, no. 8 (September 2002), www.zmag.org/ZMag/articles/sep02tokar.html.

32. Craig Sams, *The Little Food Book: You Are What You Eat* (New York: Disinformation, 2004), 97.

33. Jen Ross, "Paying the Price for Growth," *The Toronto Star*, January 8, 2005, F5.

34. Kristin Collins, "State: Women Faced Exposure to Toxins in Fields," *Raleigh*

News & Observer, March 12, 2006, www.newsobserver.com/1188/story/417424.html.

35. Simon Head, "Inside the Leviathan," *The New York Review of Books* 51, no. 20 (December 16, 2004), www.nybooks.com/articles/17647.

36. U.S. House of Representatives Committee on Education and the Workforce Democratic Staff Report, *Everyday Low Wages: The Hidden Price We All Pay for Wal-Mart* (February 16, 2004), www.mindfully.org/Industry/2004/Wal-Mart-Labor-Record16feb04.htm.

37. Carolyn Demitri and Catherine Green, *Recent Growth Patterns in the U.S. Organic Foods Market* (Washington, DC: USDA Economic Research Service, September 2002), www.ers.usda.gov/publications/aib777/aib777.pdf.

38. Michael Pollan, "Naturally: How Organic Became a Marketing Niche and a Multibillion-Dollar Industry," *New York Times Magazine*, May 13, 2001, 32.

39. Michael Sligh (at a workshop titled "Who Owns Organic?" at Carolina Farm Stewards Association, Asheville, NC, November 2004).

40. The foodshed is a concept analogous to a watershed, meaning the whole land area contributing to the supply in one case of food and in the other of water.

41. Lisa M. Heldke, *Exotic Appetites: Ruminations of a Food Adventurer* (New York and London: Routledge, 2003), 171.

42. Mark Winston Griffith, "The 'Food Justice' Movement: Trying to Break the Food Chains," *Gotham Gazette* (December 2003), www.gothamgazette.com/article//20031218/20/808.

43. www.peoplesgrocery.org, accessed Spring 2005.

44. "Seattle Bans Soda & Junk Food from Schools," news release from Seattle Public Schools, September 3, 2004, posted online by the Organic Consumers Association, www.organicconsumers.org/school/seattleban090604.cfm.

45. Margot Roosevelt, "What's Cooking on Campus: Locally Grown Food Is the Latest Student Cause," *Time*, November 14, 2005, 62.

46. Community Food Security Coalition, Farmtocollege.org, "About Farm to College" (the table "Characteristics of farm-to-college programs"), www.farm-tocollege.org/about.htm, accessed May 25, 2006.

47. Michael Ableman, *On Good Land: The Autobiography of an Urban Farm* (San Francisco: Chronicle Books, 1998), 113.

48. Gary Paul Nabhan, *Coming Home to Eat* (New York: W. W. Norton, 2002), 46.

49. Ibid., 141–42.

50. Alisa Smith and J. B. MacKinnon, "Living on the Hundred-Mile Diet," *The Tyee*, June 28, 2005, www.thetyee.ca/Life/2005/06/28/HundredMileDiet.

51. RyeBuyLocalGuy, "Whole Foods—Not So Heaven-like" (blog post, September 16, 2005), www.vancomm.com/blc2004/2005/09/whole-foods-not-so-heaven-like.html.

52. Peter M. Rosset, "Cuba: A Successful Case Study of Sustainable Agriculture" in *Hungry for Profit: The Agribusiness Threat to Farmers, Food and the Environment*, ed. Fred Magdoff, John Bellamy Foster, and Frederick H. Buttel (New York: Monthly Review Press, 2000), 204.

53. Sol Kinnis, "Out of the Rubble: Agriculture in Havana, Cuba," in *Urban Wilds: Gardeners' Stories of the Struggle for Land and Justice*, ed. Cleo Woelfle-Erskine (Oakland, CA: water/under/ground publications, 2001), 22.

54. Marcos Nieto and Ricardo Delgado, "Cuban Agriculture and Food Security" in *Sustainable Agriculture and Resistance*, ed. Fernando Funes, Luis Garcia, Martin Bourque, Nilda Perez, and Peter Rosset (Oakland, CA: Food First, 2002), 45.

55. Quoted by Peter Lamborn Wilson, "Avant Gardening," in *Avant Gardening: Ecological Struggle in the City and the World*, ed. Peter Lamborn Wilson and Bill Weinberg (New York: Autonomedia, 1999), 16.

56. Chris and Laura, *Organic Gardening: A D.I.Y. Guide* (Columbus, OH: E. G. Smith Press, date unknown), 30.

57. Cleo Woelfle-Erskine, ed., *Urban Wilds: Gardeners' Stories of the Struggle for Land and Justice*, 2nd ed. (Oakland, CA: water/under/ground publications, 2001), 8.

58. Wilson, "Avant Gardening," 10.

59. Kingsolver, "Lily's Chickens," 114–15.

60. *Webster's Collegiate Dictionary*, 5th ed., 1946.

61. Susun S. Weed, *Wise Woman Herbal: Healing Wise* (Woodstock, NY: Ash Tree, 1989), 119.

Chapter 2

1. Quoted in Nabhan, *Coming Home to Eat*, 149.

2. ETC Group, "Global Seed Industry Concentration–2005," *Communiqué* 90 (September/October 2005), www.etcgroup.org/article.asp?newsid=524.

3. Helke Ferrie, "Schmeiser vs. Monsanto," http://percyschmeiser.com/Ferrie.htm.

4. Vandana Shiva, "The Indian Seed Act and Patent Act: Sowing the Seeds of Dictatorship" (February 14, 2005), Znet, www.zmag.org/content/print_article.cfm?itemID=7249&sectionID=56.

5. ETC Group, "Canadian Government to Unleash Terminator Bombshell at UN Meeting: All-out Push for Commercialisation of Sterile Seed Technology" (February 7, 2005), www.etcgroup.org/article.asp?newsid=498

6. Wilson, "Avant Gardening," 17.

7. Stephen Leahy, "Canada: Monsanto Victory Plants Seed of Privatisation" (October 5, 2004), Inter Press Service, http://ipsnews.net/interna.asp?idnews=25740.

8. Shiva, "The Indian Seed Act and Patent Act: Sowing the Seeds of Dictatorship."

9. Coalition Against Biopiracy, "Captain Hook Awards for Biopiracy 2006," www.captainhookawards.org/winners/2006_pirates, accessed June 21, 2006.

10. ETC Group, "Whatever Happened to the Enola Bean Patent Challenge?" (December 21, 2005), www.etcgroup.org/documents/GenotypeEnola05.pdf.

11. Editorial, "TRIPS and the Legal Protection of Plants," *Biotechnology and Development Monitor* no. 34 (1998), 2.

12. Shiva, "The Indian Seed Act and Patent Act: Sowing the Seeds of Dictatorship."

13. Ibid.

14. Coalition Provisional Authority, Order 81: Patent, Industrial Design, Undisclosed Information, Integrated Circuits and Plant Variety Law, April 26, 2004, www.cpa-iraq.org/regulations/20040426_CPAORD_81_Patents_Law.pdf.

15. Greg Palast, "Adventure Capitalism" (October 27, 2004), TomPaine.com, www.tompaine.com/articles/adventure_capitalism.php?dateid=20050321.

16. Food and Agriculture Organization of the United Nations Newsroom, "Rebuilding Iraq's Collapsed Seed Industry" (August 8, 2005), www.fao.org/newsroom/en/news/2005/107246/index.html.

17. Chris Davenport, "Iraq's Hidden Enemy: Biocolonialism in Babylon," *The ACTivist Magazine* (June 22, 2005), http://reclaimthecommons.net/article.php?id=210.

18. Cary Fowler and Pat Mooney, *Shattering: Food, Politics, and the Loss of Genetic Diversity* (Tucson: University of Arizona Press, 1990), 87.

19. Norman C. Ellstrand, "When Transgenes Wander, Should We Worry?" *Plant Physiology* 125 (2001), 1543–45, quoted in *Food Safety Review* (Spring 2002), 1.

20. Leahy, "Canada: Monsanto Victory Plants Seed of Privatisation."

21. Ian Johnston, "Green Body's Fury at 'Superweed' in Field of GM Crops," *The Scotsman*, July 26, 2005, http://news.scotsman.com/scitech.cfm?id=1682082005.

22. Mae-Wan Ho, interview, "A GM-Free World: Leading Geneticist Exposes the Bad Science of Biotech," *Acres USA* (November 2004), 26.

23. Jeffrey Smith, "US Government Proposal Puts Food Supply at Risk," *Spilling the Beans* (January 2005), www.seedsofdeception.com/Public/Newsletter/Jan05USProposalPutsFoodatRisk/index.cfm.

24. Stephen Leahy, "Challenges 2004–2005: 'Pharma Crops' Threaten Food Safety" (December 30, 2004), Inter Press Service, www.ipsnews.net/interna.asp?idnews=26866.

25. Smith, "US Government Proposal Puts Food Supply at Risk."

26. Friends of the Earth International, "U.S. Plans to Allow Experimental GM Crops to Contaminate Food" (November 23, 2004), www.foei.org/media/2004/1123.html.

27. Fowler and Mooney, *Shattering*, 76.

28. "Farmers Reject GM Food Crops," *Kenya Times*, August 25, 2004, www.indymedia.org/or/2004/08/3315.shtml.

29. Fowler and Mooney, *Shattering*, 20.

30. Dan Jason, *Save Our Seeds, Save Ourselves* (Ganges, Salt Spring Island, BC: self-published, circa 2000), 3.

31. Robert Johnston, Jr., *Growing Garden Seeds: A Manual for Gardeners and Small Farmers* (Winslow, ME: Johnny's Selected Seeds, 1983), 1.

32. Jason, *Save Our Seeds, Save Ourselves*, 4.

33. Action Group on Erosion, Technology and Concentration (ETC Group), "Gene Giants," *Communiqué* (March/April 1999), www.etcgroup.org/article.asp?newsid=180.

34. Fowler and Mooney, *Shattering*, 217.

35. Michel and Jude Fanton, *The Seed Savers' Handbook for Australia and New Zealand* (Byron Bay, New South Wales, Australia: The Seed Savers' Network, 1993), 14.

36. Ibid, 10.

37. www.seedsavers.org/Aboutus.asp.

38. Shiva, *Tomorrow's Biodiversity*, 137.

39. Carol Deppe, *Breed Your Own Vegetable Varieties: The Gardener's and Farmer's Guide to Plant Breeding and Seed Saving* (White River Junction, VT: Chelsea Green, 2000), xv.

40. Paul Elias, "Feds Fine Two Biotech Companies for Seed Gaffes" (December 1, 2004), www.ebfarm.com/News/NewsStories/BiotechFines120104.aspx.

41. Colin Macilwain, "US Launches Probe into Sales of Unapproved Transgenic Corn," *Nature* (March 22, 2005), www.nature.com/news/2005/050321/full/nature03570.html.

42. Editorial, "Don't Rely on Uncle Sam," *Nature* 434, (April 14, 2005), 807.

43. Kurt Eichenwald, Gina Kolata, and Melody Petersen, "Biotechnology Food: From the Lab to a Debacle," *New York Times*, January 25, 2001, A1.

44. Memorandum from Dr. James Maryanksi, biotechnology coordinator, to the director of the Center for Applied Nutrition, "FDA Task Group on Food Biotechnology: Progress Report 2," August 15, 1991, www.biointegrity.org/FDAdocs/22/view1.html.

45. Comments from Dr. Linda Kahl, FDA compliance officer, to Dr. James Maryanski, FDA biotechnology coordinator, about the Federal Register document "Statement of Policy: Foods from Genetically Modified Plants," January 8, 1992, www.biointegrity.org/FDAdocs/01/view1.html.

46. Steven Druker, "How the U.S. Food and Drug Administration Approved Genetically Engineered Foods Despite the Deaths One Had Caused and the Warnings of its own Scientists About Their Unique Risks," Alliance for Bio-Integrity, www.biointegrity.org/ext-summary.html.

47. The Pew Initiative on Food and Biotechnology, "Factsheet: Genetically Modified Crops in the United States" (August 2004), www.pewagbiotech.org/resources/factsheets/crops.

48. Jeffrey M. Smith, "US Government Proposal Puts Food Supply at Risk."

49. Paul S. Mead, Laurence Slutsker, Vance Dietz, Linda F. McCaig, Joseph S. Bresee, Craig Shapiro, Patricia M. Griffin, and Robert V. Tauxe, "Food-Related Illness and Death in the United States," *Emerging Infectious Diseases Journal* 5, no. 5 (September–October 1999),

www.cdc.gov/ncidod/EID/vol5no5/mead.htm.

50. Jeffrey M. Smith, *Seeds of Deception: Exposing Industry and Government Lies about the Safety of the Genetically Engineered Foods You're Eating* (Fairfield, IA: Yes! Books, 2003), 39.

51. Ibid., 13.

52. Jeffrey M. Smith, "Most Offspring Died When Mother Rats Ate Genetically Engineered Soy," *Spilling the Beans* (October 2005), www.seedsofdeception.com/Public/Newsletter/Oct05RatsDieWhenMothersE atGMSoy/index.cfm.

53. Eyal Press and Jennifer Waashburn, "The Kept University," *Atlantic Monthly* (March 2000), 39–54, cited in Smith, *Seeds of Deception*, 41.

54. Smith, "U.S. Government Proposal Puts Food Supply at Risk."

55. Smith, *Seeds of Deception*, 163.

56. Ibid., 166.

57. Ibid., 168.

58. U.S. Environmental Protection Agency, "Funding Opportunities," http://es.epa.gov/ncer/rfa/2005/2005_star_biotech.html.

59. Pew Initiative on Food and Biotechnology, "Factsheet: Genetically Modified Crops in the United States" (August 2004), www.pewagbiotech.org/resources/factsheets/display.php3?FactsheetID=2.

60. Pew Initiative on Food and Biotechnology, "Public Sentiment about Genetically Modified Food" (November 2005), http://pewagbiotech.org/research/2005update/1.php.

61. The Council of Canadians, "GM Food Aid—Case Study: Zambia," www.cana-dians.org/display_document.htm?COC_token=:COC_token&id=1091&isdoc=1&catid=375.

62. Wangari Maathai, "The Linkage between Patenting of Life Forms, Genetic Engineering and Food Insecurity" (May 28, 1998), Genet, www.genet-info.org/-documents/AfricaGMOsPatents.pdf.

63. Greenpeace, "Asians Call for Ban on GE Rice" (October 14, 2005), Scoop, www.scoop.co.nz/stories/WO0510/S00279.htm.

64. Associated Press, "Mexican Farmers Protest Genetically Modified Corn Imports" (October 29, 2004), www.newfarm.org/international/news/110104/110204/gm_protest.shtml.

65. GE Free Maine has published *Town by Town: Bringing the Debate over Genetically Engineered Crops to Your Community* (August 2004), which is available online at www.gefreemaine.org/townbytownguide.pdf.

66. "Alaska Wins One for GMO Labeling" (August 19, 2005), Supermarket Guru, http://supermarketguru.com/page.cfm/15743.

67. Heike Dongowski, "Greenpeace in Hamburg Soyabean Protest," *Lloyd's List International* (November 8, 1996).

68. René Riesel, "Statement to the Agen Court," February 3, 1998, translated by Ken Knabb, www.notbored.org/agen.html.

69. Agence France Presse, "Activists' Destruction of GM Crops Was Justified: French Court" (December 9, 2005), www.agbioworld.org/newsletter_wm/ index.php?caseid=archive&newsid=2456.

70. Agence France Presse, "French Activist Bové Jailed for Destroying GM Crops" (November 15, 2005), www.archives.foodsafetynetwork.ca: 16080/agnet/2005/11-2005/agnet.nov.15.htm.

71. Luther Tweeten, "Agroterrorism" (2005), www.farmpolicy.com/Tweeten%20doc.pdf.

72. Agent Apple, "The Robert Shapiro Incident: A Strange and Terrible Saga: An Eyewitness Account," in the Biotic Baking Brigade, *Pie Any Means Necessary* (Oakland, CA: AK Press, 2004), 50–51.

73. Justin Gillis, "Clone-Generated Milk, Meat May Be Approved: Favorable FDA Ruling Seen as Imminent," *Washington Post*, October 6, 2005, A1.

74. James Owen, "Animals' Sexual Changes Linked to Waste, Chemicals" (March 1, 2004), National Geographic News, http://news.nationalgeographic. com/news/2004/03/0301_040301_genderbender.html.

75. Shiva, *Tomorrow's Biodiversity*, 30.

76. Renée Loux Underkoffler, *Living Cuisine: The Art and Spirit of Raw Foods* (New York: Avery, 2003), 211.

Chapter 3

1. Malcolm X, "Message to the Grass Roots," November 10, 1963, Detroit, Michigan, text online at www.thespeechsite.com/famous/MalcolmX-2.htm; quoted in Woelfle-Erskine, *Urban Wilds*.

2. "The True Levellers Standard Advanced: Or, The State of Community Opened, and Presented to the Sons of Men" (1649), www.diggers.org/diggers/tlsa.htm.

3. Anders Corr, *No Trespassing: Squatting, Rent Strikes and Land Struggles Worldwide* (Cambridge: South End Press, 1999), 193.

4. Ward Churchill, *Acts of Rebellion: The Ward Churchill Reader* (New York: Routledge, 2003), 141.

5. Winona LaDuke, "Voices from White Earth: Gaa-waabaabiganikaag," *Thirteenth Annual E. F. Schumacher Lectures*, October 1993, Yale University, online at www.smallisbeautiful.org/publications/laduke_93.html.

6. Ibid.

7. Ibid.

8. Churchill, *Acts of Rebellion*, 284.

9. Corr, *No Trespassing*, 2.

10. Angus Wright and Wendy Wolford, *To Inherit the Earth: The Landless Movement and the Struggle for a New Brazil* (Oakland: Food First, 2003), 74.

11. Ibid., 264.

12. Stephen Schlesinger and Stephen Kinzer, *Bitter Fruit: The Untold Story of the American Coup in Guatemala* (New York: Anchor Books, 1983), 40, 50.

13. Ibid., 55.

14. Thais Leon, "Chavez Gives Land Titles to the Indigenous," Associated Press, August 9, 2005, www.washingtonpost.com/wp-dyn/content/article/2005/08/09/AR2005080901454.html.

15. George A. Collier, with Elizabeth Lowery Quaratiello, *Basta!: Land and the Zapatista Rebellion in Chiapas* (Oakland: Food First, 1999), 46.

16. National Agricultural Statistics Service, US Department of Agriculture, *2002 Census of Agriculture*, Table 1, "Historical Highlights: 2002 and Earlier Census Years," United States Data, 6.

17. U.S. Census Bureau, *Statistical Abstract of the United States* (1950 Edition), 561, www2.census.gov/prod2/statcomp/documents/1950-08.pdf.

18. Pesticide Action Network Updates Service, "Subsidies Increase for Industrial Agriculture" (November 11, 2004), www.panna.org/resources/panups/panup_20041111.dv.html

19. Lee Rood, "On New Ground," *Des Moines Register*, July 24, 2005, www.dmregister.com/apps/pbcs.dll/article?AID=/20050724/BUSINESS01/507240348/1030.

20. Ableman, *On Good Land*, 120.

21. Ibid., 50.

22. Ibid.

23. Ibid., 57.

24. Ibid., 136.

25. U.S. Census Bureau, *Statistical Abstract of the United States* (2006), Chart 796: "Farm Operators – Tenure and Characteristics," www.census.gov/compendia/statab/tables/06s0796.xls.

26. Lee Rood, "Turning Over the Soil," *Des Moines Register*, July 17, 2005, http://desmoinesregister.com/apps/pbcs.dll/article?AID=/20050717/BUSINESS01/507170367/1030.

27. Brian Halweil, "This Old Barn, This New Money," *World Watch* (July/August 2003).

28. Heldke, *Exotic Appetites*, 212–13.

29. U.S. Census Bureau, *Statistical Abstract of the United States*, (2006) Chart 796: "Farm Operators – Tenure and Characteristics," www.census.gov/compendia/statab/tables/06s0796.xls.

30. Anuradha Mittal, "The Last Plantation," *Food First Backgrounder* 6, no. 1 (Winter 2000), 1.

31. Quoted in Howard Zinn, *A People's History of the United States* (New York: HarperCollins, 1995), 193.

32. Ibid., 204.

33. Donald J. Broussard Jr., "Lychings," www.ucs.louisiana.edu/~djb8243/Lynchings.html.

34. "Minority Family Farmers Face Extinction," *Farm Aid News & Views* (February 1997), www.ibiblio.org/ecolandtech/permaculture/mailarchives/sanet2/temp/msg00252.html www.farmaid.org.

35. Environmental Working Group, "Obstruction of Justice," www.ewg.org/reports/blackfarmers/.

36. Environmental Working Group, "USDA Settlement Fails Black Farmers," www.ewg.org/reports/blackfarmers/.

37. Mike Tierney, "Black Farmers Angry at Feds: Group Wants to Resurrect Claims Process," *Atlanta Journal Constitution*, May 5, 2005, E1.

38. "City Dwellers are Growing Food in Surprising Numbers!" *Urban Agricultural Notes,* (November 2002), www.cityfarmer.org/40percent.html#toronto.

39. Margaret Armar-Klemesu, "Urban Agriculture and Food Security, Nutrition and Health," in *Growing Cities Growing Food; Urban Agriculture on the Policy Agenda* (Resource Centre on Urban Agriculture and Forestry (RUAF), 2000), www.ruaf.org/system/files?file=Theme4.PDF

40. Jon Lamb, "Food, Poverty and Ecology: Cuba & Venezuela Lead the Way," *Green Left Weekly*, February 2, 2005, www.greenleft.org.au/back/2005/613/613p12.htm.

41. Periurban refers to the urban perimeter, the less densely settled areas directly surrounding cities.

42. Rachel Nugent, editor, *Discussion paper for FAO-ETC/RUAF electronic conference "Urban and Periurban Agriculture on the Policy Agenda"* (Food and Agriculture Organization of the United Nations: August-September 2000), www.fao.org/urbanag/Paper1-e.htm.

43. Patricia H. Hynes, *A Patch of Eden: America's Inner City Gardens* (White River Junction, VT: Chelsea Green Publishing, 1996), 31.

44. Ibid, 12-13.

45. American Community Gardening Association, *National Community Gardening Survey: 1996*, www.communitygarden.org/CGsurvey96part2.pdf.

46. Brad Lancaster, "Street Orchards for Community Security," *Permaculture Activist* 54 (Winter 2004-5), 41.

47. Bill Finch, "Chickens Are Useful Pets," *Mobile Register*, April 26, 2002, www.al.com/specialreport/mobileregister/?urban.html.

48. Andrea del Moral, "Down on the Canadian Industrial Farm," in Woelfle-Erskine, *Urban Wilds*, 32.

49. Woelfle-Erskine, *Urban Wilds*, 68.

50. Ibid., 71.

51. Sarah Ferguson, "A Brief History of Grassroots Greening on the Lower East Side," in *Avant Gardening: Ecological Struggle in the City and the World*, ed. Peter Lamborn Wilson and Bill Weinberg (New York: Autonomedia, 1999), 83.

52. Nicole Itano, "Hungry Zimbabweans Grow Food Where They Can," *Independent Online* (April 15, 2005), www.iol.co.za/index.php?set_id= 1&click_id=68&art_id=qw1112713562176B255.

53. "Food from the Graveyard," News24.com, November 11, 2004, www.news24.com/News24/Africa/Features/0,,2-11-37_1619485,00.html.

54. Ibid.

55. "Bronx United Gardeners: We're Here to Stay" in Woelfle-Erskine, *Urban Wilds*, 43.

56. Ferguson, "A Brief History of Grassroots Greening on the Lower East Side," 88.

57. Anne Raver, "City Rejects $2 Million Offer for Gardens," *New York Times*, April 23, 1999, B3.

58. Anne Raver, "Auction Plan For Gardens Stirs Tensions," *New York Times*, Jan 11, 1999, B1.

59. Douglas Martin, "City Takeover Looms for Gardens on Vacant Lots," *New York Times*, May 1, 1998, B1.

60. More Gardens! Coalition, *How to Save Your Community Garden*, pamphlet (circa 2000), 2.

61. Dan Barry, "Garden-Lovers Arrested at City Hall Sit-In," *New York Times*, Feb 25, 1999, B8.

62. Barry, "Giuliani Seeks Deal to Sell 63 Gardens to Land Group and End Suits," *New York Times*, May 12, 1999, B1.

63. Dean Kuipers, "Trouble in the Garden," *LA City Beat* (January 26, 2005) www.lacitybeat.com/article.php?id=3200&IssueNum=138.

64. Tom Philpott, "Community Farming in LA: Neoliberalism at the Garden Gate," *Counterpunch*, March 16, 2006, www.counterpunch.org/philpott03162006.html.

65. South Central Farmers, "Newsflash: We're Taking Back the Farm!", www.southcentralfarmers.com (accessed June 25, 2006).

66. Jen Ross, "Paying the Price for Growth," *The Toronto Star*, January 8, 2005, F5.

67. Kadi Hodges, "FLOC Pact in North Carolina 'Historic': Agreement With Growers Calls For Better Wages, Conditions" in *Toledo Blade*, September 17, 2004, www.toledoblade.com/apps/pbcs.dll/article?AID=/20040917/BUSI-NESS07/409170372.

68. Ibid.

69. Coalition of Immokalee Workers, "Victory at Taco Bell," www.ciw-online.org/agreementanalysis.html.

70. Ibid.

71. Katherine Ellison, "Can Great Coffee Save the Jungle?" *Smithsonian*, June 2004, 102.

72. Luis Hernandez Navarro, "To Die A Little: Migration and Coffee in Mexico and Central America," a report of the Interhemispheric Resource Center (December 15, 2004), www.americas.irc-online.org/reports/2004/0412coffee_body.html.

73. Peter Rosset, "Food Sovereignty: Global Rallying Cry of Farmer Movements," *Food First Backgrounder* 9, no. 4 (Fall 2003), 1.

74. Karen Brandon, "New Technology Likely To Impact Some California Farmers," *LA Times Magazine*, January 1, 2002.

75. Peter Holmes, *The Energetics of Western Herbs*, Revised Third Edition (Boulder, Colorado: Snow Lotus Press, 1998), 841.

Chapter 4

1. The Slow Food Manifesto, www.slowfoodusa.org/about/manifesto.html.

2. Carlo Petrini, Speech at the W.K. Kellogg Foundation Conference, April 28, 2005, www.slowfoodusa.org/events/carlo_petrini_speech.html.

3. July 2005 invitation from Slow Food USA to a dinner with Carlo Petrini at the restaurant Blue Hill in New York City.

4. Carlo Petrini, "The New Gastronomy of Food Communities," *The Snail* (Slow Food USA newsletter), Fall 2005, 3.

5. John Hooper, "Peasant Farmers of the World Unite!" *The Guardian*, October 20, 2004, www.guardian.co.uk/italy/story/0,12576,1331314,00.html.

6. Carlo Petrini, Opening Speech at Terra Madre, October 20, 2004, www.slow-foodusa.org/events/petrini_speech.html.

7. Carlo Petrini, "The New Gastronomy of Food Communities," *The Snail* (Slow Food USA newsletter), Fall 2005, 3.

8. Carlo Petrini, "Food and Folk," *Slow: The International Herald of Tastes* (2005, Number 3), 4.

9. Vandana Shiva, "Terra Madre v. Terra Nullius," *Slow: The International Herald of Tastes* (2005, Number 3), 6.´

10. Elizabeth Weise, "There's One Flaw in the Pawpaw," *USA Today*, November 28, 2005, 9D, www.usatoday.com/news/health/2005-11-28-pawpaw-foodies_x.htm#.

11. Timothy Le Riche, "Geneticist Warns and Challenges Students," *The Edmonton Sun*, October 28, 2005, 63.

12. Hope Shand, *Human Nature: Agricultural Biodiversity and Farm-based Food Security* (Rural Advancement Foundation International, December 1997), www.etcgroup.org/documents/other_human.pdf.

13. Makalé Faber, "Springing Forth a Renewal of America's Food Traditions," *The Snail* (Slow Food USA newsletter), Fall 2005, 11.

14. Carlo Petrini, Speech at the W.K. Kellogg Foundation Conference, April 28, 2005, www.slowfoodusa.org/events/carlo_petrini_speech.html.

15. Ibid.

16. Corby Krummer, "White Earth Land Recovery Project," www.slowfood.com/img_sito/PREMIO/vincitori2003/pagine_en/USA_03.html

17. Winona LaDuke, National Public Radio Morning Edition (November 12, 2004).

18. White Earth Land Recovery Project, "Anishinaabeg Culture and the History of Manoomin," www.savewildrice.org/default.asp?active_page_id=31.

19. Albert Jenks, quoted by Winona LaDuke, "Wild Rice and Ethics," *Cultural Survival Quarterly* 28, no. 3 (Fall 2004),15.

20. Winona LaDuke, "The Political Economy of Wild Rice Indigenous Heritage and University Research," *Multinational Monitor* 25, no. 4 (April 2004), www.multinationalmonitor.org/mm2004/04012004/april04corp4.html.

21. Krummer, "White Earth Land Recovery Project."

22. Nabhan, *Coming Home to Eat*, 247.

23. Ibid, 260.

24. Ibid, 293.

25. Gary Paul Nabhan, *Why Some Like It Hot: Food, Genes, and Cultural Diversity* (Washington: Island Press, 2004), 168.

26. Ibid, 184.

27. Frank Bruni, "Chewing the Fat While It's Fresh," *New York Times*, November 3, 2004, F1.

28. Ibid.

29. Marla Cone, "Dozens of Words for Snow, None for Pollution," *Mother Jones*, January 2005, 47.

30. Patricia Gadsby, "The Inuit Paradox: How Can People Who Gorge on Fat and Rarely See a Vegetable Be Healthier Than We Are?", *Discover*, October 2004, 54.

31. Robert McClure, "Bush Administration Proposes 80% Cutback in Protected Salmon Habitat," *Seattle Post-Intelligencer*, December 1, 2004, http://seattlepi.nwsource.com/local/201848_salmon01.html.

32. Winona LaDuke, *All Our Relations: Native Struggles for Land and Life* (Cambridge, MA: South End Press, 1999), 1.

33. Blaine Harden, "Tribe Fights Dams to Get Diet Back," *Washington Post*, January 30, 2005, A3, www.washingtonpost.com/wp-dyn/articles/A47525-2005Jan29.html.

34. Village Earth Pine Ridge Project Blog, "Being the Buffalo" (October 6, 2005), www.villageearth.org/pages/Projects/Pine_Ridge/pineridgeblog/2005/10/being-buffalo-article-in-rocky.html

35. LaDuke, *All Our Relations*, 143–44.

36. Ibid., 160.

37. Carlo Petrini, Speech at the W.K. Kellogg Foundation Conference, April 28, 2005, www.slowfoodusa.org/events/carlo_petrini_speech.html.

38. Yaroslav Trofimov, "As a Cheese Turns, So Turns This Tale of Many a Maggot," *Wall Street Journal*, April 23, 2000, 1.

39. "Sardinia's Liveliest Pecorino," *Saveur*, August 2003, 86.

40. Dev Raj, "Officials 'Helpless' as Spurious Oil Kills 50: Opens the Door to Canola Trade," Inter Press Service, September 6, 1998, www.gene.ch/gentech/1998/Sep-Nov/msg00018.html.

41. Vandana Shiva, "The Mustard Oil Conspiracy," *The Ecologist*, June, 2001, 27, www.findarticles.com/p/articles/mi_m2465/is_5_31/ai_76285485.

42. Vandana Shiva, "The Law For Food Facism: The Proposed Food Safety & Standards Bill, 2005," *ZNet*, February 21, 2005, www.zmag.org/content/print_article.cfm?itemID=7289&sectionID=66.

43. William Branigin, Mike Allen and John Mintz, "Tommy Thompson Resigns From HHS," *Washington Post*, December 3, 2004, www.washingtonpost.com/wp-dyn/articles/A31377-2004Dec3.html.

44. Richard Morgan, "Government Tries to Squelch Alert on Milk Terror Threat," *Discover*, January 2006, 48.

45. Vandana Shiva, "The Law For Food Facism: The Proposed Food Safety & Standards Bill, 2005," *Znet,* February 21, 2005, www.zmag.org/content/showarticle.cfm?ItemID=7289

46. Ibid.

47. Association for the Study of Food and Society Listserv, August 22, 2005.

48. Amy Rose, "It's Not Business As Usual At Farmers' Market," *The Greeneville Sun*, August 1, 2005, www.greene.xtn.net/index.php?table=news&template=news.view.subscriber&newsid=123190.

49. Nabhan, *Coming Home to Eat*, 125.

50. Barbara McMahon, "Italy's DIY Food Fundis," *Mail and Guardian*, July 8, 2005, www.mg.co.za/articlePage.aspx?articleid=244926&area=/insight/insight__escape/#.

51. Janelle Brown, "Restaurants On the Fringe, And Thriving," *New York Times*, March 12, 2003, F1.

52. Janine DeFao, "Guerilla Gourmet," *San Francisco Chronicle*, January 22, 2006, A1.

53. Jim Leff, online posting at www.chowhound.com/boards/general8/messages/14416.html.

54. Nabhan, *Coming Home to Eat*, 259.

55. Jessica Prentice, "Stirring the Cauldron" (November 2004), www.stirringthecauldron.com/2004/m11_snow_moon.php.

56. Harold McGee, *On Food and Cooking: The Science and Lore of the Kitchen* (New York: Scribner, 2004), 603.

Chapter 5

1. "Food Irradiation," U.S. Centers for Disease Control Division of Bacterial and Mycotic Diseases, www.cdc.gov/ncidod/dbmd/diseaseinfo/foodirradiation.htm.

2. John E. Peck, "Nuking Food for Profit," *Z Magazine*, February 2003, http://zmagsite.zmag.org/Feb2003/peck0203.html

3. Public Citizen Critical Mass Energy and Environment Program, The Cancer Prevention Coalition, and Global Resource Action Center for the Environment, "A Broken Record: How the FDA Legalized – and Continues to Legalize – Food Irradiation Without Testing It for Safety" (October 2000), 11, www.citizen.org/documents/brokenrecordfinal.PDF

4. Peck, "Nuking Food for Profit."

5. www.organicpastures.com.

6. Don P. Blayney and Alden C. Manchester, "Large Companies Active in Changing Dairy Industry," *FoodReview* 23, no. 2 (May-August 2000), 9.

7. Shiv Chopra et. al, "Gaps Analysis," Health Canada, April 21, 1998, cited in Smith, *Seeds of Deception*, 84.

8. Union of Concerned Scientists, "Greener Pastures: How Grass-Fed Beef and Milk Contribute to Healthy Eating," March 8, 2006, www.ucsusa.org/food_ and_environment/sustainable_food/greener-pastures.html.

9. Ron Schmid, *The Untold Story of Milk: Green Pastures, Contented Cows, and Raw Dairy Foods* (Washington, DC: New Trends Publishing, 2003), 315.

10. Ibid., 32.

11. Ibid., 54.

12. Ibid., 58.

13. Laura LaFay, "The Milk Maneuvers: Why is Gov. Warner's Pro-Pasteurization Stance Causing Such a Commotion?" *Style Weekly* (Richmond, VA), December 29, 2004, www.styleweekly.com/article.asp?idarticle=9612.

14. Lina Gutherz Straus, *Disease in Milk, The Remedy Pasteurization: The Life Work of Nathan Straus* (New York: Dutton, 1917), 214, cited in Schmid, *The Untold Story of Milk*, 67.

15. Frederick Kaufman, "Contraband: Psst! Got Milk?," *The New Yorker,* November 29, 2004, 62.

16. Sally Fallon, "The Politics and Economics of Food," Keynote Address at the Northeast Organic Farming Association Conference (Ahmerst, Massachusetts, August, 2003), www.westonaprice.org/farming/polecon foods.html

17. Campaign for Real Milk, "What's Happening With Real Milk?" www.realmilk.com/happening.html.

18. Panel on raw milk activism at the 2005 conference of the Weston A. Price Foundation.

19. Campaign for Real Milk, "Update from Tim Wightman" (March 18, 2004), www.realmilk.com/update-wi.html.

20. USDA National Agricultural Statistics Service, "Tennessee Data – Dairy Milk Cows by Size Groups: Operations," http://151.121.3.33:8080/QuickStats/PullData_US.

21. Steve Jenkins, *Cheese Primer* (New York: Workman, 1996), xxvi.

22. Remy Grappin and Eric Beuvier, Institut National de la Recherche Agronomique (I.N.R.A.), Station de Recherches en Technologie et Analyses Laitieres in Pouligny, France, quoted by Jean Garsuault, President of L'Institut International du Fromage, "The Raw Milk Debate In The European Union," www.vtcheese.com/vtcheese/rawmilk_files/rawmilk3.html

23. Ibid.

24. "We Want to Live," http://home.earthlink.net/~welive/index.html

Chapter 6

1. Annemarie Colbin, *Food and Healing: How What You Eat Determines Your Health, Your Well-being, and the Quality of Your Life* (New York: Ballantine Books, 1986), 10.

2. Frank M. Torti, Jr. et. al., "Survey of Nutrition Education in U.S. Medical Schools – An Instructor-Based Analysis," 2000, www.med-ed-online.org/res00023.htm.

3. *The U.S. Market for Nutritional Supplements: Vitamins, Minerals and Dietary Supplements*, 5th Edition (Packaged Facts, 2004), www.packagedfacts,com/pub/977844.html.

4. Centers for Disease Control and Prevention, *National Report on Human Exposure to Environmental Chemicals*, July 2005, www.cdc.gov/exposurereport/.

5. Environmental Working Group, "Body Burden—The Pollution in Newborns" (July 14, 2005), www.ewg.org/reports/bodyburden2/execsumm.php.

6. Sandra Steingraber, "Organic Food as Good Prenatal Care: Agricultural Threats to Pregnancy, Breast Milk and Infant Development," keynote address at Eco-Farm Conference in Asilomar, California (January 20, 2005), www.newfarm.org/features/2005/0905/ecofarmkey/steingraber.shtml.

7. U.S. Environmental Protection Agency, *Guidelines for Carcinogen Risk Assessment and Supplemental Guidance for Assessing Susceptibility from Early-Life Exposure to Carcinogens*, March 2005, http://cfpub.epa.gov/ncea/raf/recordisplay.cfm?deid=116283.

8. USDA Economic Research Service, "Food CPI, Prices, and Expenditures: Expenditures as a Share of Disposable Income," www.ers.usda.gov/Briefing/CPIFoodAndExpenditures/Data/; and Centers for Medicare & Medicaid Services, "National Health Expenditure Data: Historical," www.cms.hhs.gov/NationalHealthExpendData/02_NationalHealthAccountsHistorical.asp

9. E. Frazão, "High Costs of Poor Eating Patterns in the United States" in E. Frazão, ed., *America's Eating Habits: Changes and Consequences* (Washington, DC: USDA, 1999, 5-32, cited in Nestle, *Food Politics*, 7.

10. Centers for Disease Control and Prevention, "Overweight and Obesity, Economic Consequences," http://198.246.96.2/NCCDPHP/dnpa/obesity/economic_consequences.htm.

11. Barbara Starfield, "Is U.S. Health Really the Best in the World?" *Journal of the American Medical Association* 284, no. 4 (July 26, 2000), 483-5, www.mercola.com/2000/jul/30/doctors_death.htm.

12. Gary Null PhD, Carolyn Dean MD ND, Martin Feldman MD, Debora Rasio MD, and Dorothy Smith PhD, "Death by Medicine" (October 2003), available online at www.newmediaexplorer.org/sepp/Death%20by%20Medicine%20Nov%2027.doc.

13. "Pharmaceuticals In Our Water Supplies," *Arizona Water Resources* (July–August 2000), www.ag.arizona.edu/AZWATER/awr/july00/feature1.html.

14. The AIDS Coalition to Unleash Power (ACT UP) defines itself as "a diverse, non-partisan group of individuals united in anger and committed to direct action to end the AIDS crisis." We used loud, confrontational tactics to demand action on AIDS, and in the midst of much despair over illness and death, we found solidarity and forged ahead with a vision of the end of the crisis and a belief that a better world is possible.

15. Barbara Ehrenreich and Deirdre English, *Witches, Midwives and Nurses* (New York: Feminist Press, 1973), 17, quoted in Starhawk, "The Burning Times: Notes on a Crucial Period of History," appendix to *Dreaming the Dark: Magic, Sex and Politics* (Boston: Beacon Press, 1988), 203.

16. Starhawk, "The Burning Times: Notes on a Crucial Period of History," appendix to *Dreaming the Dark: Magic, Sex and Politics* (Boston: Beacon Press, 1988), 199.

17. "Katuah Medics Presents a Wilderness First Responder Course for Activists" (2005), www.medic.democracyuprising.org/index.php.

18. Weed, *Wise Woman Herbal*, x.

19. "U.S. Life Expectancy Expected to Drop for First Time in History as Effect of Obesity," *Health Talk* (March 17, 2005), www.healthtalk.ca/obesity_life_031705_399312.php.

20. Helen H. Jensen and John C. Beghin, "U.S. Sweetener Consumption Trends and Dietary Guidelines," *Iowa Ag Review Online* (Winter 2005), www.card.iastate.edu/iowa_ag_review/winter_05/article5.aspx.

21. U.S. Department of Agriculture Economic Research Service, "Sweetener Consumption in the United States: Distribution by Demographic and Product Characteristics," August 2005 www.ers.usda.gov/Publications/SSS/aug05/sss24301.pdf.

22. Linda Joyce Forristal, "The Murky World of High Fructose Corn Syrup," *Wise Traditions* (Weston A. Price Foundation, Fall 2001), www.weston-aprice.org/motherlinda/hfcs.html.

23. George A Bray, Samara Joy Nielsen, and Barry M Popkin, "Consumption of High-Fructose Corn Syrup in Beverages May Play a Role in the Epidemic of Obesity," *American Journal of Clinical Nutrition* 79, no. 4 (2004), 537.

24. Mary G. Enig, PhD and Sally Fallon, "The Oiling of America," first published in *Nexus Magazine*, December 1998-March 1999. www.westonaprice.org/knowyourfats/oiling.html.

25. Mary Enig, PhD, and Sally Fallon, "The Skinny on Fats," www.westonaprice. org/knowyourfats/skinny.html.

26. Marc Santora, "Hold That Fat, New York Asks Its Restaurants," *New York Times*, August 11, 2005, A1.

27. Nicholas von Hoffman, "Eating Ourselves to Death," *The Nation*, February 6, 2006, www.thenation.com/doc/20060206/vonhoffman.

28. National Center for Health Statistics, "Health, United States, 2004," www.cdc.gov/nchs/data/hus/hus04.pdf.

29. Harvard University School of Public Health, "Study Finds Increased Consumption of Sugar-Sweetened Beverages Promotes Childhood Obesity," press release (February 15, 2001), www.hsph.harvard.edu/press/releases/press02152001.html.

30. Sams, *The Little Food Book*, 40.

31. Ibid., 41.

32. National Diabetes Information Clearinghouse, National Diabetes Statistics, "Total Prevalence of Diabetes by Race/Ethnicity Among People Aged 20 Years or Older, United States, 2002", www.diabetes.niddk.nih.gov/dm/pubs/statistics/.

33. Nestle, *Food Politics*, 22.

34. "U.S. Soft Drink Sales Up Slightly in 2004," news release from Beverage Marketing Corporation (March 14, 2005), www.beveragemarketing.com/news2uu.htm.

35. Nestle, *Food Politics*, 211.

36. J. Wynns, "Yes: Selling Students to Advertisers Sends the Wrong Message in the Classroom" in *Advertising Age*, June 7, 1999, 26, as cited in Nestle, *Food Politics*, 188.

37. Nestle, *Food Politics*, 206.

38. Michele Simon, "Big Food's 'Health Education,'" *San Francisco Chronicle*, September 7, 2005, B9.

39. McSpotlight Press Release, February 12, 2003, www.mcspotlight.org/media/press/releases/msc021203.html

40. Dani Veracity, "The Great Direct-to-Consumer Prescription Drug Advertising Con," *News Target*, July 31, 2005, www.newstarget.com/010315.html.

41. Arnold S. Relman and Marcia Angell, "America's Other Drug Problem: How the Drug Industry Distorts Medicine and Politics," *The New Republic*, December 16, 2002, 27.

42. Ibid., 36.

43. Martin T. Gahart, Louise M. Duhamel, Anne Dievier, and Roseanne Price, "Examining The FDA's Oversight Of Direct-To-Consumer Advertising," *Health Affairs*, February 26, 2003, 121.

44. Online Lawyer Source, "Number of Estimated Vioxx Prescriptions Increases," www.onlinelawyersource.com/news/vioxx-prescriptions.html.

45. www.merck.com/about/.

46. Anna Wilde Mathews and Barbara Martinez, "Warning Signs: E-Mails Suggest Merck Knew Vioxx's Dangers at Early Stage," *Wall Street Journal*, November 1, 2004, A1.

Chapter 7

1. Winona LaDuke, *All Our Relations: Native Struggles for Land and Life* (Cambridge: South End Press, 1999), 197.

2. See my discussion of sugar and the fermented stimulants in *Wild Fermentation*, 22-26.

3. Fowler and Mooney, *Shattering*, 177.

4. Ibid., 179.

5. D. Pimentel, et. al., Bioscience 47 (1997) cited by the South African Department of Environmental Affairs and Tourism, "Invasive Species Regulations," www.invasive.species.sanbi.org/.

6. National Aeronautics and Space Administration Office of Earth Science and the U.S. Geological Survey, "Invasive Species Forecasting System: Background" (April 23, 2004), www.bp.gsfc.nasa.gov/isfs_science.html.

7. Alan Burdick, "The Truth About Invasive Species," *Discover*, May 2005, 40.

8. Stephen Jay Gould, "An Evolutionary Perspective on Strengths, Fallacies, and Confusions in the Concept of Native Plants," in Joachim Wolschke-Bulmahn, editor, *Nature and Ideology: Natural Garden Design in the Twentieth Century* (Washington, D.C.: Dumbarton Oaks Research Library and Collection, 1997), 19, www.doaks.org/Nature/natur002.pdf.

9. Michael Pollan, "Against Nativism," *The New York Times Magazine*, May 15, 1994, 55.

10. Patricia Leigh Brown, "By the Bay, Old Dunes Vie With Exotic Trees," *New York Times*, March 9, 2003, A24.

11. David I. Theodoropoulos, *Invasion Biology: Critique of a Pseudoscience* (Blythe, California: Avvar Books, 2003), 88.

12. Pollan, "Against Nativism," 54.

13. G. Groening and J. Wolschke-Bulmahn, "Some Notes on the Mania for Native Plants in Germany," *Landscape Journal* 11 (1992), 116-126, quoted in Janet Marinelli, "Natives Revival—Is Native-plant Gardening Linked to Fascism?", *Plants & Gardens News* 15, no. 2 (Summer 2000), www.bbg.org/gar2/topics/wildflower/1995fa_native.html.

14. Pollan, "Against Nativism," 54.

15. Stephen Jay Gould, "An Evolutionary Perspective on Strengths, Fallacies, and Confusions in the Concept of Native Plants," 19.

16. Theodoropoulos, *Invasion Biology*, 176.

17. Canadian Food Inspection Agency, "Weed Seed Order 2005," *Canada Gazette* 139, no. 9, part 1 (February 26, 2005), www.canadagazette.gc.ca/partI/2005/20050226/html/regle1-e.html.

18. Massachusetts Department of Agricultural Resources, "Massachusetts Prohibited Plant List" (December 12, 2005), www.mass.gov/agr/farmproducts/proposed_prohibited_plant_list_v12-12-05.htm.

19. New South Wales Department of Primary Industries, "Resolving Conflicts in Weed Control: Roles and Responsibilities for Noxious Weed Control," www.agric.nsw.gov.au/reader/weed-legislation/weeds-conflict.pdf?MIvalObj= 25764&doctype=document&MItypeObj=application/pdf&name=/weeds-conflict.pdf.

20. South Africa Department of Environmental Affairs and Tourism, "Guidelines for the Listing Process for Regulations for the National Environmental Management: Biodiversity Act, Act No. 10 of 2004," www.invasive.species.sanbi.org/regulations/Guidelines.pdf.

21. U.S. Department of Agriculture Animal and Plant Health Inspection Service Plant Protection and Quarantine "Issue Group: Risk Assessment," www.safe-guarding.org/getcomments.cfm?RecID=108.

22. No White List Coalition, "What is the White List?," www.geocities.com/nowhitelist/whtlist.html.

23. No White List Coalition, "FAQ," www.geocities.com/nowhitelist/faq.html.

24. Theodoropoulos, *Invasion Biology,* 141.

25. Charles Lewis, *Green Nature—Human Nature: The Meaning of Plants in Our Lives* (Urbana and Chicago: 1996), 124f, quoted in Joachim Wolschke-Bulmahn, "The Search for 'Ecological Goodness' among Garden Historians," Michel Conan, editor, *Perspectives on Garden Histories* (Washington, D.C.: Dumbarton Oaks Research Library and Collection, 1999), 180, www.doaks.org/Perspectives/perspec08.pdf.

26. Theodoropoulos, *Invasion Biology,* 141.

27. United Nations Office of Drugs and Crime, *World Drug Report 2005,* 84, www.unodc.org/unodc/en/world_drug_report.html.

28. Ibid., 286-307.

29. "Tennessee's eradicated marijuana crop for 1999 yielded plants valued at $628,226,000 which surpassed all other legitimate cash crops individually with the closest being tobacco at $217,429,000." U.S. Office of National Drug Control Policy, "High-Intensity Drug Trafficking Areas, Appalachia HIDTA, www.ncjrs.gov/ondcppubs/publications/enforce/hidta2001/appl-fs.html.

30. Martin Booth, *Cannabis: A History* (New York: St. Martin's Press, 2003), 159.

31. Ibid., 32-34.

32. Ibid., 93.

33. Ibid., 99.

34. Headline reproduced (without date) in Jack Herer, *The Emperor Wears No Clothes* (Van Nuys, California: HEMP Publishing, 1990), 24.

35. Ibid., 24.

36. Booth, *Cannabis,* 149.

37. Ibid., 135.

38. Henry J. Anslinger, "Marijuana—Assassin of Youth," *The American Magazine,* 1937, reproduced in William Daniel Drake, Jr., *The Connoisseur's Handbook of Marijuana* (San Francisco: Straight Arrow Books, 1971), 133.

39. Booth, *Cannabis,* 146.

40. Herer, *The Emperor Wears No Clothes,* 25.

41. Booth, *Cannabis,* 155; Herer, *The Emperor Wears No Clothes,* 25.

42. Jon B. Gettman, *Crimes of Indiscretion: Marijuana Arrests in the United States* (Washington, DC: National Organization for the Reform of Marijuana Laws, 2005), 23, www.norml.org/pdf_files/NORML_Crimes_of_Indiscretion.pdf.

43. Ibid., 56-7.

44. Ryan S. King and Marc Mauer, *The War on Marijuana: The Transformation of the War on Drugs in the 1990s*, (Washington, DC: The Sentencing Project, May 2005), 23, www.sentencingproject.org/pdfs/waronmarijuana.pdf.

45. Gettman, *Crimes of Indiscretion*, 82.

46. Ibid., 92.

47. King and Mauer, *The War on Marijuana*, 27.

48. Jeffrey A. Miron, *The Budgetary Implications of Marijuana Prohibition* (Washington, DC: Marijuana Policy Project, June 2005), 8-11, www.prohibitioncosts.org/mironreport.html.

49. Ibid., 15-16.

50. Milton Friedman et. al., "An Open Letter to the President, Congress, Governors, and State Legislatures," June 2005, www.prohibitioncosts.org/endorsers.html.

51. Rasmussen, D.W. and Benson, B.L., *The Economic Anatomy of a Drug War: Criminal Justice in the Commons* (Lanham, MD: Rowman and Littlefield, 1994), 135.

52. Jeffrey A. Miron, *Federal Marijuana Policy: A Preliminary Assessment* (Washington, DC: Taxpayers for Common Sense, June 2005), 17, www.taxpayer.net/drugreform/mironreport.pdf.

53. U.S. Department of Health and Human Services, Substance Abuse and Mental Health Services Administration, *National Survey on Drug Use and Health* (2002), cited in Gettman, *Crimes of Indiscretion*, 9.

54. Michael Pollan, "How Pot Has Grown," *New York Times Magazine*, February 19, 1995, 32, www.lectlaw.com/files/drg17.htm; Duncan Campbell, "With Pot and Porn Outstripping Corn, America's Black Economy is Flying High," *The Guardian*, May 2, 2003, www.guardian.co.uk/usa/story/0,12271,947880,00.htm

55. Johnston, L.D., O'Malley, P.M., Bachman, J.G., and Schulenberg, J.E., *Monitoring the Future: National Survey Results on Drug Use, 1975-2003. Volume I: Secondary School Students*, (Bethesda, MD: National Institute on Drug Abuse, 2004; NIH Publication No. 04-5507), Table 9-6, cited in King and Mauer, *The War on Marijuana*, 7.

56. Booth, *Cannabis*, 253.

57. Michael Pollan, *The Botany of Desire* (New York: Random House, 2001), 129.

58. Booth, *Cannabis*, 58.

59. Pollan, *The Botany of Desire*, 174.

60. www.gwpharm.com/research_cri.asp.

61. The Yippies were a group of political hippies, sometimes known as the Youth International Party, not a traditional political party at all, but rather a motley anarchic group of flamboyant activists, best remembered for their role in the huge demonstrations at the 1968 Democratic National Convention in Chicago. Their most famous member was author Abbie Hoffman.

62. Canadian Hemp Trade Alliance estimate, cited in Donna Leinwand, "Industrial Hemp Support Takes Root," *USA Today*, November 22, 2005, 3A, www.usatoday.com/news/nation/2005-11-22-hemp-crop_x.htm.

63. Bob Egelko, "U.S. Won't Try to Ban Hemp Foods, Oils," San Francisco Chronicle, September 28, 2004, B-4, http://sfgate.com/cgi-bin/article.cgi?file=/chronicle/archive/2004/09/28/BAGVO8VTND1.DTL

64. Wade Davis, *One River: Explorations and Discoveries in the Amazon Rainforest* (New York: Simon & Schuster, 1996), 419.

65. Ibid., 416.

66. Ibid., 419.

67. Michael Pollan, "Opium Made Easy: One Gardener's Encounter with the War on Drugs," *Harper's Magazine*, April 1997, 58.

68. Federal Controlled Substances Act of 1970, Section 841, cited in Pollan, "Opium Made Easy," 45.

69. Pollan, "Opium Made Easy," 43.

70. Ibid., 35.

71. Louisiana Act 159 of 2005, www.legis.state.la.us/billdata/streamdocument.asp?did=318544.

72. Weed, *Wise Woman Herbal*, 70.

73. Theodoropoulos, *Invasion Biology*, 179.

74. Nicolas Monardes, 1574, translated by Frampton, 1577, cited in Charlotte Erichsen-Brown, *Medicinal and Other Uses of North American Plants* (New York: Dover, 1979), 103.

75. Peter Holmes, *The Energetics of Western Herbs* Revised Third Edition (Boulder, Colorado: Snow Lotus Press, 1998), 356.

Chapter 8

1. Wendell Berry, "The Pleasures of Eating" in Wendell Berry, *What Are People For?* (New York: North Point Press, 1990), 151.

2. Michael Stumo, "In Firm Control: Industrial Concentration in the U.S. Livestock Market," *Multinational Monitor*, July/August 2000, www.multinationalmonitor.org/mm2000/00july-aug/stumo.html.

3. Andrew Martin, "Audit: USDA Blocks Real Probes, Records Fake Ones," *Chicago Tribune*, January 19, 2006, 9.

4. William Heffernan, Mary Hendrickson, and Robert Gronski, *Report to the National Farmers Union: Consolidation in the Food and Agriculture System* (Columbia, MO: National Farmers Union, 1999), 4, www.nfu.org/wp-content/uploads/2006/03/1999.pdf.

5. Stephanie Simon, "A Killing Floor Chronicle: A Down-and-Out Former Poultry Worker's Online Memoirs of his Gruesome Job Have Electrified Animal-Rights Activists Worldwide," *Los Angeles Times*, December 8, 2003, 1, www.commondreams.org/cgi-bin/print.cgi?file=/headlines03/1208-07.htm.

6. Virgil Butler, "Inside the Mind of a Killer" (August 31, 2003), excerpted from his blog at www.cyberactivist.blogspot.com/2003/08/inside-mind-of-killer.html.

7. Upton Sinclair, *The Jungle* (New York: Signet Classics, 1960), 39-41.

8. Howard Lyman statement upon dismissal of "false disparagement" charges, February 29th, 1998, on his "New Mad Cowboy" Web site, www.mad-cowboy.com/01_BookOP.000.html.

9. Donald G. McNeil, Jr. and Alexei Barrionuevo, "For Months, Agriculture Department Delayed Announcing Result of Mad Cow Test," *New York Times*, June 26, 2005, A16.

10. Amanda Griscom Little, "Old Big Brother Had a Farm," *Grist* (March 6, 2006), www.grist.org/news/muck/2006/03/10/griscom-little/index.html.

11. Ibid.

12. Pythagoras, as quoted by Ovid, according to Jon Wynne-Tyson, *The Extended Circle: A Commonplace Book of Animal Rights* (Pub Group West, 1988), cited online at www.answers.com/topic/pythagoras.

13. Vegetarian Society UK, "21st Century Vegetarian—Through the Ages," www.vegsoc.org/news/2000/21cv/ages.html.

14. Frances Moore Lappé, *Diet for a Small Planet* (New York: Ballantine Books, 1971), 6.

15. Alisa Smith and J.B. MacKinnon, "Wanted: A Perfectly Local Chicken," *The Tyee*, July 13, 2005, www.thetyee.ca/Life/2005/07/13/LocalChicken.

16. Miguel Bustillo, "In San Joaquin Valley, Cows Pass Cars as Polluters," *Los Angeles Times*, August 2, 2005, 1, www.latimes.com/news/local/la-me-cows2aug02,0,5709626.story?coll=la-home-headlines%20

17. Bloodroot Collective, *The Political Palate: A Feminist Vegetarian Cookbook* (Bridgeport, Connecticut: Sanguinaria, 1980), xi.

18. Carol J. Adams, *The Sexual Politics of Meat: A Feminist-Vegetarian Critical Theory* (New York: Continuum, 1990), 47.

19. Ibid., 187.

20. Mary Enig, *Know Your Fats* (Silver Spring, Maryland: Bethesda Press, 2000), 100.

21. Mary Enig and Sally Fallon, *Eat Fat, Lose Fat* (New York: Hudson Street Press, 2005), 42.

22. Ibid., 24.

23. Gina Kolata, "Low-Fat Diet Does Not Cut Health Risks, Study Finds," *New York Times*, February 8, 2006, A1.

24. Enig and Fallon, *Eat Fat, Lose Fat*, 43.

25. Alan Watts, *Does It Matter? Essays on Man's Relationship to Materiality* (New York, Vintage Books, 1968, 26.

26. Ibid., 27.

27. Sandy Wilkens, Slaughterhouse Human Resources Director, in John Bowe, et. al., *Gig: Americans Talk About Their Jobs* (New York: Three Rivers Press, 2000), 49.

28. Mark Shipley, Personal correspondence, June 2006.

29. Richard Manning, "The Oil We Eat: Following the Food Chain Back to Iraq," *Harper's Magazine*, February 2004, 45.

30. Joel Salatin, *Holy Cows and Hog Heaven: The Food Buyer's Guide to Farm Friendly Food* (Swoope, Virginia: Polyface, Inc., 2004), 22.

31. Ibid., 105.

32. Detailed in their newsletters posted online at www.peacefulpastures.com.

33. Jenny Drake, "The Government vs. Peaceful Pastures Round #3." *Peaceful Pastures Press* (January 2003), www.peacefulpastures.com.

34. Will Winter, "Mom's Dairy vs. the Supreme Court," *Acres USA*, April 2005, 19.

35. Lance Gay, "Toxic Gas Hides Meat Spoilage, Firm Says," *Detroit News*, November 17, 2005, www.detnews.com/2005/business/0511/17/A10-384898.htm.

36. Salatin, *Holy Cows and Hog Heaven*, 117.

37. Paul Pitchford, *Healing with Whole Foods*, Revised Edition (Berkeley, California: North Atlantic Books, 1993), 256.

38. Sally Fallon with Mary G. Enig, *Nourishing Traditions: The Cookbook that Challenges Politically Correct Nutrition and the Diet Dictocrats* (Washington, DC: New Trends, 1999), 123.

Chapter 9

1. Warren J. Belasco, *Appetite for Change* (New York: Pantheon, 1989), 119,

2. Frances Moore Lappé and Joseph Collins with Cary Fowler, *Food First: Beyond the Myth of Scarcity* (New York: Ballantine, 1977), 17.

3. Elizabeth Becker, "Number of Hungry Rising, U.N. Says," *New York Times*, December 8, 2004, A5.

4. U.S. Department of Agriculture Economic Research Service, *Household Food Security in the United States, 2004*, "Table 1: Prevalence of Food Security, Food Insecurity, and Food Insecurity with Hunger by Year," 6, www.ers.usda.gov/publications/err11/err11b.pdf.

5. "Industrial Agriculture Wastes 50% of Food," *Food Production Daily*, November 25, 2004, http://foodproductiondaily.com/news/ng.asp?id=56340&n=dh330&c=tzlvsrxy-wshqwyj; "U.S. Wastes $14 Billion in Food & Crops Every Year," *Agribusiness Examiner* 410 (June 20, 2005).

6. U.S. Environmental Protection Agency, "Municipal Solid Waste Generation, Recycling, and Disposal in the United States: Facts and Figures for 2003," www.epa.gov/epaoswer/non-hw/muncpl/pubs/msw05rpt.pdf.

7. C.T. Butler and Keith McHenry, *Food Not Bombs* (Tucson, Arizona: See Sharp Press, 2000), 80.

8. Ibid., 3-4.

9. Lauren Rosa and Chris Crass, "Food Not Bombs Turns 20," *Clamor*, October/November 2000.

10. Anonymous, *Evasion* (Atlanta, GA: CrimethInc. Workers' Collective, 2002), 80.

11. Dave, *Dumpsterland* #11, May, 2002, available from dumpsterland@riseup.net.

12. "Roadkill Census: Weather is Most Significant Factor in Numbers Observed," *Farmers and Wildlife* 7, no. 1 (Winter 2001), 6, www.asi.ksu.edu/DesktopModules/ViewDocument.aspx?DocumentID=1734.

13. Bret Liebendorfer, "The Real Roadkill Café," *Columbus Alive*, March 16, 2005, www.columbusalive.com/2005/20050316/031605/03160513.html.

14. Terra, *Feral Forager* 4, circa 2003, available from Wildroots Collective, P.O. Box 1485, Asheville, NC 28802, www.wildroots.org.

15. Laurel Luddite and Skunkly Munkly, *Fire and Ice* (Apeshit Press, 2004), 164.

16. Green Anarchy and the Wildroots Collective, *Rewilding: A Primer for a Balanced Existence Amid the Ruins of Civilization*, Back to Basics vol. 3, 9.

17. Terra, *Feral Forager*, 5.

18. Nabhan, *Coming Home to Eat*, 142.

19. Green Anarchy and the Wildroots Collective, *Rewilding*, 4.

20. Woelfle-Erskine, *Urban Wilds*, 20.

21. Tamara Jones, "The Man Who Ate Manhattan," Associated Press report, April 1, 1986, asap.ap.org/data/interactives/_lifestyles/urban_forager/.

22. Alan Muskat, *Wild Mushrooms: A Taste of Enchantment*, Fourth Edition (Asheville, North Carolina: Self-published, 2004), 35.

23. Anonymous, *Beyond Agriculture* (zine), no date.

24. Euell Gibbons, *Stalking the Healthful Herbs* (New York: David McKay Company, 1966), 282.

25. John Zerzan, "Agriculture—Essence of Civilization," *Fifth Estate* 23, no. 2 (Summer 1988), 17.

26. Joe Hollis, "Paradise Gardening," http://mountaingardensherbs.com/about.html#.

27. Holmes, *The Energetics of Western Herbs*, 705.

28. Weed, *Wise Woman Herbal*, 181.

29. Holmes, *The Energetics of Western Herbs*, 441.

30. Frances Cerra Whittelsey, "Fuel For Thought," *Smithsonian Magazine*, September 2005, 30.

31. Lyle Estill, *Biodiesel Power: The Passion, the People, and the Politics of the Next Renewable Fuel* (Gabriola Island, British Columbia: New Society, 2005), 1.

32. Ibid.

33. Greg Pahl, *Biodiesel: Growing a New Energy Economy* (White River Junction, VT: Chelsea Green, 2005), 51.

34. Maria "Mark" Alovert, *Biodiesel Homebrew Guide*, Edition 10, January 3, 2005 (self-published), www.localb100.com.

35. Estill, *Biodiesel Power*, 25.

36. Ibid., 14.

37. Peter J. Howe, "From Tasty to Toasty: Used Cooking Oil Heats a Diner," *Boston Globe,* January 21, 2006, A1.

38. J.I. Rodale, Editor, *Encyclopedia of Organic Gardening* (Emmaus, PA: Rodale, 1959), 211.

39. California Integrated Waste Management Board, "Frequently Asked Questions: Food Scrap Management," www.ciwmb.ca.gov/foodwaste/FAQ.htm; also www.organicconsumers.org/organic/compost110504.cfm.

40. Woelfle-Erskine, *Urban Wilds,* 102.

41. Ibid., 21.

42. Michelle Locke, "Citywide Composting of Food Wastes in San Francisco Sets National Model," Associated Press, November 3, 2004, www.organic-consumers.org/organic/compost110504.cfm

43. Joseph Jenkins, *The Humanure Handbook,* Third Edition (Grove City, PA: Joseph Jenkins, Inc., 2005), 8.

44. Seyed Mohammad Kazem Hosseini Asl MD and Seyed Davood Hosseini MD, "Determination of the Mean Daily Stool Weight, Frequency of Defecation and Bowel Transit Time: Assessment of 1000 Healthy Subjects," *Archives of Iranian Medicine* 3, no. 4 (October 2000), www.ams.ac.ir/AIM/0034/asl0034.html.

45. "Excrement Happens," *Rachel's Environmental & Health Weekly* no. 644 (April 1, 1999), www.purewatergazette.net/excrementhappens.htm.

46. Jenkins, *Humanure Handbook,* 15.

47. Ibid., 231.

48. Ibid., 8.

49. Ibid., 198.

50. Joseph Jenkins on Jenkins Publishing Message Board, "Humanure Legality Ontario," June 4, 2004, www.jenkinspublishing.com/messages/ messages/4/1205.html?1087093339.

Chapter 10

1. United Nations Educational, Scientific and Cultural Organization World Water Assessment Programme, "Securing the Food Supply," www.unesco.org/water/wwap/facts_figures/food_supply.shtml.

2. Mark Briscoe, "Water: The Overtapped Resource," in Andrew Kimbrell, editor, *The Fatal Harvest Reader: The Tragedy of Industrial Agriculture* (Washington, DC: Island Press, 2002), 190.

3. "The State of the Planet: Vanishing Wetlands," *Journey to Planet Earth,* www.pbs.org/journeytoplanetearth/stateoftheplanet/index_wetlands.html.

4. High Plains Underground Water Conservation District Number 1, "The Ogallala Aquifer," www.hpwd.com/the_ogallala.asp.

5. United Nations Educational, Scientific and Cultural Organization World Water Assessment Programme, "Securing the Food Supply," www.unesco.org/water/wwap/facts_figures/food_supply.shtml.

6. Robert Glennon, "The Perils of Groundwater Pumping," *Issues in Science and Technology*, Fall 2002, www.issues.org/issues/19.1/glennon.htm.

7. Lester R. Brown, "World Creating Food Bubble Economy Based on Unsustainable Use of Water," Earth Policy Institute Update 22 (March 13, 2003), www.earth-policy.org/Updates/Update22.htm.

8. Shawn Tully, "Water, Water Everywhere," *Fortune*, May 15, 2000, 344.

9. *Water Privatization Fiascos: Broken Promises and Social Turmoil* (Public Citizen, March 2003), 1, www.foodandwaterwatch.org/publications/reports/water-privatization-fiascoes-broken-promises-and-social-turmoil.

10. Ibid., 3.

11. Ibid., 5; and Jim Shultz, "The Blue Revolution," in Anita Roddick with Brooke Shelby Biggs, *Troubled Water: Saints, Sinners, Truths and Lies about the Global Water Crisis* (Chichester, West Sussex, UK: Anita Roddick Books, 2004),22-26.

12. Beverage Marketing Corporation, *2005 Market Report*, www.bottledwater.org/public/BWFactsHome_main.htm.

13. Abid Aslam, "Bottled Water: Nectar of the Frauds?," *The Progressive Populist*, Febuary 4, 2006, http://us.oneworld.net/article/view/126829/1/.

14. Natural Resources Defense Council, "Bottled Water: Pure Drink or Pure Hype?" March 1999, www.nrdc.org/water/drinking/bw/bwinx.asp.

15. Sierra Club Water Privatization Task Force of the Corporate Accountability Committee, "Bottled Water: Learning the Facts" brochure (circa 2003).

16. Suzanna Brabant, "Caught Between a Rock and a Hard Place," *Macon County Times*, March 23, 2004, www.maconcountytimes.com/articles/2004/03/23/news/newsa.txt.

17. Natural Resources Defense Council, "Bottled Water: Pure Drink or Pure Hype?"

18. "Coca-Cola Responsible for Decline in Groundwater Table in Rajasthan," *The Hindu*, June 17, 2004, www.indiaresource.org/news/2004/1020.html.

19. "Coca-Cola Crisis in India," India Resource Center, www.indiaresource.org/campaigns/coke/index.html.

20. "Health Effects of Chlorine in Drinking Water," www.pure-earth.com/chlorine.html.

21. Murray N. Rothbard, "Fluoridation Revisited," *The New American*, December 14, 1992, www.thenewamerican.com/departments/feature/2001/121492.htm.

22. Joel Griffiths, "Fluoride: Industry's Toxic Coup," *Food & Water Journal*, Summer 1998, www.nofluoride.com/food&water.htm.

23. J. William Hirzy, Ph.D, "Why EPA Headquarters' Union of Scientists Opposes Fluoridation," Chapter 280 of the National Treasury Employees Union, www.nteu280.org/Issues/Fluoride/NTEU280-Fluoride.htm.

24. Catherine Clyne, "Life is Not a Spectator Sport: The Satya Interview with Diane Wilson," *Satya*, November 2002, www.satyamag.com/nov02/wilson.html.

25. Ibid.

26. Diane Wilson, "The Art of Misbehavin'," in Medea Benjamin and Jodie Evans, *Stop the Next War Now: Effective Responses to Violence and Terrorism* (Maui, HI: Inner Ocean, 2005), 72.

27. Woelfle-Erskine, *Urban Wilds*, 93.

28. Pitchford, *Healing with Whole Foods*, 89.

Epilogue

1. Shiva, *Tomorrow's Biodiversity*, 121.

2. Alexander Cockburn, "Travels with Sainath, Being an Indian Diary, First of Three Parts: Why Indian Farmers Kill Themselves; Why Lange's Photographs are Phony," *Counterpunch* (August 4, 2005), www.counterpunch.org/cockburn08042005.html.

3. Alexander Cockburn, "Travels with Sainath, Being an Indian Diary, Third of Three Parts: The Rise and Fall of Chandrababu Naidu, Western Poster Boy; Parrots that Read Tarot; a Brothel in Mumbai; How the British Destroyed India," *Counterpunch* (August 6-8, 2005), www.counterpunch.org/cockburn08062005.html.

4. John D. Ragland and Alan L. Berman, "Farm Crisis and Suicide: Dying on the Vine?," *Omega: Journal of Death and Dying* 22, no. 3 (1990-91), 180.

5. "Farmer's Suicide Linked to Crisis," *New Zealand Herald*, March 15, 2001.

6. LaDuke, *All Our Relations*, 200.

7. *Korea AgraFood*, April 2003, quoted by Anuradha Mittal, "A Farmer's Suicide: A Farmer's Message," www.earthisland.org/project/newsPage2.cfm?newsID=472&pageID=177&subSiteID=4.

Index